Statistical Modeling for Biomedical Researchers

A Simple Introduction to the Analysis of Complex Data

This text will enable biomedical researchers to use a number of advanced statistical methods that have proven valuable in medical research. It is intended for people who have had an introductory course in biostatistics. A statistical software package (Stata) is used to avoid mathematics beyond the high school level. The emphasis is on understanding the assumptions underlying each method, using exploratory techniques to determine the most appropriate method, and presenting results in a way that will be readily understood by clinical colleagues. Numerous real examples from the medical literature are used to illustrate these techniques. Graphical methods are used extensively. Topics covered include linear regression, logistic regression, Poisson regression, survival analysis, fixed-effects analysis of variance, and repeated-measures analysis of variance. Each method is introduced in its simplest form and is then extended to cover situations in which multiple explanatory variables are collected on each study subject.

Educated at McGill University, and the Johns Hopkins University, Bill Dupont is currently Professor and Director of the Division of Biostatistics at Vanderbilt University School of Medicine. He is best known for his work on the epidemiology of breast cancer, but has also published papers on power calculations, the estimation of animal abundance, the foundations of statistical inference, and other topics.

Statistical Modeling for Biomedical Researchers

A Simple Introduction to the Analysis of Complex Data

William D. Dupont

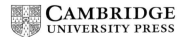

CAMBRIDGE
UNIVERSITY PRESS

PUBLISHED BY THE PRESS SYNDICATE OF THE UNIVERSITY OF CAMBRIDGE
The Pitt Building, Trumpington Street, Cambridge, United Kingdom

CAMBRIDGE UNIVERSITY PRESS
The Edinburgh Building, Cambridge CB2 2RU, UK
40 West 20th Street, New York, NY 10011-4211, USA
477 Williamstown Road, Port Melbourne, VIC 3207, Australia
Ruiz de Alarcón 13, 28014 Madrid, Spain
Dock House, The Waterfront, Cape Town 8001, South Africa

http://www.cambridge.org

First published 2002

Printed in the United Kingdom at the University Press, Cambridge

Typefaces Minion 10.5/14 pt and Formata BQ   *System* LaTeX 2_ε [TB]

A catalogue record for this book is available from the British Library

Library of Congress Cataloguing in Publication data

Dupont, William D. (William Dudley), 1946–
Statistical modeling for biomedical researchers / William D. Dupont.
     p.   cm.
Includes bibliographical references and index.
ISBN 0 521 65578 1 (pb.)
1. Medicine – Research – Statistical methods – Mathematical models.   I. Title.
R853.M3 D865   2002
610′.7′27 – dc21   2002073487

ISBN 0 521 82061 8 hardback
ISBN 0 521 65578 1 paperback

Contents

2   Simple Linear Regression   34

3   Multiple Linear Regression   72

4   **Simple Logistic Regression**   **108**

5   Multiple Logistic Regression   143

Preface

The purpose of this text is to enable biomedical researchers to use a number of advanced statistical methods that have proven valuable in medical research. The past thirty years have seen an explosive growth in the development of biostatistics. As with so many aspects of our world, this growth has been strongly influenced by the development of inexpensive, powerful computers and the sophisticated software that has been written to run them. This has allowed the development of computationally intensive methods that can effectively model complex biomedical data sets. It has also made it easy to explore these data sets, to discover how variables are interrelated and to select appropriate statistical models for analysis. Indeed, just as the microscope revealed new worlds to the eighteenth century, modern statistical software permits us to see interrelationships in large complex data sets that would have been missed in previous eras. Also, modern statistical software has made it vastly easier for investigators to perform their own statistical analyses. Although very sophisticated mathematics underlies modern statistics, it is not necessary to understand this mathematics to properly analyze your data with modern statistical software. What is necessary is to understand the assumptions required by each method, how to determine whether these assumptions are adequately met for your data, how to select the best model, and how to interpret the results of your analyses. The goal of this text is to allow investigators to effectively use some of the most valuable multivariate methods without requiring an understanding of more than high school algebra. Much mathematical detail is avoided by focusing on the use of a specific statistical software package.

This text grew out of my second semester course in biostatistics that I teach in our Masters of Public Health program at the Vanderbilt University Medical School. All of the students take introductory courses in biostatistics and epidemiology prior to mine. Although this text is self-contained, I strongly recommend that readers acquire good introductory texts in biostatistics and epidemiology as companions to this one. Many excellent texts are available on these topics. At Vanderbilt we are currently using Pagano and Gauvreau (2000) for biostatistics and Hennekens and Buring (1987) for epidemiology.

The statistical software used in this text is Stata (2001). It was chosen for the breadth and depth of its statistical methods, for its ease of use, and for its excellent documentation. There are several other excellent packages available on the market. However, the aim of this text is to teach biostatistics through a specific software package, and length restrictions make it impractical to use more than one package. If you have not yet invested a lot of time learning a different package, Stata is an excellent choice for you to consider. If you are already attached to a different package, you may still find it easier to learn Stata than to master or teach the material covered here from other textbooks.

The topics covered in this text are linear regression, logistic regression, Poisson regression, survival analysis, and analysis of variance. Each topic is covered in two chapters: one introduces the topic with simple univariate examples and the other covers more complex multivariate models. The text makes extensive use of a number of real data sets. They all may be downloaded from my web site at *www.mc.vanderbilt.edu/prevmed/wddtext*. This site also contains complete log files of all analyses discussed in this text.

I would like to thank Gordon R. Bernard, Jeffrey Brent, Norman E. Breslow, Graeme Eisenhofer, Cary P. Gross, Daniel Levy, Steven M. Greenberg, Fritz F. Parl, Paul Sorlie, Wayne A. Ray, and Alastair J. J. Wood for allowing me to use their data to illustrate the methods described in this text. I am grateful to William Gould and the employees of Stata Corporation for publishing their elegant and powerful statistical software and for providing excellent documentation. I would also like to thank the students in our Master of Public Health program who have taken my course. Their energy, intelligence and enthusiasm have greatly enhanced my enjoyment in preparing this material. Their criticisms and suggestions have profoundly influenced this work. I am grateful to David L. Page, my friend and colleague of 24 years, with whom I have learnt much about the art of teaching epidemiology and biostatistics to clinicians. My appreciation goes to Sarah K. Meredith for introducing me to Cambridge University Press, to Peter Silver, Frances Nex, Lucille Murby, Jane Williams and their colleagues at Cambridge University Press for producing this beautiful book, to William Schaffner, my chairman, who encouraged and facilitated my spending the time needed to complete this work, to W. Dale Plummer for technical support, to Patrick G. Arbogast for proofreading the entire manuscript, and to my mother and sisters for their support during six critical months of this project. Finally, I am especially grateful to my wife and family for their love and support, and for their cheerful tolerance of the countless hours that I spent on this project.

W.D.D.
Quebec, Canada

Disclaimer: The opinions expressed in this text are my own and do not necessarily reflect those of the authors acknowledged in this preface, their employers or funding institutions. This includes the National Heart, Lung, and Blood Institute, National Institutes of Health, Department of Health and Human Services, USA.

Introduction

This text is primarily concerned with the interrelationships between multiple variables that are collected on study subjects. For example, we may be interested in how age, blood pressure, serum cholesterol, body mass index and gender affect a patient's risk of coronary heart disease. The methods that we will discuss involve descriptive and inferential statistics. In descriptive statistics, our goal is to understand and summarize the data that we have actually collected. This can be a nontrivial task in a large database with many variables. In inferential statistics, we seek to draw conclusions about patients in the population at large from the information collected on the specific patients in our database. This requires first choosing an appropriate model that can explain the variation in our collected data and then using this model to estimate the accuracy of our results. The purpose of this chapter is to review some elementary statistical concepts that we will need in subsequent chapters.

1.1. Algebraic Notation

This text assumes that the reader is familiar with high school algebra. In this section we review notation that may be unfamiliar to some readers.

- We use parentheses to indicate the order of multiplication and addition; brackets are used to indicate the arguments of functions. Thus, $a(b+c)$ equals the product of a and $b+c$, while $a[b+c]$ equals the value of the function a evaluated at $b+c$.
- The function $\log[x]$ denotes the natural logarithm of x. You may have seen this function referred to as either $\ln[x]$ or $\log_e[x]$ elsewhere.
- The constant $e = 2.718\ldots$ is the base of the natural logarithm.
- The function $\exp[x] = e^x$ is the constant e raised to the power x.
- The function

$$\text{sign}[x] = \begin{cases} 1: \text{if } x \geq 0 \\ -1: \text{if } x < 0 \end{cases}.$$

- The absolute value of x is written $|x|$ and equals

$$\text{sign}\,[x]\,x = \begin{cases} x: \text{if } x \geq 0 \\ -x: \text{if } x < 0 \end{cases}.$$

- The expression $\int_a^b f\,[x]\,dx$ denotes the area under the curve $f\,[x]$ between a and b. That is, it is the region bounded by the function $f\,[x]$ and the x-axis and by vertical lines drawn between $f\,[x]$ and the x-axis at $x = a$ and $x = b$. With the exception of the occasional use of this notation, no calculus is used in this text.

Suppose that we have measured the weights of three patients. Let $x_1 = 70$, $x_2 = 60$ and $x_3 = 80$ denote the weight of the first, second and third patient, respectively.

- We use the Greek letter Σ to denote summation. For example,

$$\sum_{i=1}^{3} x_i = x_1 + x_2 + x_3 = 70 + 60 + 80 = 210.$$

When the summation index is unambiguous we will drop the subscript and superscript on the summation sign. Thus, $\sum x_i$ also equals $x_1 + x_2 + x_3$.

- We use the Greek letter Π to denote multiplication. For example,

$$\prod_{i=1}^{3} x_i = \prod x_i = x_1 x_2 x_3 = 70 \times 60 \times 80 = 336\,000.$$

- We use braces to denote sets of values; $\{i: x_i > 65\}$ is the set of integers for which the inequality to the right of the colon is true. Since $x_i > 65$ for the first and third patient, $\{i: x_i > 65\} = \{1, 3\}$ = the integers one and three. The summation

$$\sum_{\{i: x_i > 65\}} x_i = x_1 + x_3 = 70 + 80 = 150.$$

The product

$$\prod_{\{i: x_i > 65\}} x_i = 70 \times 80 = 5600.$$

1.2. Descriptive Statistics

1.2.1. Dot Plot

Suppose that we have a sample of n observations of some variable. A **dot plot** is a graph in which each observation is represented with a dot on the

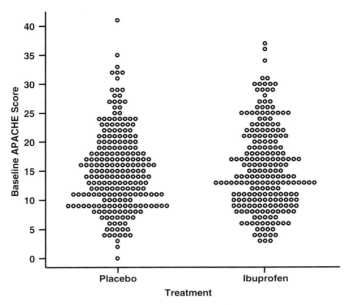

Figure 1.1   Dot plot of baseline APACHE score subdivided by treatment (Bernard et al., 1997).

y-axis. Dot plots are often subdivided by some grouping variable in order to permit a comparison of the observations between the two groups. For example, Bernard et al. (1997) performed a randomized clinical trial to assess the effect of intravenous ibuprofen on mortality in patients with sepsis. People with sepsis have severe systemic bacterial infections that may be due to a wide number of causes. Sepsis is a life threatening condition. However, the mortal risk varies considerably from patient to patient. One measure of a patient's mortal risk is the Acute Physiology and Chronic Health Evaluation (APACHE) score (Bernard et al., 1997). This score is a composite measure of the patient's degree of morbidity that was collected just prior to recruitment into the study. Since this score is highly correlated with survival, it was important that the treatment and control groups be comparable with respect to baseline APACHE score. Figure 1.1 shows a dot plot of the baseline APACHE scores for study subjects subdivided by treatment group. This plot indicates that the treatment and placebo groups are comparable with respect to baseline APACHE score.

1.2.2. Sample Mean

The **sample mean** $\bar{x}$ for a variable is its average value for all patients in the sample. Let x_i denote the value of a variable for the ith study subject

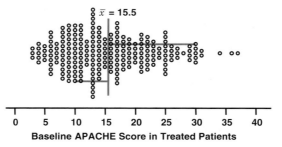

$\bar{x} = 15.5$

Baseline APACHE Score in Treated Patients

Figure 1.2

Dot plot for treated patients in the Ibuprofen in Sepsis study. The vertical line marks the sample mean, while the length of the horizontal lines indicates the residuals for patients with APACHE scores of 10 and 30.

$(i = 1, 2, \ldots, n)$. Then the sample mean is

$$\bar{x} = \sum_{i=1}^{n} x_i/n = (x_1 + x_2 + \cdots + x_n)/n, \tag{1.1}$$

where n is the number of patients in the sample. In Figure 1.2 the vertical line marks the mean baseline APACHE score for treated patients. This mean equals 15.5. The mean is a measure of central tendency of the x_is in the sample.

1.2.3. Residual

The **residual** for the ith study subject is the difference $x_i - \bar{x}$. In Figure 1.2 the length of the horizontal lines show the residuals for patients with APACHE scores of 10 and 30. These residuals equal $10 - 15.5 = -5.5$ and $30 - 15.5 = 14.5$, respectively.

1.2.4. Sample Variance

We need to be able to measure the variability of values in a sample. If there is little variability, then all of the values will be near the mean and the residuals will be small. If there is great variability, then many of the residuals will be large. An obvious measure of sample variability is the average absolute value of the residuals, $\sum |x_i - \bar{x}|/n$. This statistic is not commonly used because it is difficult to work with mathematically. A more mathematician-friendly measure of variability is the **sample variance**, which is

$$s^2 = \sum (x_i - \bar{x})^2/(n - 1). \tag{1.2}$$

You can think of s^2 as being the average squared residual. (We divide the sum of the squared residuals by $n - 1$ rather than n for arcane mathematical reasons that are not worth explaining at this point.) Note that the greater the variability of the sample, the greater the average squared residual and hence, the greater the sample variance.

1.2.5. Sample Standard Deviation

The **sample standard deviation** s is the square root of the sample variance. Note that s is measured in the same units as x_i. For the treated patients in Figure 1.1 the variance and standard deviation of the APACHE score are 52.7 and 7.26, respectively.

1.2.6. Percentile and Median

Percentiles are most easily defined by an example; the 75th **percentile** is that value that is greater or equal to 75% of the observations in the sample. The **median** is the 50th percentile, which is another measure of central tendency.

1.2.7. Box Plot

Dot plots provide all of the information in a sample on a given variable. They are ineffective, however, if the sample is too large and may require more space than is desirable. The mean and standard deviation give a terse description of the central tendency and variability of the sample, but omit details of the data structure that may be important. A useful way of summarizing the data that provides a sense of the data structure is the **box plot** (also called the **box-and-whiskers** plot). Figure 1.3 shows such plots for the APACHE data in each treatment group. In each plot, the sides of the box mark the 25th and 75th percentiles, which are also called the **quartiles**. The vertical line in the middle of the box marks the median. The width of the box is called

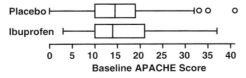

Figure 1.3   Box plots of APACHE scores of patients receiving placebo and ibuprofen in the Ibuprofen in Sepsis study.

the **interquartile range**. The middle 50% of the observations lie within this range. The vertical bars at either end of the plot mark the most extreme observations that are not more than 1.5 times the interquartile range from their adjacent quartiles. Any values beyond these bars are plotted separately as in the dot plot. They are called **outliers** and merit special consideration because they may have undue influence on some of our analyses. Figure 1.3 captures much of the information in Figure 1.1 in less space.

For both treated and control patients the largest APACHE scores are farther from the median than are the smallest scores. For treated subjects the upper quartile is farther from the median than is the lower quartile. Data sets in which the observations are more stretched out on one side of the median than the other are called **skewed**. They are **skewed to the right** if values above the median are more dispersed than are values below. They are **skewed to the left** when the converse is true. Box plots are particularly valuable when we wish to compare the distributions of a variable in different groups of patients, as in Figure 1.3. Although the median APACHE values are very similar in treated and control patients, the treated patients have a slightly more skewed distribution. (It should be noted that some authors use slightly different definitions for the outer bars of a box plot. The definition given here is that of Cleveland (1993).)

1.2.8. Histogram

This is a graphic method of displaying the distribution of a variable. The range of observations is divided into equal intervals; a bar is drawn above each interval that indicates the proportion of the data in the interval. Figure 1.4 shows a histogram of APACHE scores in control patients. This graph also shows that the data is skewed to the right.

1.2.9. Scatter Plot

It is often useful to understand the relationship between two variables that are measured on a group of patients. A **scatter plot** displays these values as points in a two-dimensional graph: the x-axis shows the values of one variable and the y-axis shows the other. For example, Brent et al. (1999) measured baseline plasma glycolate and arterial pH on 18 patients admitted for ethylene glycol poisoning. A scatter plot of plasma glycolate versus arterial pH for these patients is plotted in Figure 1.5. Each circle on this graph shows the plasma glycolate and arterial pH for a study subject. The black dot represents two

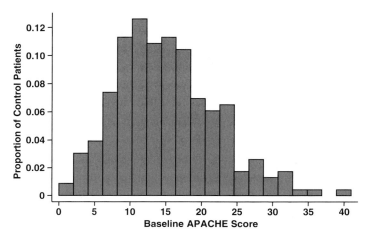

Figure 1.4   Histogram of APACHE scores among control patients in the Ibuprofen in Sepsis trial.

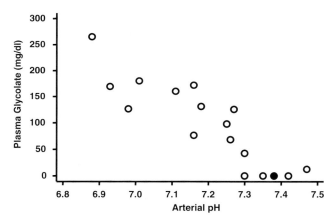

Figure 1.5   Scatter plot of baseline plasma glycolate vs. arterial pH in 18 patients with ethylene glycol poisoning (Brent et al., 1999).

patients with identical values of these variables. Note that patients with high glycolate levels tended to have low pHs, and that glycolate levels tended to decline with increasing pH.

1.3. The Stata Statistical Software Package

The worked examples in this text are performed using Stata (2001). This software comes with excellent documentation. At a minimum, I suggest you read their *Getting Started* manual. This text is not intended to replicate the Stata documentation, although it does explain the use of those commands needed in this text. The Appendix provides a list of these commands and the section number where the command is first explained.

1.3.1. Downloading Data from My Web Site

An important feature of this text is the use of real data sets to illustrate methods in biostatistics. These data sets are located at *www.mc.vanderbilt.edu/ prevmed/wddtext/wddtext*. In the examples, I assume that you have downloaded the data into a folder on your C drive called *WDDtext*. I suggest that you create such a folder now. (Of course the location and name of the folder is up to you but if you use a different name you will have to modify the file address in my examples.) Next, use your web browser to go to *www.mc.vanderbilt.edu/prevmed/wddtext/wddtext* and click on the blue underlined text that says Data Sets. A page of data sets will appear. Click on 1.3.2.Sepsis. A dialog box will ask where you wish to download the sepsis data set. Enter *C:/WDDtext* and click the download button. A Stata data set called *1.3.2.Sepsis.dta* will be copied to your *WDDtext* folder. Purchase a license for *Intercooled Stata Release 7* for your computer and install it following the directions in the *Getting Started* manual. You are now ready to start analyzing data with Stata.

When you launch the Stata program you will see a screen with three windows. These are the Stata Command window where you will type your commands, the Stata Results window where output is written, and the Review window where previous commands are stored. A Stata command is executed when you press the Enter key at the end of a line in the command window. Each command is echoed back in the Results window followed by the resulting output or error message. Graphic output appears in a separate Stata Graph window. In the examples given in this text, I have adopted the following conventions: all Stata commands and output are written in a typewriter font (all letters have the same width). Commands are written in bold face while output is written in regular type. On command lines, variable names and labels and other text chosen by the user are italicized; command names and options that must be entered as is are not. Highlighted output is discussed in the comments following each example. Numbers in braces on the right margin refer to comments that are given at the end of the example. Comments in the middle of an example are in braces and are written in a proportionally spaced font.

1.3.2. Creating Dot Plots with Stata

The following example shows the contents of the Results window after entering a series of commands in the Command window. Before replicating this example on your computer, you must first download *1.3.2.Sepsis.dta* as described in the preceding section.

```
. * Examine the Stata data set 1.3.2.Sepsis.dta. Create a dot plot of     {1}
. * baseline APACHE scores in treated and untreated patients
. *
. use C:\WDDtext\1.3.2.Sepsis.dta                                          {2}

. describe                                                                 {3}

Contains data from C:\WDDtext\1.3.2.Sepsis.dta
 obs:            455
vars:             2                          16 Apr 2002 15:36
size:         5,460   (99.4% of memory free)
-----------------------------------------------------------------
   1. treat      float    %9.0g      treatment  Treatment
   2. apache     float    %9.0g                 Baseline APACHE Score
-----------------------------------------------------------------
Sorted by:

. list treat apache in 1/3                                                 {4}

         treat       apache
1.      Placebo          27
2. Ibuprofen           14
3.      Placebo          33                                                {5}

. edit                                                                     {6}

. dotplot apache, by(treat) center                                        {7}
```
{Graph omitted. See Figure 1.8}

Comments

1 Command lines that start with an asterisk (*) are treated as comments and are ignored by Stata.

2 The *use* command specifies the name of a Stata data set that is to be used in subsequent Stata commands. This data set is loaded into memory where it may be analyzed or modified. In Section 4.21 we will illustrate how to create a new data set using Stata.

3 The *describe* command provides some basic information about the current data set. The *1.3.2.Sepsis* data set contains 454 observations. There are two variables called *treat* and *apache*. The labels assigned to these variables are *Treatment* and *Baseline APACHE Score*.

4 The *list* command gives the values of the specified variables; *in 1/3* restricts this listing to the first through third observations in the file.

5 At this point the Review, Variables, Results, and Command windows should look like those in Figure 1.6. (The size of these windows has been changed to fit in this figure.) Note that if you click on any command in

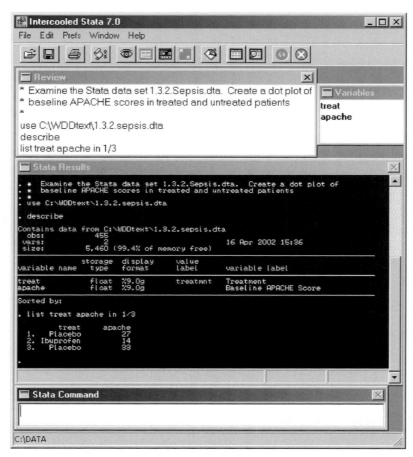

Figure 1.6   The Stata Review, Variables, Results, and Command windows are shown immediately after the *list* command is given in Example 1.3.2. The shapes and sizes of these windows have been altered to fit in this figure.

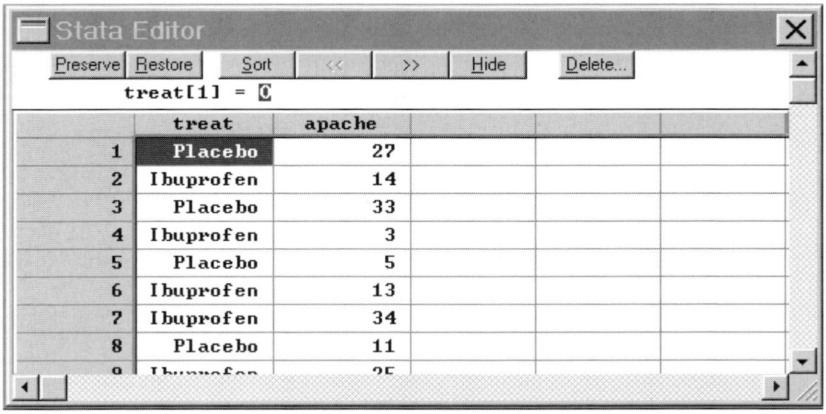

Figure 1.7   The Stata Editor shows the individual values of the data set, with one row per patient and one column per variable.

the Review window it will appear in the Command window where you can edit and re-execute it. This is particularly useful for fixing command errors. When entering variables in a command you may either type them directly or click on the desired variable from the Variables window. The latter method avoids spelling mistakes.

6 Typing *edit* opens the Stata Editor window (there is a button on the toolbar that does this as well). This command permits you to review or edit the current data set. Figure 1.7 shows this window, which presents the data in a spreadsheet format with one row per patient and one column per variable.

7 This *dotplot* command generates the graph shown in Figure 1.8. This figure appears in its own Graph window. A separate dotplot of the APACHE variable is displayed for each value of the *treat* variable; *center* draws the dots centered over each treatment value. Stata graphs can either be saved as separate files or cut and pasted into a graphics editor for additional modification (see the File and Edit menus, respectively).

1.3.3. Stata Command Syntax

Stata requires that your commands comply with its grammatical rules. For the most part, Stata will provide helpful error messages when you type something wrong (see Section 1.3.4). There are, however, a few instances where you may be confused by its response to your input.

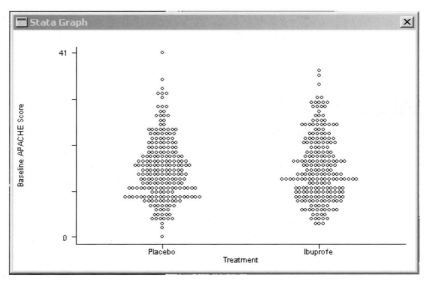

Figure 1.8   This figure shows the Stata Graph window after the *dotplot* command in Example 1.3.2. The dot plot in this window is similar to Figure 1.1. We will explain how to improve the appearance of such graphs in subsequent examples.

Punctuation   The first thing to check if Stata gives a confusing error message is your punctuation. Stata commands are modified by **qualifiers** and **options**. Qualifiers precede options; there must be a comma between the last qualifier and the first option. For example, in the command

```
dotplot apache, by(treat) center
```

the variable *apache* is a qualifier while *by(treat)* and *center* are options. Without the comma, Stata will not recognize *by(treat)* or *center* as valid options to the *dotplot* command. In general, qualifiers apply to most commands while options are more specific to the individual command. A qualifier that precedes the command is called a **command prefix**. Most command prefixes must be separated from the subsequent command by a colon. See the Stata reference manuals or the Appendix for further details.

Capitalization   Stata variables and commands are case sensitive. That is, Stata considers *age* and *Age* to be two distinct variables. In general, I recommend that you always use lower case variables. Sometimes Stata will create variables for you that contain upper case letters. You must use the correct capitalization when referring to these variables.

Abbreviations   Some commands and options may be abbreviated. The minimum acceptable abbreviation is underlined in the Stata reference manuals.

1.3.4. Obtaining Interactive Help from Stata

Stata has an extensive interactive help facility that is fully described in the *Getting Started* and *User's Guide* manuals (Stata, 2001). I have found the following features to be particularly useful.

- If you type *help command* in the Stata Command window, Stata will provide instructions on syntax for the specified command. For example, *help dotplot* will generate instructions on how to create a dotplot with Stata.

- Typing *search word* will provide a table of contents from the Stata database that relates to the word you have specified. You may then click on any command in this table to receive instructions on its use. For example, *search plot* will give a table of contents of all commands that provide plots, one of which is the *dotplot* command.

- When you make an error specifying a Stata command, Stata will provide a terse error message followed by the code *r(#)*, where *#* is some error number. If you then type *search r(#)* you will get a more detailed description of your error. For example, the command *dotplt apache* generates the error message *unrecognized command: dotplt* followed by the error code *r(199)*. Typing *search r(199)* generates a message suggesting that the most likely reason why Stata did not recognize this command was because of a typographical error (*i.e. dotplt* was misspelt).

1.3.5. Stata Log Files

You can keep a permanent record of your commands and Stata's responses in a log file. This is a simple text file that you can edit with any word processor or text editor. You can cut and paste commands from a log file back into the Command window to replicate old analyses. In the next example we illustrate the creation of a log file. You will find log files from each example in this text at *www.mc.vanderbilt.edu/prevmed/wddtext*.

1.3.6. Displaying Other Descriptive Statistics with Stata

The following log file and comments demonstrate how to use Stata to obtain the other descriptive statistics discussed above.

```
. log using C:\WDDtext\1.3.6.Sepsis.log                              {1}
. * 1.3.6.Sepsis.log
. *
. * Calculate the sample mean, median, variance and standard deviation
. * for the baseline APACHE score in each treatment group. Draw box plots
. * and histograms of APACHE score for treated and control patients.
. *
. use C:\WDDtext\1.3.2.Sepsis.dta

. sort treat                                                         {2}

. by treat: summarize apache, detail                                {3}

-> treat=  Placebo
                     Baseline APACHE Score
-----------------------------------------------------------------
          Percentiles      Smallest
  1%            3               0
  5%            5               2
 10%            7               3        Obs                  230
 25%           10               4        Sum of Wgt.          230
 50%           14.5                      Mean            15.18696
                              Largest    Std. Dev.       6.922831
 75%           19              32
 90%           24              33        Variance        47.92559
 95%           28              35        Skewness        .6143051
 99%           33              41        Kurtosis        3.383043

-> treat=Ibuprofen
                     Baseline APACHE Score
-----------------------------------------------------------------
          Percentiles      Smallest
  1%            3               3
  5%            5               3
 10%            7               3        Obs                  224
 25%           10               4        Sum of Wgt.          224
 50%           14                        Mean            15.47768
                              Largest    Std. Dev.       7.261882
 75%           21              31
 90%           25              34        Variance        52.73493
 95%           29              36        Skewness        .5233335
 99%           34              37        Kurtosis        2.664936
```

```
. graph apache, box by(treat)                                           {4}
```
{Graph omitted. See Figure 1.3}
```
. graph apache, bin(20)                                                 {5}
```
{Graph omitted. See Figure 1.4}
```
. by treat: graph apache, bin(20)                                       {6}
```
{Graph omitted.}
```
-> treat=  Placebo
-> treat=Ibuprofen

.   log close                                                           {7}
```

Comments

1 The *log using* command creates a log file of the subsequent Stata session. This file, called *1.3.6.Sepsis.log* will be written in the *WDDtext* folder. There is also a button on the Stata toolbar that permits you to open, close and suspend log files.

2 The *sort* command sorts the data by the values of *treat*, thereby grouping all of the patients on each treatment together.

3 The *summarize* command provides some simple statistics on the *apache* variable calculated across the entire data set. With the *detail* option these include means, medians and other statistics. The command prefix *by treat*: subdivides the data set into as many subgroups as there are distinct values of *treat*, and then calculates the summary statistics for each subgroup. In this example, the two values of *treat* are *Placebo* and *Ibuprofen*. For patients on ibuprofen, the mean APACHE score is 15.48 with variance 52.73 and standard deviation 7.26; their interquartile range is from 10 to 21. The data must be sorted by *treat* prior to this command.

4 The *graph* command produces a wide variety of graphics. With the *box* option Stata draws box plots for the *apache* variable that are similar to those in Figure 1.3. The *by(treat)* option tells Stata that we want a box plot for each treatment drawn in a single graph. (The command *by treat*: *graph apache, box* would have produced two separate graphs: the first graph would have had a single box plot for the placebo patients while the second graph would be for the ibuprofen group.)

5 With the *bin*(20) option, the *graph* command produces a histogram of APACHE scores with the APACHE data grouped into 20 evenly spaced bins, and one bar per bin.

6 Adding the *by treat*: prefix to the preceding command causes two separate histograms to be produced which give the distribution of APACHE scores

in patients receiving placebo and ibuprofen, respectively. The first of these graphs is similar to Figure 1.4.

7 This command closes the log file *C:\WDDtext\1.3.2.Sepsis.dta*. You can also do this by clicking the *Close/Suspend Log* button and choosing *Close log file*.

1.4. Inferential Statistics

In medical research we are interested in drawing valid conclusions about all patients who meet certain criteria. For example, we would like to know if treating septic patients with ibuprofen improves their chances of survival. The **target population** consists of all patients, both past and future, to whom we would like our conclusions to apply. We select a sample of these subjects and observe their outcome or attributes. We then seek to infer conclusions about the target population from the observations in our sample.

The typical response of subjects in our sample may differ from that of the target population due to chance variation in subject response or to bias in the way that the sample was selected. For example, if tall people are more likely to be selected than short people, it will be difficult to draw valid conclusions about the average height of the target population from the heights of people in the sample. An **unbiased sample** is one in which each member of the target population is equally likely to be included in the sample. Suppose that we select an unbiased sample of patients from the target population and measure some attribute of each patient. We say that this attribute is a **random variable** drawn from the target population. The observations in a sample are mutually **independent** if the probability that an individual is selected is unaffected by the selection of any other individual in the sample. In this text we will assume that we observe unbiased samples of independent observations and will focus on assessing the extent to which our results may be inaccurate due to chance. Of course, choosing an unbiased sample is much easier said than done. Indeed, implementing an unbiased study design is usually much harder than assessing the effects of chance in a properly selected sample. There are, however, many excellent epidemiology texts that cover this topic. I strongly recommend that you peruse such a text if you are unfamiliar with this subject (see, for example, Hennekens and Buring, 1987).

1.4.1. Probability Density Function

Suppose that we could measure the value of a continuous variable on each member of a target population (for example, their height). The distribution

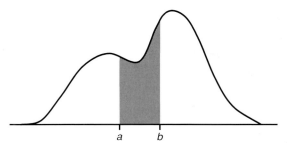

Figure 1.9   Probability density function for a random variable in a hypothetical population. The probability that a member of the population has a value of the variable in the interval (*a, b*) equals the area of the shaded region.

of this variable throughout the population is characterized by its probability density function. Figure 1.9 gives an example of such a function. The *x*-axis of this figure gives the range of values that the variable may take in the population. The **probability density function** is the uniquely defined curve that has the following property: For any interval (a,b) on the *x*-axis, the probability that a member of the population has a value of the variable in the interval (a,b) equals the area under the curve over this interval. In Figure 1.9 this is the area of the shaded region. It follows that the total area under the curve must equal one since each member of the population must have some value of the variable.

1.4.2. Mean, Variance and Standard Deviation

The **mean** of a random variable is its average value in the target population. Its **variance** is the average squared difference between the variable and its mean. Its **standard deviation** is the square root of its variance. The key distinction between these terms and the analogous sample mean, sample variance and sample standard deviation is that the former are unknown attributes of a target population, while the latter can be calculated from a known sample. We denote the mean, variance and standard deviation of a variable by μ, σ^2 and σ, respectively. In general, unknown attributes of a target population are called **parameters** and are denoted by Greek letters. Functions of the values in a sample, such as $\bar{x}$, s^2 and s, are called **statistics** and are denoted by Roman letters or Greek letters covered by a hat. (For example, $\hat{\beta}$ might denote a statistic that estimates a parameter β.) We will often refer to $\bar{x}$, s^2 and s as the mean, variance and standard deviation of the sample when it is obvious from the context that we are

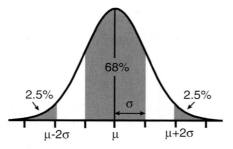

Figure 1.10   Probability density function for a normal distribution with mean μ and standard deviation σ. Sixty-eight percent of observations from such a distribution will lie within one standard deviation of the mean. Only 5% of observations will lie more than two standard deviations from the mean.

talking about a statistic from an observed sample rather than a population parameter.

1.4.3. Normal Distribution

The distribution of values for random variables from many target populations can be adequately described by a **normal distribution**. The probability density function for a normal distribution is shown in Figure 1.10. Each normal distribution is uniquely defined by its mean and standard deviation. The normal probability density function is a symmetric bell shaped curve that is centered on its mean. Sixty-eight percent of the values of a normally distributed variable lie within one standard deviation of its mean; 95% of these values lie within 1.96 standard deviations of its mean.

1.4.4. Expected Value

Suppose that we conduct a series of identical experiments, each of which consist of observing an unbiased sample of independent observations from a target population and calculating a statistic. The **expected value** of the statistic is its average value from a very large number of these experiments. If the target population has a normal distribution with mean μ and standard deviation σ, then the expected value of $\bar{x}$ is μ and the expected value of s^2 is σ^2. We express these relationships algebraically as $E[\bar{x}] = \mu$ and $E[s^2] = \sigma^2$. A statistic is an **unbiased estimate** of a parameter if its expected value equals the parameter. For example $\bar{x}$ is an unbiased estimate of μ since $E[\bar{x}] = \mu$. (The reason why the denominator of equation (1.2) is $n - 1$ rather than n is to make s^2 an unbiased estimator of σ^2.)

1.4.5. Standard Error

As the sample size n increases, the variation in $\bar{x}$ from experiment to experiment decreases. This is because the effects of large and small values in each sample tend to cancel each other out. The standard deviation of $\bar{x}$ in this hypothetical population of repeated experiments is called the **standard error**, and equals $\sigma/\sqrt{n}$. If the target population has a normal distribution, so will $\bar{x}$. Moreover, the distribution of $\bar{x}$ converges to normality as n gets large even if the target population has a non-normal distribution. Hence, unless the target population has a badly skewed distribution, we can usually treat $\bar{x}$ as having a normal distribution with mean μ and standard deviation $\sigma/\sqrt{n}$.

1.4.6. Null Hypothesis, Alternative Hypothesis and *P* Value

The **null hypothesis** is one that we usually hope to disprove and which permits us to completely specify the distribution of a relevant test statistic. The null hypothesis is contrasted with the **alternative hypothesis** that includes all possible distributions except the null. Suppose that we observe an unbiased sample of size n and mean $\bar{x}$ from a target population with mean μ and standard deviation σ. For now, let us make the rather unrealistic assumption that σ is known. We might consider the null hypothesis that $\mu = 0$ versus the alternative hypothesis that $\mu \neq 0$. If the null hypothesis is true, then the distribution of $\bar{x}$ will be as in Figure 1.11 and $\bar{x}$ should be near zero. The farther $\bar{x}$ is from zero the less credible the null hypothesis. The ***P*** **value** is the probability of obtaining a sample mean that is at least as unlikely under the null hypothesis as the observed value $\bar{x}$. That is, it is the probability of obtaining a sample mean greater than $|\bar{x}|$ or less than $-|\bar{x}|$. This probability equals the area of the shaded region in Figure 1.11. When the P value is small, then either the null hypothesis is false or we have observed an unlikely event. By convention, if $P < 0.05$ we claim that our result provides statistically significant evidence against the null hypothesis in favor of the alternative hypothesis; $\bar{x}$ is then said to provide evidence against the null hypothesis at the 5% level of significance. The P value indicated in Figure 1.11 is called a **two-sided** or **two-tailed** P value because the **critical region** of values deemed less credible than $\bar{x}$ includes values less than $-|\bar{x}|$ as well as those greater than $|\bar{x}|$. Recall that the standard error of $\bar{x}$ is $\sigma/\sqrt{n}$.

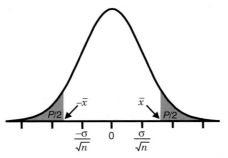

Figure 1.11   The *P* value associated with the null hypothesis that $\mu = 0$ is given by the area of the shaded region. This is the probability that the sample mean will be greater than $|\bar{x}|$ or less than $-|\bar{x}|$ when the null hypothesis is true.

The absolute value of $\bar{x}$ must exceed 1.96 standard errors to have $P < 0.05$. In Figure 1.11, $\bar{x}$ lies between 1 and 2 standard errors. Hence, in this example $\bar{x}$ is not significantly different from zero. If we were testing some other null hypothesis, say $\mu = \mu_0$, then the distribution of $\bar{x}$ would be centered over μ_0 and we would reject this null hypothesis if $|\bar{x} - \mu_0| > 1.96\,\sigma/\sqrt{n}$.

1.4.7. 95% Confidence Interval

In the preceding example, we were unable to reject at the 5% level of significance all null hypotheses $\mu = \mu_0$ such that $|\bar{x} - \mu_0| < 1.96\,\sigma/\sqrt{n}$. A **95% confidence interval** for a parameter consists of all possible values of the parameter that cannot be rejected at the 5% significance level given the observed sample. In this example, this interval is

$$\bar{x} - 1.96\,\sigma/\sqrt{n} \leq \mu \leq \bar{x} + 1.96\,\sigma/\sqrt{n}.$$

In this and most other examples involving normal distributions, the probability that $\bar{x} - 1.96\,\sigma/\sqrt{n} \leq \mu \leq \bar{x} + 1.96\,\sigma/\sqrt{n}$ equals 0.95. In other words, the true parameter will lie within the confidence interval in 95% of similar experiments. This interval, $\bar{x} \pm 1.96\,\sigma/\sqrt{n}$, provides a measure of the accuracy with which we can estimate μ from our sample. Note that this accuracy increases as $\sqrt{n}$ increases and decreases with increasing σ.

Many textbooks define the 95% confidence interval to be an interval that includes the parameter with 95% certainty. These two definitions, however, are not always equivalent, particularly in epidemiologic statistics involving discrete distributions. This has led most modern epidemiologists to prefer the definition given here. It can be shown that the probability that a 95%

confidence interval, as defined here, includes its parameter is at least 95%. Rothman and Greenland (1998) discuss this issue in greater detail.

1.4.8. Statistical Power

If we reject the null hypothesis when it is true we make a **Type I error**. The probability of making a Type I error is denoted by α, and is the **significance level** of the test. For example, if we reject the null hypothesis when $P < 0.05$, then $\alpha = 0.05$ is the probability of making a Type I error. If we do not reject the null hypothesis when the alternative hypothesis is true we make a **Type II error**. The probability of making a Type II error is denoted by β. The **power** of the test is the probability of correctly accepting the alternative hypothesis when it is true. This probability equals $1 - \beta$. It is only possible to derive the power for alternative hypotheses that completely specify the distribution of the test statistic. However, we can plot **power curves** that show the power of the test as a function of the different values of the parameter under the alternative hypothesis. Figure 1.12 shows the power curves for the example introduced in Section 1.4.6. Separate curves are drawn for sample sizes of $n = 1$, 10, 100 and 1000 as a function of the mean μ_a under different alternative hypotheses. The power is always near α for values of μ_a that are very close to the null ($\mu_0 = 0$). This is because the probability of accepting an alternative hypothesis that is virtually identical to the null equals the probability of falsely rejecting the null hypothesis, which equals α. The greater the distance between the alternative and null hypotheses the greater

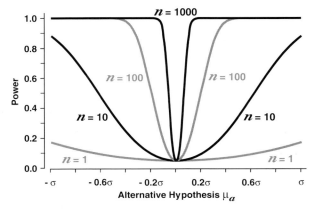

Figure 1.12   Power curves for samples of size 1, 10, 100, and 1000. The null hypothesis is $\mu_0 = 0$. The alternative hypothesis is expressed in terms of σ, which in this example is assumed to be known.

the power, and the rate at which the power rises increases with increasing sample size. Regardless of the sample size, the power eventually approaches 1 (certainty) as the magnitude of μ_a gets sufficiently large. Note that the larger n results in greater ability to correctly reject the null hypothesis in favor of any specific true alternative hypothesis. For example, the power associated with $\mu_a = 0.2\ \sigma$ is 0.055, 0.097, 0.516, and 1.00 when $n = 1$, 10, 100, and 1000, respectively.

Power calculations are particularly useful when designing a study to ensure that the sample size is large enough to detect alternative hypotheses that are clinically important. There are several good software packages available for calculating statistical power. One of these is the *PS* program (Dupont and Plummer, 1990, 1998). This is a self-documented interactive program that produces power and sample size graphs and calculations for most of the commonly used study designs. It is freely available and can be downloaded from the web at *www.mc.vanderbilt.edu/prevmed/ps*.

1.4.9. The *z* and Student's *t* Distributions

There are several distributions of special statistics for which we will need to calculate confidence intervals and *P* values. Two of these are the *z* and *t* distributions. The *z* or **standardized normal distribution** is the normal distribution with mean $\mu = 0$ and standard deviation $\sigma = 1$. If each observation x_i in a sample has a normal distribution with mean μ and standard deviation σ, then $(x_i - \mu)/\sigma$ will have a standardized normal distribution. In addition, if the n observations in the sample are independent, then $(\bar{x} - \mu)/(\sigma/\sqrt{n})$ also has a standard normal distribution.

The examples given in the last three sections are rather artificial in that it is unusual to know the true standard deviation of the target population. However, we can estimate σ by the sample standard deviation s. Moreover, $(\bar{x} - \mu)/(s/\sqrt{n})$ has a completely specified distribution. This is a **Student's t distribution**, which is one of a family of bell shaped distributions that are symmetric about zero. Each such distribution is indexed by an integer called its **degrees of freedom**. The statistic $t_{n-1} = (\bar{x} - \mu)/(s/\sqrt{n})$ has a *t* distribution with $n - 1$ degrees of freedom. Figure 1.13 shows the probability density functions for *t* distributions with one, three and ten degrees of freedom. As the degrees of freedom increase the probability density function converges towards the standard normal distribution, which is also shown in this figure. The standard deviation of a *t* statistic is greater than that of the standard normal distribution due to imprecision in s as an estimate of σ. As the sample size increases s becomes a more and more accurate estimate of σ and t_{n-1} converges to z.

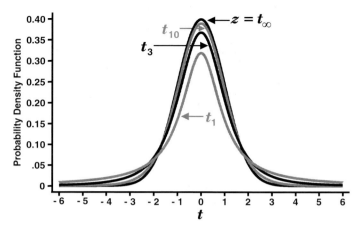

Figure 1.13   Probability density functions for t distributions with 1, 3 and 10 degrees of freedom. These distributions converge to the standard normal distribution as the number of degrees of freedom gets large.

Suppose that z has a standard normal distribution. Let z_α be the **100 α%** **critical value** that is exceeded by z with probability α. (For example, $z_{0.025} = 1.96$ is the 2.5% critical value that is exceeded by z with probability 0.025.) Algebraically, we write this relationship as

$$\alpha = \Pr[z > z_\alpha].$$

If z has a standard normal distribution under the null hypothesis, then we can reject this hypothesis at the 100 α% significance level if $z > z_{\alpha/2}$ or $z < -z_{\alpha/2}$. Similarly, let t_{df} be a t statistic with df degrees of freedom. We define $t_{df,\alpha}$ to be the 100 α% critical value that is exceeded by t_{df} with probability α.

1.4.10. Paired t Test

Suppose that normally distributed responses x_{i1} and x_{i2} are measured before and after treatment on the ith member of an independent sample of n patients. We wish to test the null hypothesis that the treatment has no effect on the mean patient response. Let $d_i = x_{i1} - x_{i2}$ be the change in response for the ith patient. Then under the null hypothesis, d_i has a normal distribution with mean 0 and some unknown standard deviation σ_d. Let $\bar{d}$ and s_d be the sample mean and standard deviation of the differences d_i. Then $s_d/\sqrt{n}$ estimates the standard error of $\bar{d}$. Under the null hypothesis

$$\bar{d}/(s_d/\sqrt{n}) \tag{1.3}$$

has a t distribution with $n - 1$ degrees of freedom. The P value associated with this statistic is

$$P = \Pr[t_{n-1} < -|\bar{d}/(s_d/\sqrt{n})| \text{ or } t_{n-1} > |\bar{d}/(s_d/\sqrt{n})|], \qquad (1.4)$$

where t_{n-1} has a t distribution with $n - 1$ degrees of freedom.

The 95% confidence interval for the true change in response associated with treatment is

$$\bar{d} \pm t_{n-1,\,0.025}(s_d/\sqrt{n}). \qquad (1.5)$$

Example

In the Ibuprofen in Sepsis study, the body temperature of all study subjects was recorded at baseline and after two hours of therapy. All patients received standard care for sepsis. In addition, patients who were randomized to the intervention group received intravenous ibuprofen. There were $n = 208$ patients in the intervention group who had their temperatures recorded at both of these times. The average drop in temperature for these patients is $\bar{d} = 0.8845°$ F. The sample standard deviation of these differences is $s_d = 1.2425$. The estimated standard error of $\bar{d}$ is $s_d/\sqrt{n} = 1.2425/\sqrt{208} = 0.086\,15$, and the t statistic equals $0.8845/0.086\,15 = 10.27$ with 207 degrees of freedom. The two-sided P value associated with this test is $<0.000\,05$. This provides overwhelming evidence that the drop in temperature in the first two hours of treatment was not due to chance. The 95% confidence interval for the true mean drop in temperature among septic patients treated with ibuprofen is $\bar{d} \pm t_{n-1,\,0.025}(s_d/\sqrt{n}) = 0.8845 \pm 1.971 \times 0.086\,15 = (0.71, 1.05)$. Note that the critical value $t_{207,0.025} = 1.971$ is close to $z_{0.025} = 1.960$. This is due to the fact that a t distribution with 207 degrees of freedom is almost identical to the standard normal distribution.

1.4.11. Performing Paired t Tests with Stata

The following Stata log file shows the derivation of the statistics from the example in the preceding section.

```
. * 1.4.11.Sepsis.log

. *

. * Perform paired t test of temperature change by 2 hours

. * in septic patients receiving ibuprofen.

. *

. use C:\WDDtext\1.4.11.Sepsis.dta
```

```
. codebook treat                                                    {1}

treat ---------------------------------------------------- Treatment
                type:   numeric (float)
                label:  treatmnt

               range:   [0,1]                   units:   1
       unique values:   2              coded missing:   0 / 455

          tabulation:   Freq.    Numeric   Label
                          231        0     Placebo
                          224        1     Ibuprofen
```

```
. keep if treat==1                                                  {2}
( 231 observations deleted)
```

```
. codebook temp0   temp1                                            {3}
temp0 ---------------------------------------------- Baseline temperature
                                                      {Output omitted}
       unique values:   96           coded missing: 0 / 224
                                                      {Output omitted}
temp1 ---------------------------------------------- Temperature after 2 hours
                                                      {Output omitted}
       unique values:   78           coded missing: 16 / 224
                                                      {Output omitted}
```

```
. ttest temp0 = temp1                                               {4}
Paired t test
------------------------------------------------------------------------------
Variable |   Obs      Mean     Std. Err.    Std. Dev.   [95% Conf. Interval]
---------+--------------------------------------------------------------------
   temp0 |   208   100.4056   .1493624     2.154135    100.1111      100.7
   temp1 |   208   99.52106   .1285554     1.854052    99.26761    99.7745
---------+--------------------------------------------------------------------
    diff |   208   .8845193   .0861504     1.242479    .7146746   1.054364
------------------------------------------------------------------------------
            Ho: mean(temp0 - temp1) = mean(diff) = 0

 Ha: mean(diff) <  0       Ha: mean(diff) ~= 0       Ha: mean(diff) > 0
     t = 10.2672               t =   10.2672             t =   10.2672
 P < t =  1.0000          P > |t| =   0.0000        P > t =   0.0000
```

Comments

1 This *codebook* command provides information on the variable *treat*. It indicates that *treat* is a numeric variable that takes the values zero and

one. The value labels *Placebo* and *Ibuprofen* are assigned to these numeric values. (See Section 4.21 for an explanation of how to assign value labels to numeric variables.) Stata uses these labels whenever possible. However, when we wish to specify a value of *treat* in a Stata command we must use its numeric value.

2 The *keep* command is used to designate either observations or variables that are to be kept in the data set. When used with the qualifier *if logical_expression* this command keeps all records for which *logical_expression* is true; *treat==1* is a logical expression that is true if *treat* equals 1. Hence, this command keeps all records for which *treat* equals 1. That is, it keeps the records of all patients receiving ibuprofen. Stata indicates that 231 observations have been deleted, which are the records of the 231 placebo patients.

Logical expressions can be constructed in Stata using "and" (&), "or" (|) or "not" (~) operators. For example, *treat* ~= 0 & (*apache* >= 30 | *temp0* < 96) is true for all patients for whom *treat* is not equal to 0 and either *apache* $\geq$ 30 or *temp0* < 96; otherwise it is false. The expression ~(*fruit* == "apple") is true whenever (*fruit* == "apple") is false. That is, it is true when *fruit* takes any value other than "apple".

3 The patient's body temperature at baseline and after two hours of therapy are recorded in the *temp0* and *temp1* variables, respectively. This *codebook* command indicates that while all ibuprofen patients have a recorded baseline temperature, there are 16 patients for whom the 2 hour temperature is missing. Hence there are $n = 224 - 16 = 208$ patients in the ibuprofen group who had their temperatures recorded at both times.

4 The *ttest* command performs independent and paired t tests. The qualifier *temp0 = temp1* specifies that a paired test of these two variables is to be performed. In the notation of the Section 1.4.10 x_{i1} and x_{i2} denote *temp0* and *temp1*, respectively. The mean change in temperature is $\bar{d} = 0.8845$, $s_d = 1.242$, $n = 224 - 16 = 208$, $s_d/\sqrt{n} = 0.086\,15$, and the t statistic equals 10.27 with 207 degrees of freedom. The two-sided P value associated with this test is $<0.000\,05$ (see last row of output). The 95% confidence interval for the true drop in temperature is $(0.715, 1.054)$.

1.4.12. Independent t Test Using a Pooled Standard Error Estimate

Suppose that we have two independent samples of size n_0 and n_1 from normal populations with means μ_0 and μ_1 and standard deviations both equal to σ. Let $\bar{x}_0$, $\bar{x}_1$, s_0 and s_1 be the means and standard deviations from these two samples. Then a pooled estimate of σ from both samples is

$$s_p = \sqrt{\left((n_0 - 1)s_0^2 + (n_1 - 1)s_1^2\right) / (n_0 + n_1 - 2)}, \tag{1.6}$$

and the estimated standard error of $(\bar{x}_0 - \bar{x}_1)$ is

$$s_p \sqrt{\frac{1}{n_0} + \frac{1}{n_1}}.$$

Under the null hypothesis that $\mu_0 = \mu_1$,

$$t_{n_0+n_1-2} = (\bar{x}_0 - \bar{x}_1) \left/ \left(s_p \sqrt{\frac{1}{n_0} + \frac{1}{n_1}} \right) \right. \tag{1.7}$$

has a t distribution with $n_0 + n_1 - 2$ degrees of freedom. A 95% confidence interval for $\mu_0 - \mu_1$ is therefore

$$(\bar{x}_0 - \bar{x}_1) \pm t_{n_0+n_1-2,\ 0.025} \left(s_p \sqrt{\frac{1}{n_0} + \frac{1}{n_1}} \right). \tag{1.8}$$

Example

In the previous two sections we showed that the observed drop in temperature in septic patients treated with ibuprofen could not be explained by chance fluctuations. Of course, this does not prove that ibuprofen caused the temperature drop since there are many other factors associated with treatment in an intensive care unit (ICU) that could cause this change. To show a causal relationship between ibuprofen treatment and temperature we need to compare temperature change in treated and untreated patients. In the Ibuprofen in Sepsis study there were $n_0 = 212$ patients in the control group and $n_1 = 208$ patients in the ibuprofen group who had temperature readings at baseline and after two hours. The average drop in temperature in these two groups was $\bar{x}_0 = 0.3120$ and $\bar{x}_1 = 0.8845°$ F with standard deviations $s_0 = 1.0705$ and $s_1 = 1.2425$, respectively. (Note that temperatures fall in both groups, although the average reduction is greater in the ibuprofen group than in the control group.) The pooled estimate of the standard deviation is

$$s_p = \sqrt{\frac{(212 - 1) \times 1.0705^2 + (208 - 1) \times 1.2425^2}{212 + 208 - 2}} = 1.1589.$$

The estimated standard error of

$\bar{x}_0 - \bar{x}_1$ is $1.1589 \times \sqrt{(1/212) + (1/208)} = 0.1131,$

and

$t = (0.3120 - 0.8845)/0.1131 = -5.062$

has a t distribution with $212 + 208 - 2 = 418$ degrees of freedom. The two-sided P value associated with the null hypothesis of equal temperature drops in the two patient groups is $P < 0.000\,05$. This result, together with the fact that these data come from a double-blinded randomized clinical trial provides convincing evidence of the antipyretic effects of ibuprofen in septic patients. A 95% confidence interval for the true difference in temperature reduction associated with the placebo and treatment groups is $(0.3120 - 0.8845) \pm 1.9657 \times 0.1131 = -0.5725 \pm 0.2223 = (-0.79, -0.35)$, where $t_{418,0.025} = 1.9657$ is the 2.5% critical value for a t statistic with 418 degrees of freedom. In other words, the likely average true reduction in temperature due to ibuprofen, and above and beyond that due to other therapy on the ICU, is between 0.35 and 0.79° F.

1.4.13. Independent t Test using Separate Standard Error Estimates

Sometimes we wish to compare groups that have markedly different standard error estimates. In this case it makes sense to abandon the assumption that both groups share a common standard deviation σ. Let

$$t_\nu = (\bar{x}_0 - \bar{x}_1) \bigg/ \left(\sqrt{\frac{s_0^2}{n_0} + \frac{s_1^2}{n_1}} \right). \tag{1.9}$$

Then t_ν will have an approximately t distribution with

$$\nu = \frac{\left(s_0^2/n_0 + s_1^2/n_1\right)^2}{s_0^4 \big/ \left(n_0^2\,(n_0 - 1)\right) \; + \; s_1^4 \big/ \left(n_1^2\,(n_1 - 1)\right)} \tag{1.10}$$

degrees of freedom (Satterthwaite, 1946). The analogous 95% confidence interval associated with this test is

$$(\bar{x}_0 - \bar{x}_1) \pm t_{\nu,\,0.025} \left(\sqrt{\frac{s_0^2}{n_0} + \frac{s_1^2}{n_1}} \right). \tag{1.11}$$

This test is less powerful than the test with the pooled standard error estimate and should only be used when the assumption of identical standard errors in the two groups appears unreasonable.

1.4.14. Independent t tests using Stata

The following log file and comments illustrate how to perform independent t tests with Stata.

```
. * 1.4.14.Sepsis.log
. *
. * Perform an independent t test comparing change in temperature
. * from baseline after two hours in the ibuprofen group compared
. * to that in the control group.
. *
. use C:\WDDtext\1.4.11.Sepsis.dta

. generate tempdif = temp0 - temp1                                    {1}

(35 missing values generated)

. *
. * Assume equal standard deviations in the two groups
. *
. ttest tempdif, by(treat)                                           {2}


Two-sample t test with equal variances
---------------------------------------------------------------------------
  Group |   Obs       Mean      Std. Err.    Std. Dev.   [95% Conf. Interval]
--------+------------------------------------------------------------------
 Placebo |  212    .3119811     .0735218    1.070494    .1670496   .4569125
Ibuprofe |  208    .8845193     .0861504    1.242479    .7146746   1.054364
--------+------------------------------------------------------------------
combined |  420    .5955238     .0581846    1.192429    .4811538   .7098938
--------+------------------------------------------------------------------
    diff |        -.5725383     .1130981               -.7948502  -.3502263
---------------------------------------------------------------------------
Degrees of freedom: 418

             Ho: mean (Placebo) - mean (Ibuprofe) = diff = 0

    Ha: diff < 0              Ha: diff ~= 0              Ha: diff > 0
     t =  -5.0623              t =  -5.0623              t =  -5.0623
   P < t =   0.0000         P > |t| =   0.0000         P > t =   1.0000


. *
. * Assume unequal standard deviations in the two groups
. *
. ttest tempdif, by(treat) unequal                                  {3}
```

```
Two-sample t test with unequal variances
-------------------------------------------------------------------------------
   Group |   Obs       Mean    Std. Err.      Std. Dev.     [95% Conf.   Interval]
---------+---------------------------------------------------------------------
 Placebo |   212    .3119811    .0735218       1.070494     .1670496    .4569125
Ibuprofe |   208    .8845193    .0861504       1.242479     .7146746    1.054364
---------+---------------------------------------------------------------------
combined |   420    .5955238    .0581846       1.192429     .4811538    .7098938
---------+---------------------------------------------------------------------
    diff |        −.5725383    .1132579                     −.7951823   −.3498942
-------------------------------------------------------------------------------
Satterthwaite's degrees of freedom:  406.688

               Ho: mean(Placebo) − mean(Ibuprofe) = diff = 0

    Ha: diff < 0                Ha: diff ~= 0                Ha:  diff > 0
      t =  −5.0552                t =  −5.0552                t =  −5.0552
  P < t =   0.0000           P > |t| =   0.0000           P > t =   1.0000
```

Comments

1 The *generate* command calculates the values of new variables from old ones. In this example *tempdif* is set equal to the difference between the patient's baseline temperature (*temp0*) and his or her temperature two hours later (*temp1*). When either *temp0* or *temp1* are missing so is *tempdif*. There are 35 records where this occurs.

    Note that Stata distinguishes between *apple* = 1, which assigns the value 1 to *apple*, and *apple* == 1, which is a logical expression that is true if *apple* equals 1 and false otherwise.

2 This form of the *ttest* command performs an independent *t* test comparing *tempdif* in the two groups of patients defined by the values of *treat*. The highlighted values in this output correspond to those in the example in Section 1.4.12.

3 The *unequal* option causes Satterthwaite's *t* test for groups with unequal standard deviations to be performed. In this example, the standard deviations in the two groups are similar and the sample sizes are large. Hence, it is not surprising that this test gives very similar results to the test that assumes equal standard deviations. Note that the approximate degrees of freedom are reduced by about 11 and the absolute value of the *t* statistic drops from 5.062 to 5.055. Hence, in this example, the loss in power due to not assuming equal standard deviations is trivial.

1.4.15. The Chi-Squared Distribution

Another important standard distribution that we will use is the **chi-squared** distribution. Let $z_1, z_2, \ldots, z_n$ denote n mutually independent variables that have standard normal distributions. Then $\chi_n^2 = \sum z_i^2$ has a chi-squared distribution with n degrees of freedom. The probability density functions for chi-squared distributions with one though six degrees of freedom are plotted in Figure 1.14. We will use this distribution for testing certain null hypotheses involving one or more parameters. A chi-squared statistic always takes a positive value. Low values of this statistic are consistent with the null hypothesis while high values provide evidence that it is false. The expected value of a chi-squared statistic under the null hypothesis equals its degrees of freedom. The P value associated with an observed value of χ_n^2 is the probability that a chi-squared distribution with n degrees of freedom will exceed this value. Note that with the t distribution we reject the null hypothesis if t is either very large or very small. With the chi-squared distribution we only reject the null hypothesis when χ_n^2 is large.

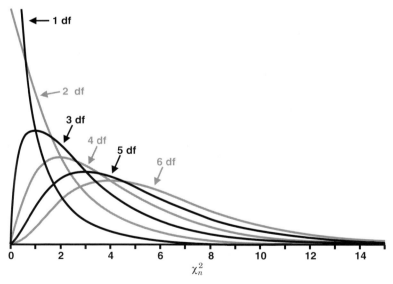

Figure 1.14   Probability density functions for the chi-squared distributions with one through six degrees of freedom (df). High values of a chi-squared statistic provide evidence against the null hypothesis of interest. The expected value of a chi-squared statistic equals its degrees of freedom.

1.5. Additional Reading

At the end of each chapter I have referenced textbooks that cover additional material that may be of interest to readers. I have selected texts that I have found helpful in writing this book or that may appeal to readers with varying levels of mathematical and statistical backgrounds. These references are by no means exhaustive. There are many other excellent texts that cover the same material that are not listed here.

Pagano and Gauvreau (2000) is an excellent all round introductory text in biostatistics.

Armitage and Berry (1994) is another well written introductory text. It covers some material in greater detail than Pagano and Gauvreau (2000).

Hennekens and Buring (1987) is an excellent introductory text in epidemiology.

Rothman and Greenland (1998) is a more advanced epidemiology text. It has an excellent section on the definition of confidence intervals and on the foundations of statistical inference as they apply to epidemiology.

Stata (2001) is mandatory reading for anyone who wishes to use the Stata statistical package for his or her analyses.

Bernard et al. (1997) conducted a randomized clinical trial of ibuprofen in patients with sepsis. We use data from this study to illustrate a number of important methods for analyzing medical data.

Brent et al. (1999) studied patients with ethylene glycol poisoning. We use data from this study to illustrate elementary methods of analyzing bivariate data.

Student (1908) is the original reference on t tests. It was written by W.S. Gosset under the pen name "Student" because his employer, an Irish brewer, thought that he should be spending his time attending to the quality of their brew rather than writing papers in academic journals.

Satterthwaite (1946) is the original reference for the t test with unequal variances.

1.6. Exercises

The following questions relate to the *1.4.11.Sepsis.dta* data set from my web site, which you should download onto your computer.

1 List the names and labels of all variables in the *1.4.11.Sepsis.dta* data set.

2 What are the numeric values of the *race* variable? Which races do these numeric codes represent? Can you answer this question without opening the data editor?

3 List the APACHE score and baseline temperature of the six patients with the lowest APACHE scores. List the APACHE score, fate and ID number of all black patients whose APACHE score is 35 or greater.

4 Draw dot plots of baseline temperature in black and white patients. Draw these plots on a single graph. Do not include people of other races. Where does Stata obtain the title of the y-axis of your dot plot?

5 Draw box plots of temperature at two hours in treated and untreated patients.

6 Consider treated patients whose race is recorded as "other". Test whether these patients' baseline temperature is significantly different from their temperature after two hours. What is the P value associated with this test? How many degrees of freedom does it have? What is a 95% confidence interval for the true change in temperature among this group of subjects?

7 Test whether baseline APACHE score is different in treated and untreated patients. What is the P value associated with this test? How many degrees of freedom does it have? What is a 95% confidence interval for the true difference in APACHE score between treated and untreated patients. Why is this test important in a clinical trial of the efficacy of ibuprofen in septic patients?

2

Simple Linear Regression

There is often an approximately linear relationship between two variables associated with study subjects. Simple linear regression is used to predict one of these variables given the other. We assume that the relationship between these variables can be described by a linear function of one variable plus an error term. We use a sample of observations to estimate the slope and y-intercept of this function and the standard deviation of the error term.

2.1. Sample Covariance

Figure 2.1 shows the scatter plot of plasma glycolate vs. arterial pH in patients with ethylene glycol poisoning (see Section 1.2.9). These variables are negatively correlated in that the glycolate levels tend to decrease with increasing pH. Note, however, that there is some individual variation in this relationship, with different glycolate levels in patients with similar pH levels. In Figure 2.1 the sample mean glycolate and pH values are indicated by the horizontal and vertical lines at $\bar{y} = 90.44$ and $\bar{x} = 7.21$, respectively. Dashed lines show the glycolate and pH residuals for three of these patients. For example, one of the patients has glycolate and pH values of 265.24 and 6.88, respectively. The glycolate and pH residuals for this patient are $265.24 - 90.44 = 174.8$ and $6.88 - 7.21 = -0.33$. The product of these residuals is $174.8 \times (-0.33) = -57.7$. If we divide Figure 2.1 into four quadrants defined by the two sample means, then all observations in the upper left or lower right quadrants will have a product of residuals that is negative. All observations in the lower left and upper right quadrants will have a positive product of residuals. Since glycolate levels tend to fall with increasing pH levels, most observations are in the upper left or lower right quadrants and have a negative product of residuals. For this reason the sum of these products, $\sum (x_i - \bar{x})(y_i - \bar{y})$, will be negative. The **sample covariance** is

$$s_{xy} = \sum (x_i - \bar{x})(y_i - \bar{y})/(n - 1), \tag{2.1}$$

which can be thought of as the average product of residuals. In the poison example, there are $n = 18$ patients, and the sample covariance is

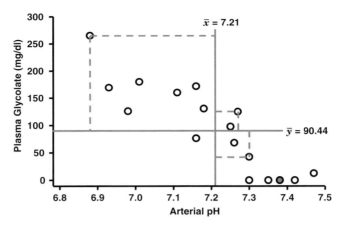

Figure 2.1 Scatter plot of plasma glycolate vs. arterial pH in patients with ethylene gly-col poisoning. The dashed lines show the glycolate and pH residuals for three patients (Brent et al., 1999).

$s_{xy} = -211.26/17 = -12.43$. Note that if there is no relationship between values of the two variables then there will be roughly equal numbers of obser-vations in the four quadrants. In this case, the sum of products of residuals will tend to cancel each other out, giving a small sample covariance. If there is a positive relationship between x_i and y_i then most observations will lie in the lower left or upper right quadrants and s_{xy} will be positive.

2.2. Sample Correlation Coefficient

It is often useful to be able to quantify the extent to which one variable can be used to predict the value of another. The sample covariance measures this relationship to some extent but is also affected by the variability of the observations. A better measure of this association is the sample correlation coefficient, which is adjusted for the variability of the two variables. If s_x and s_y denote the standard deviation of x_i and y_i then

$$r = \frac{s_{xy}}{s_x s_y} \tag{2.2}$$

is the **sample correlation coefficient** between x_i and y_i. In the poison exam-ple $s_x = 0.1731$, $s_y = 80.58$ and $r = -12.43/(0.1731 \times 80.58) = -0.891$. The correlation coefficient can take values from -1 to 1; $r = 1$ implies that the points of a scatter plot of x_i and y_i fall on a straight line with a positive slope; $r = 0$ implies no relationship between x_i and y_i while $r = -1$ im-plies a strict linear relationship with negative slope. The closer r is to ± 1 the

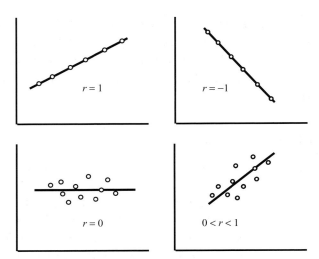

Figure 2.2   Correlation coefficients for four different scatter plots. The closer the points are to lying on a straight line, the closer r is to 1 or −1.

more accurately the values of one variable can be predicted by a linear function of the other (see Figure 2.2).

2.3. Population Covariance and Correlation Coefficient

Suppose that two variables x and y describe attributes of members of some target population. Let μ_x, μ_y, σ_x and σ_y denote the population means and standard deviations for these variables. Then a patient with variable values x_i and y_i will have a residual product equal to $(x_i - \mu_x)(y_i - \mu_y)$. The **population covariance**, σ_{xy}, is the mean residual product for all members of the population. If we observe x_i and y_i on an unbiased sample of n patients from the target population then

$$E[s_{xy}] = \sigma_{xy}. \tag{2.3}$$

The reason why the denominator of s_{xy} in equation (2.1) is $n - 1$ rather than n is to make equation (2.3) true.

The **population correlation coefficient** is $\rho = \sigma_{xy}/(\sigma_x\sigma_y)$, which is estimated by the sample correlation coefficient r. The key difference between ρ and r and s_{xy} and σ_{xy} is that ρ and σ_{xy} are unknown parameters of the target population while r and s_{xy} are known statistics that are calculated from a known sample. We will often omit the adjective "population" or "sample" when it is clear from the context whether we are talking about a known statistic or an unknown parameter.

The population correlation coefficient also lies between ± 1. Variables are said to be positively or negatively **correlated** if ρ is positive or negative. Normally distributed variables are said to be **independent** if $\rho = 0$. In this case knowing the value of one variable for a patient tells us nothing about the likely value of the other.

2.4. Conditional Expectation

Suppose that x and y are variables that can be measured on patients from some population. We observe an unbiased, mutually independent sample of patients from this population. Let x_i and y_i be the values of x and y for the ith patient in this sample. The expected value of y_i, denoted $E[y_i]$, is the average value of y in the population. The **conditional expectation** of y_i given x_i is the average value of y in the subpopulation whose value of x equals x_i. We denote this conditional expectation $E[y_i \mid x_i]$. For example, suppose that half of a population are men, and that $x = 1$ for men and $x = 2$ for women. Let y denote a subject's weight. Suppose that the average weight of men and women in the population is 80 and 60 kg, respectively. Then $E[y_i \mid x_i = 1] = 80$ is the expected weight of the ith sampled subject given that he is a man. $E[y_i \mid x_i = 2] = 60$ is the expected weight of ith sampled subject given that she is a woman, and $E[y_i] = 70$ is the expected weight of the ith subject without considering his or her sex.

2.5. Simple Linear Regression Model

There is often an approximately linear relationship between variables from a population. Simple linear regression allows us to quantify such relationships. As with most inferential statistics, we first assume a statistical model for the data and then estimate the parameters of the model from an unbiased sample of observations. Suppose that we observe an unbiased sample of n patients from a population, with x_i and y_i representing the values of two variables measured on the ith patient. The **simple linear regression model** assumes that

$$y_i = \alpha + \beta x_i + \varepsilon_i, \tag{2.4}$$

where
- (i) α and β are unknown parameters of the population,
- (ii) ε_i has a normal distribution with mean 0 and standard deviation σ, and
- (iii) the values of ε_i are mutually independent.

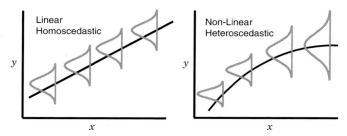

Figure 2.3

Schematic diagrams depicting a simple linear model (left) and a non-linear model with heteroscedastic errors (right). The linear model assumes that the expected value of *y* given *x* is a linear function of *x* and that the error terms are independent and have a constant standard deviation.

That is, the value of ε_i for any one patient is unaffected by the values of any other. ε_i is called the **error** for the ith patient; σ and σ^2 are called the **error standard deviation** and **error variance**, respectively.

It can be shown for any statistics u and v and any constant c that $E[u + v] = E[u] + E[v]$, $E[cu] = cE[u]$ and $E[c] = c$. Suppose that we hold x_i fixed. That is, we restrict our attention to a subpopulation of patients with a specific value of x_i. Then the expected value of y_i given x_i for this subpopulation is

$$E[y_i \mid x_i] = E[\alpha + \beta x_i \mid x_i] + E[\varepsilon_i \mid x_i] = \alpha + \beta x_i + 0 = \alpha + \beta x_i. \quad (2.5)$$

Thus, the expected value of y_i given x_i is $E[y_i \mid x_i] = \alpha + \beta x_i$, and the response y_i equals the sum of a deterministic linear component $\alpha + \beta x_i$ plus a random error component ε_i. Two explicit assumptions of the model are that the expected response y_i is a linear function of x_i and that the standard deviation of ε_i is a constant that does not depend on x_i. Models that have the latter property are called **homoscedastic**. The left panel of Figure 2.3 shows a schematic representation of the linear model. The expected value of y given x is represented by the straight line while the homoscedastic errors are indicated by identical normal probability density functions. The right panel of Figure 2.3 violates the linear model in that the expected value of y is a non-linear function of x, and y has **heteroscedastic** error terms whose standard error increases with increasing x.

2.6. Fitting the Linear Regression Model

Let us return to the ethylene glycol poisoning example introduced in Section 1.2.9. We wish to fit the linear model $E[y_i \mid x_i] = \alpha + \beta x_i$, where $E[y_i \mid x_i]$

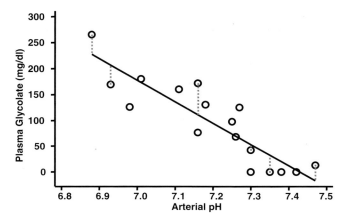

Figure 2.4   The estimated linear regression line is chosen so as to minimize the sum of squared residuals between the observed and expected value of the y variable. The gray dotted lines show the lengths of six of these residuals.

is the expected glycolate value of a patient whose arterial pH is x_i. Let a and b be estimates of α and β. Then $\hat{y}_i = a + bx_i$ is an estimate of $E[y_i \mid x_i]$. The **residual** of y_i given x_i is $y_i - \hat{y}_i$, the difference between the observed value of y_i and its estimated expected value. The dotted lines in Figure 2.4 show these residuals for six of these study subjects. A line that gives a good fit to the data will come as close to as many of the observations as possible. For this reason, we choose as our estimates of α and β those values of a and b that minimize the sum of squared residuals for all patients in the observed sample. It can be shown that these estimates are

$$b = r s_y / s_x \tag{2.6}$$

and

$$a = \bar{y} - b\bar{x}. \tag{2.7}$$

The statistic

$$\hat{y}[x] = a + bx \tag{2.8}$$

is called the **least squares estimate** of $\alpha + \beta x$, and equation (2.8) defines the **linear regression line** of y_i against x_i. It can also be shown that $\hat{y}_i = \hat{y}[x_i]$ is an unbiased estimate of $\alpha + \beta x_i$. Substituting equation (2.7) into equation (2.8) gives us $\hat{y}[x] - \bar{y} = b(x - \bar{x})$. Hence, the linear regression line always passes through the point $(\bar{x}, \bar{y})$. Since

$b = rs_y/s_x$ the slope of the regression line approaches zero as r approaches zero. Thus, if x and y are independent and n is large then r will be very close to zero since $r \cong \rho = 0$, and the regression line will be approximately $\hat{y}(x) = \bar{y}$. This makes sense since if x and y are independent then x is of no value in predicting y. On the other hand, if $r = 1$, then the observations lie on the linear regression line (all the residuals are zero). The slope of this line equals s_y/s_x, which is the variation of y_i relative to the variation of x_i.

Note that we have used the term *residual* in two slightly different ways. In general, the residual for an observation is the difference between the observation and its estimated expected value. When we are looking at a single variable y_i the residual of y_i is $y_i - \bar{y}$, since $\bar{y}$ is our best estimate of $E[y_i]$. This is the definition of residual that we have used prior to this section. When we have two variables and wish to predict y_i in terms of x_i then the residual of y_i is $y_i - \hat{y}_i$, where $\hat{y}_i$ is our best estimate of $E[y_i \mid x_i]$. It is usually clear from the context which type of residual we are talking about.

2.7. Historical Trivia: Origin of the Term *Regression*

When $s_y = s_x$, the slope of the linear regression curve is r and $\hat{y}[x] - \bar{y} = r(x - \bar{x})$, which is less than $x - \bar{x}$ whenever $0 < r < 1$ and $x > \bar{x}$. Francis Galton, a 19th century scientist with an interest in eugenics, studied patterns of inheritance of all sorts of attributes. He found, for example, that the sons of tall men tended to be shorter than their fathers, and that this pattern occurred for most of the variables that he studied. He called this phenomenon regression towards the mean, and the origin of the term *linear regression* is from his work. Regression towards the mean will be observed whenever the linear model is valid, the correlation between x and y is between –1 and 1, and the standard deviation of the x and y variables are equal. Had he run his regressions the other way he would have also discovered that the fathers of tall men also tend to be shorter than their sons.

Note that the regression line of x on y is not the inverse of the regression line of y on x unless $r = \pm 1$. The reason for this asymmetry is that when we regress y on x we are minimizing the squared residuals of y compared to $\hat{y}[x]$ while when we regress x on y we are minimizing the squared residuals of x compared to $\hat{x}[y]$. Figure 2.5 shows the linear regression lines of y on x and x on y for a positively correlated set of data.

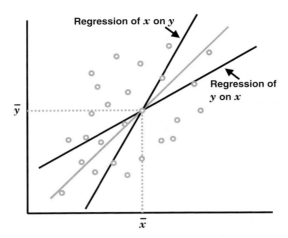

Regression of x on y

Regression of y on x

Figure 2.5   Plot of linear regression lines of y on x and x on y for a positively correlated set of data. These plots are not inverses of each other because of the presence of the correlation coefficient in equation (2.6).

2.8. Determining the Accuracy of Linear Regression Estimates

In the linear regression model, the error term ε_i has a normal distribution with mean 0 and standard deviation σ. We estimate the error variance σ^2 by

$$s^2 = \sum (y_i - \hat{y}_i)^2/(n-2). \tag{2.9}$$

The denominator of equation (2.9) is reduced by two in order to make s^2 an unbiased estimate of σ^2. For large n, s^2 is very close to the average squared residual of y_i. This statistic, s^2, is often called the **mean squared error**, or **MSE**; s is called the **root MSE**.

The variance of b can be shown to be

$$\sigma^2 / \sum (x_i - \bar{x})^2 \tag{2.10}$$

and the standard error of b is

$$\sigma / \sqrt{\sum (x_i - \bar{x})^2} = \sigma/(s_x\sqrt{n-1}). \tag{2.11}$$

This implies that the precision with which we can estimate b
 (i) decreases as σ, the standard deviation of ε_i, increases,
 (ii) increases as the square root of the sample size increases, and
 (iii) increases as the estimated standard deviation of the x variable increases.
The reason why s_x appears in equation (2.11) can be explained intuitively by looking at Figure 2.6. The panels on this figure depict linear regression

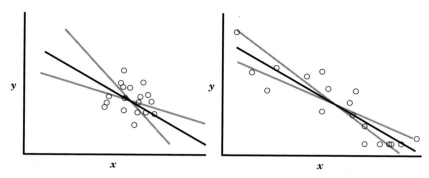

Figure 2.6   The standard error of *b* is affected by the range of the observed values of *x* as well as by the sample size and error standard deviation σ. In both panels of this figure, the regression lines, error standard deviations and sample sizes are identical. They differ in that the range of the *x* values is greater in the right panel than in the left. This greater variation allows us to estimate the slope parameter with greater precision in the right panel.

models with identical values of α and β (indicated by black lines), identical values of σ, and identical sample sizes. They differ in that the range of the *x* variable in the left panel is less than that on the right. This implies that s_x is smaller for the data in the left panel than it is in the right. The gray lines denote possible estimates of $\alpha + \beta x$ that are compatible with the data. Note that the small range of *x* in the left panel makes the data compatible with a larger range of slope estimates than is the case for the right panel.

An unbiased estimate of the variance of *b* is

$$\text{var}[b] = s^2 / \sum (x_i - \bar{x})^2. \tag{2.12}$$

We estimate the standard error of *b* to be

$$se[b] = s/(s_x\sqrt{n-1}). \tag{2.13}$$

Under the null hypothesis that $\beta = 0$,

$$b/se[b] \tag{2.14}$$

has a *t* distribution with $n - 2$ degrees of freedom. We can use equation (2.14) to test this null hypothesis. A 95% confidence interval for β is given by

$$b \pm t_{n-2,0.025}se[b]. \tag{2.15}$$

The variance of *a* is estimated by

$$\text{var}[a] = \frac{s^2}{n} + \bar{x}^2\text{var}[b], \tag{2.16}$$

and $a/\sqrt{\mathrm{var}[a]}$ has a t distribution with $n - 2$ degrees of freedom under the null hypothesis that $a = 0$.

It is helpful to know how successful a linear regression is in explaining the variation of the y variable. We measure the total variation by the **total sum of squares** (TSS) which equals $\sum(y_i - \bar{y})^2$. The analogous variation explained by the model is the **model sum of squares** (MSS), which equals $\sum(\hat{y}_i - \bar{y})^2$. $R^2 = \mathrm{MSS/TSS}$ measures the proportion of the total variation explained by the model. It can be shown that R^2 equals the square of the correlation coefficient r (hence its name). If x and y are independent then $\hat{y}_i \cong \bar{y}$ for all i and $\sum(\hat{y}_i - \bar{y})^2 \cong 0$. If x and y are perfectly correlated, then $y_i = \hat{y}_i$ and hence $R^2 = 1$.

2.9. Ethylene Glycol Poisoning Example

For the poison data discussed in Section 1.2.9 and throughout this chapter we have that $n = 18$, $\bar{x} = 7.210\,56$, $\bar{y} = 90.44$, $s_x = 0.173\,05$, $s_y = 80.584\,88$ and $r = -0.891\,12$. Hence equations (2.6) and (2.7) give that $b = rs_y/s_x = -0.891\,12 \times 80.584\,88/0.173\,05 = -414.97$ and $a = \bar{y} - b\bar{x} = 90.44 - (-414.97 \times 7.210\,56) = 3082.6$. The estimate of σ is

$$s = \sqrt{\sum(y_i - \hat{y}_i)^2/(n-2)} = 37.693.$$

The estimated standard error of b is

$$\mathrm{se}[b] = s/(s_x\sqrt{n-1}) = 37.693/(0.173\,05\sqrt{18-1}) = 52.83.$$

To test the null hypothesis that $\beta = 0$ we calculate $t = b/\mathrm{se}[b] = -414.97/52.83 = 7.85$, which has a t distribution with 16 degrees of freedom ($P < 0.0005$). Hence, we can accept the alternative hypothesis that glycolate levels fall with increasing pH. Now $\pm t_{16, 0.025} = 2.12$. Therefore, a 95% confidence interval for b is $b \pm t_{n-2, 0.025}\mathrm{se}(b) = -414.97 \pm t_{16, 0.025} \times 52.83 = -414.97 \pm 2.12 \times 52.83 = (-527, -303)$.

2.10. 95% Confidence Interval for $y[x] = \alpha + \beta x$ Evaluated at x

Let $y[x] = \alpha + \beta x$ be the expected value of y given x. Then $y[x]$ is estimated by $\hat{y}[x] = a + bx$. The expected value of $\hat{y}[x]$ given x is $\mathrm{E}[\hat{y}[x] \mid x] = y[x]$ and the estimated variance of $\hat{y}[x]$ given x is

$$\mathrm{var}[\hat{y}[x] \mid x] = (s^2/n) + (x - \bar{x})^2\mathrm{var}[b]. \tag{2.17}$$

Since the regression line goes through the point $(\bar{x}, \bar{y})$, we have that $\hat{y}[\bar{x}] = \bar{y}$ and equation (2.17) reduces to s^2/n when $x = \bar{x}$. The farther x is from $\bar{x}$ the

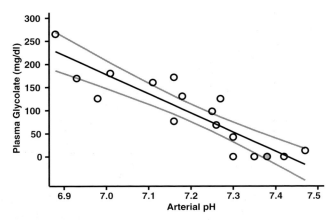

Figure 2.7   This graph shows the estimated linear regression line of plasma glycolate against arterial pH (Brent et al., 1999). The gray lines in this graph show the 95% confidence intervals for the expected glycolate response $E[\hat{y}(x) \mid x] = \alpha + \beta x$.

greater the variance of $\hat{y}[x]$ and the greater the influence of var$[b]$ in determining this variance. This reflects the fact that errors in the estimate of β are amplified as x moves away from $\bar{x}$. The 95% confidence interval for $\hat{y}[x]$ is

$$\hat{y}[x] \pm t_{n-2,0.025}\sqrt{\text{var}[\hat{y}[x] \mid x]}. \qquad (2.18)$$

For example, suppose that we wanted to estimate a 95% confidence interval for the expected glycolate level of patients with an arterial pH of 7.0 who have been poisoned by ethylene glycol. Then $\hat{y}[7.0] = a + 7.0b = 3082.6 - 7.0 \times 414.97 = 177.81$, var$[\hat{y}[7.0] \mid x = 7] = [s^2/n] + (7.0 - \bar{x})^2$ var$[b] = 37.693^2/18 + (7.0 - 7.210\,56)^2 \times 52.83^2 = 202.7$ and a 95% confidence interval for $\hat{y}(7.0)$ is $177.81 \pm 2.12\sqrt{202.7} = (148, 208)$. Figure 2.7 shows a plot of equations (2.8) and (2.18) for the poison data. Note that these confidence limits indicate the plausible degree of error in our estimate of the regression line $y[x] = \alpha + \beta x$. They do not indicate the likely range of the observed values of y_i, and indeed the observations for half of the patients lie outside these bounds. Note also that the linear regression model assumptions are false for larger pH values since the glycolate values cannot be less than zero. Nevertheless, the overall fit of the data to this linear model appears to be excellent.

2.11. 95% Prediction Interval for the Response of a New Patient

Sometimes we would like to predict the likely range of response for a new patient given her value of the x variable. Under the linear model

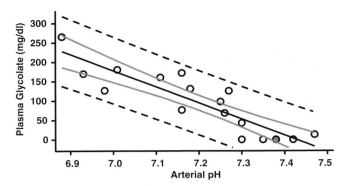

Figure 2.8   The dashed lines on this graph show 95% prediction intervals for the plasma glycolate levels of new patients based on the data from Brent et al. (1999).

we can write her response as $y[x] = \alpha + \beta x + \varepsilon_i \cong \hat{y}[x] + \varepsilon_i$. It can be shown for any two independent variables u and v with variances σ_u^2 and σ_v^2 that the variance of $u + v$ is $\sigma_u^2 + \sigma_v^2$. Hence $\text{var}[y \mid x] \cong \text{var}[\hat{y}[x] \mid x] + \text{var}[\varepsilon_i] = \text{var}[\hat{y}(x) \mid x] + \sigma^2$, and a **95% prediction interval** for y can be estimated by

$$\hat{y}[x] \pm t_{n-2,0.025}\sqrt{\text{var}[\hat{y}[x] \mid x] + s^2}. \tag{2.19}$$

That is, the probability that her response will lie in the interval given by equation (2.19) is 0.95. For example, suppose that a new patient poisoned with ethylene glycol has an arterial pH of 7.0. Then $\hat{y}[7.0] = 177.81$, $\text{var}[\hat{y}[7.0] \mid x = 7] = 202.7$, $s = 37.693$ and a 95% prediction interval for y at $x = 7.0$ is $177.81 \pm 2.12\sqrt{202.7 + 37.693^2} = (92.4, 263)$. In Figure 2.8 the dashed lines show the 95% prediction intervals for new patients poisoned by ethylene glycol. Note that we can make the 95% confidence interval for $\hat{y}[x]$ as narrow as we want by choosing a sufficiently large sample size. The lower limit on the width of the 95% prediction interval for new observations, however, is constrained by the standard deviation of ε_i for individual observations.

2.12. Simple Linear Regression with Stata

The following log file and comments illustrates how to use Stata to perform the calculations discussed in the previous sections.

```
. * 2.12.Poison.log
. *
. * Calculate the mean plasma glycolate and arterial pH levels for the
. * ethylene glycol poisoning data of Brent et al. (1999). Regress glycolate
```

```
. * levels against pH. Draw a scatter plot of glycolate against pH. Plot the
. * linear regression line on this scatter plot together with the 95%
. * confidence limits for this line and the 95% prediction intervals for new
. * patients.
. *
. use C:\WDDtext\2.12.Poison.dta, clear                                   {1}

. summarize ph glyco


Variable |   Obs      Mean    Std. Dev.    Min        Max
---------+-------------------------------------------------
      ph |    18   7.210556   .1730512   6.88        7.47
   glyco |    18     90.44   80.58488      0       265.24

. format ph %9.1g                                                        {2}

. format glyco %9.0g

. graph glyco ph, gap(4) xlabel(6.8,6.9 to 7.5) ylabel(0, 50 to 300)     {3}
> xline(7.21) yline(90.4)
```

                                        {Graph omitted. See Figure 2.1}

```
. regress glyco ph                                                       {4}


  Source |      SS      df       MS              Number of obs =     18   {5}
-------- + --------------------------           F( 1,    16) =  61.70
   Model | 87664.6947   1   87664.6947          Prob > F      = 0.0000   {7}
Residual | 22731.9877  16   1420.74923          R-squared     = 0.7941   {8}
-------- + --------------------------           Adj R-squared = 0.7812
   Total | 110396.682  17   6493.9225           Root MSE      = 37.693   {6}
------------------------------------------------------------------------
   glyco |    Coef.   Std. Err.      t     P>|t|    [95% Conf. Interval]
---------+--------------------------------------------------------------
      ph | -414.9666  52.82744   -7.855   0.000   -526.9558 -302.9775    {9}
   _cons |  3082.58   381.0188    8.090   0.000    2274.856  3890.304   {10}
------------------------------------------------------------------------

. predict yhat, xb                                                      {11}

. graph glyco yhat ph, gap(4) xlabel(6.9,7.0 to 7.5) ylabel(0, 50 to 300) {12}
> connect(.l) symbol(Oi)
```

                                        {Graph omitted. See Figure 2.4}

```
. predict std_p, stdp                                                   {13}

. display _N                                                            {14}
```

```
. display invttail(_N-2,0.025)                                          {15}

2.1199053

. generate ci_u = yhat + invttail(_N-2,0.025)*std_p                     {16}

. generate ci_l = yhat - invttail(_N-2,0.025)*std_p                     {17}

. sort ph                                                               {18}

. graph glyco yhat ci_u ci_l ph, gap(4) xlabel(6.9,7.0 to 7.5)          {19}
> ylabel(0, 50 to 300) connect(.lll) symbol(Oiii)
```
                                                {Graph omitted. See Figure 2.7.}
```
. predict std_f, stdf                                                   {20}

. generate ci_uf = yhat + invttail(_N-2,0.025)*std_f                    {21}

. generate ci_lf = yhat - invttail(_N-2,0.025)*std_f

. graph glyco yhat ci_u ci_l ci_lf ci_uf ph, gap(4) xlabel(6.9,7.0 to 7.5)  {22}
> ylabel(0, 50 to 300) connect(.lllll) symbol(Oiiiii)
```
                                                {Graph omitted. See Figure 2.8}

Comments

1 The *2.12.Poison.dta* data set contains the plasma glycolate and arterial pH levels of 18 patients admitted for ethylene glycol poisoning. These levels are stored in variables called *glyco* and *ph*, respectively. The *clear* option of the *use* command deletes any data that may have been in memory when this command was given.

2 Stata variables are associated with formats that control how they are displayed in the Stata Editor and in graphs and data output. This command assigns *ph* a general numeric format with up to nine digits and one digit after the decimal point. The next command assigns *glyco* a similar format with no digits after the decimal point. These commands will affect the appearance of the axis labels in the subsequent graph commands. They do not affect the numeric values of these variables. In the *2.12.Poison data* set both of these formats are set to %9.2g.

3 The command *graph glyco ph* draws a scatter plot of *glyco* by *ph*. The options on this command improve the visual appearance of the scatter plot; *gap(4)* places the title of the *y*-axis four spaces to the left of the *y*-axis. The *xlabel* option labels the *x*-axis from 6.8 to 7.5 in even increments 0.1 units apart. The *ylabel* options labels the *y*-axis from 0 to 300 in increments of 50. The *xline* and *yline* options draw vertical and horizontal lines at $x = 7.21$ and $y = 90.4$ respectively. The default titles of the *x*- and *y*-axes are labels assigned to the *ph* and *glyco* variables in the

2.12.Poison.dta data set. The resulting graph is similar to Figure 2.1. (In this latter figure I used a graphics editor to annotate the mean glycolate and pH values and to indicate the residuals for three data points.)

4 This command performs a linear regression of *glyco* against *ph*. That is, we fit the model $E[glyco \mid ph] = \alpha + \beta \times ph$ (see equation 2.5). The most important output from this command has been highlighted and is defined below.

5 The number of patients $n = 18$.

6 The root MSE is $s = 37.693$ (see equation 2.9). The total sum of squares is TSS = 110 396.682.

7 The model sum of squares is MSS = 87 664.6947.

8 $R^2 = MSS/TSS = 0.7941$. Hence 79% of the variation in glycolate levels is explained by this linear regression.

9 The slope estimate of β for this linear regression is $b = -414.9666$ (see equation 2.6). The estimated standard error of b is se$[b] = 52.827\,44$ (see equation 2.13). The t statistic to test the null hypothesis that $\beta = 0$ is $t = b/se[b] = -7.855$ (see equation 2.14). The P value associated with this statistic is < 0.0005. The 95% confidence interval for β is $(-526.9558, -302.9775)$ (see equation 2.15).

10 The y intercept estimate of α for this linear regression is $a = 3082.58$ (see equation 2.7).

11 The *predict* command can estimate a variety of statistics after a regression or other estimation command. (Stata refers to such commands as post estimation commands.) The *xb* option causes a new variable (in this example *yhat*) to be set equal to each patient's expected plasma glycolate level $\hat{y}[x] = a + bx$; in this equation, x is the patient's arterial pH and a and b are the parameter estimates of the linear regression (see also equation 2.8).

12 This command graphs *glyco* and *yhat* against *ph*. The *connect* and *symbol* options specify how this is to be done. There must be one character between the parentheses following the *connect* and *symbol* options for each plotted variable. The first character affects the first variable (*glyco*), the second affects the second variable (*yhat*) et cetera; *connect*(.l) specifies that the *glyco* values are not connected and the *yhat* values are connected by a straight line; *symbol*(Oi) specifies that each glyco value is indicated by a large circle but that no symbol is used for *yhat*. The net effect of this command is to produce a scatter plot of glycolate against pH together with a straight line indicating the expected glycolate levels as a function of pH. The resulting graph is similar to Figure 2.4.

Stata commands can often be too long to fit on a single line of a log file. When this happens the command wraps onto the next line.

A ">" symbol at the beginning of a line indicates the continuation of the preceding command rather than the start of a new one.

13 With the *stdp* option *predict* defines a new variable (in this example *std_p*) to be the standard error of *yhat*. That is, $std\_p = \sqrt{var[\hat{y}[x] \mid x]}$ (see equation 2.17).

14 The *display* command calculates and displays a numeric expression or constant. _N denotes the number of variables in the data set, which in this example is 18.

15 The Stata function *invttail*(n, $1 - \alpha$) calculates a critical value of size α for a t distribution with n degrees of freedom. Thus, *invttail*(_N − 2,0.025) = *invttail*(16,0.025) = $t_{16,0.025}$ = 2.119 9053.

16 The *generate* command defines a new variable in terms of old ones. Here *ci_u* is set equal to

$$\hat{y}[x] + t_{n-2,0.025}\sqrt{var[\hat{y}[x] \mid x]},$$

which is the upper bound for the 95% confidence interval for $\hat{y}[x]$ (see equation 2.18).

17 Similarly

$$ci\_l = \hat{y}[x] - t_{n-2,0.025}\sqrt{var[\hat{y}[x] \mid x]}.$$

18 This command sorts the data by *ph*. This is needed to ensure that the following graph command draws the confidence bounds correctly. The data should be sorted by the *x*-axis variable whenever a non-linear curve is to be plotted.

19 We next add the graphs of the 95% confidence intervals for $\hat{y}[x]$ to the preceding graph, which generates Figure 2.7.

20 The *stdf* option of the *predict* command defines a new variable (*std_f*) that equals the standard deviation of the response for a new patient. That is,
$$std\_f = \sqrt{var[\hat{y}[x] \mid x] + s^2}.$$

21 The next two commands define *ci_uf* and *ci_lf* to be the bounds of the 95% prediction intervals for new patients (see equation 2.19).

22 This final *graph* command adds the 95% prediction intervals to the preceding graph. It is similar to Figure 2.8.

2.13. Lowess Regression

Linear regression is a useful tool for describing a relationship that is linear, or approximately linear. It has the disadvantage that the linear relationship is assumed *a priori*. It is often useful to fit a line through a scatter plot that does not make any model assumptions. One such technique is **lowess regression**, which stands for locally weighted scatter plot smoothing (Cleveland, 1993). The idea is that each observation (x_i, y_i) is fitted to a separate linear regression line based on adjacent observations. These points are weighted so that the farther away the x value is from x_i, the less effect it has on determining the estimate of $\hat{y}_i$. The proportion of the total data set that is considered for each estimate $\hat{y}_i$ is called the **bandwidth**. In Stata, the default bandwidth is 0.8, which works well for midsize data sets. For large data sets a bandwidth of 0.3 or 0.4 usually works best; a bandwidth of 0.99 is recommended for small data sets. The wider the bandwidth the smoother the regression curve. Narrow bandwidths produce curves that are more sensitive to local perturbations in the data. Experimenting with different bandwidths helps to find a curve that is sensitive to real trends in the data without being unduly affected by random variation. The lowess method is computationally intensive on large data sets. Reducing the bandwidth will reduce the time needed to derive these curves.

The black curve in Figure 2.9 shows a lowess regression curve for the ethylene glycol poisoning data. It was drawn with a bandwidth of 0.99. The gray line in this graph marks the least squares linear regression line. These two curves are similar for pHs lower than 7.4. There is evidence of a mild departure from the linear model for the larger pH values that are associated with glycolate values at, or near, zero.

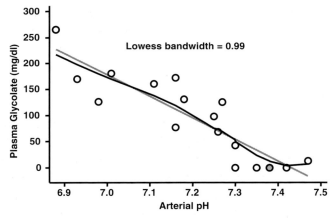

Figure 2.9   The black line shows the lowess regression curve for the ethylene glycol poisoning data (Brent 1999). This curve closely approximates the linear regression curve over most of the observed range of arterial pH.

2.14. Plotting a Lowess Regression Curve in Stata

The *2.12.Poison.log* file that was started in Section 2.12 continues as follows.

```
. * Derive a lowess regression curve for the ethylene glycol poisoning data
. * using a bandwidth of 0.99. Plot this curve together with the linear
. * regression line and a scatterplot of plasma glycolate by arterial pH
. * levels.
. *
. ksm glyco ph, lowess bwidth(.99) generate(low99glyco)                    {1}
                                                                  {Graph omitted}
. graph glyco yhat low99glyco ph, gap(4) xlabel(6.9,7.0 to 7.5)            {2}
> ylabel(0, 50 to 300) connect(.11) symbol(Oii)
                                            {Graph omitted. See Figure 2.9}
```

Comments

1 The *ksm* command with the *lowess* option derives a lowess regression curve; *ksm glyco ph, lowess* graphs this regression curve together with a scatterplot of *glyco* against *ph*. The default bandwidth for lowess regression is 0.8. To use a different bandwidth add the *bwidth(#)* option, where # is a number greater than zero and less than one. In this example I have chosen a bandwidth of 0.99. The option *generate(low99glyco)* creates an new variable called *low99glyco* that equals the value of the lowess regression curve associated with each patient's pH.

2 This command plots the lowess regression curve given by *low99glyco* together with the linear regression line and a scatter plot of *glyco* against *ph*. The resulting graph is similar to Figure 2.9.

2.15. Residual Analyses

An important advance in modern data analysis is the use of computers for exploratory data analysis. Such analyses are useful in determining whether a given model is appropriate for a given data set or whether specific observations are having an excessive influence on the conclusions of our analyses. One of these techniques is residual analysis. In linear regression the residual for the ith patient is $e_i = y_i - \hat{y}_i$ (see Section 2.6). Figure 2.10 shows a linear regression of systolic blood pressure (SBP) against body mass index (BMI) for 25 patients from the Framingham Heart Study (Levy, 1999). The solid line shows the estimated expected SBP derived from all 25 patients.

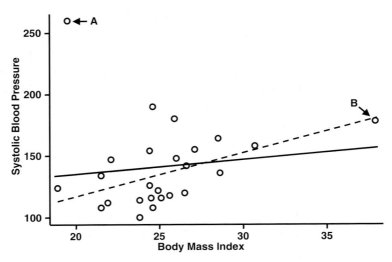

Figure 2.10

Regression of systolic blood pressure against body mass index. The solid line includes all patients in the regression. The dashed line excludes Patient A. Patient A exerts a large influence on the regression line. Patients A and B both have high leverage because they are both far from the mean body mass index. However, Patient B has little influence because her systolic blood pressure falls near the regression line.

Note that patient A has an observed SBP of 260 and an expected SBP of 134 giving a very large residual $260 - 134 = 126$. If we delete this patient from the analysis the regression line shifts to the dashed line in Figure 2.10. The solid and dashed lines in this figure have slopes of 1.19 and 3.53, respectively. Thus, the deletion of this single data point causes a three-fold increase in the regression slope. This data point is said to have great **influence** on our slope estimate. The reason for this is partly because of the large residual and partly because the patient's BMI is fairly far from the mean BMI value. Recall that the regression line is fitted by minimizing the sum of the squared residuals. Rotating the dashed line in a clockwise direction towards the solid line reduces the squared residual for patient A more than it increases the squared residuals for all other patients.

The potential for an independent variable value to influence the results is quantified by its **leverage**, which is given by the formula

$$h_j = \frac{1}{n} + \frac{(\bar{x} - x_j)^2}{\sum_i (\bar{x} - x_i)^2}. \tag{2.20}$$

The leverage is minimized when $\bar{x} = x_j$, in which case $h_j = 1/n$. A large residual with little leverage will have little effect on the parameter estimates, particularly if the sample size, n, is large. It can be shown that h_j always lies between $1/n$ and 1. Data points with high leverage will have great influence if the associated residual is large. In Figure 2.10 patient B has high leverage but little influence since the regression lines pass near the data point. This is particularly true of the regression in which patient A is omitted. Note that the leverage is determined entirely by the values of the x variable and is not affected by the y variable.

We can rewrite equation (2.17) using equation (2.20) as

$$\text{var}[\hat{y}_i \mid x_i] = s^2 h_i. \tag{2.21}$$

Hence, an alternative definition of h_i is that it is the variance of $\hat{y}_i$ given x_i expressed in units of s^2. If x is the covariate of a new patient with leverage h then the estimated variance of her predicted response y given x is

$$\text{var}[y \mid x] = s^2 (h + 1). \tag{2.22}$$

Thus, we can rewrite the 95% prediction interval for y (equation (2.19)), as

$$\hat{y}[x] \pm t_{n-2, 0.025}(s\sqrt{h + 1}). \tag{2.23}$$

We will discuss the concepts of influence and leverage in greater detail in the next chapter.

The variance of the residual e_i is

$$\text{var}[e_i] = s^2 (1 - h_i). \tag{2.24}$$

Note that high leverage reduces the variance of e_i because the data point tends to pull the regression line towards it, thereby reducing the variation of the residual. (In the extreme case when $h_i = 1$ the regression line always goes through the ith data point giving a residual of zero. Hence the variance of e_i also equals zero.) Dividing e_i by its standard deviation gives the **standardized residual** for the ith patient, which is

$$z_i = e_i / s\sqrt{1 - h_i}. \tag{2.25}$$

Large standardized residuals identify values of y_i that are outliers and are not consistent with the linear model. A problem with equation (2.25) is that a single large residual can inflate the value of s^2, which in turn will decrease the size of the standardized residuals. To avoid this problem, we usually calculate **the studentized residual**

$$t_i = e_i / s_{(i)}\sqrt{1 - h_i}, \tag{2.26}$$

where $s_{(i)}$ denotes the root MSE estimate of σ with the ith case deleted (t_i is sometimes referred to as the **jackknife residual**). If the linear model is

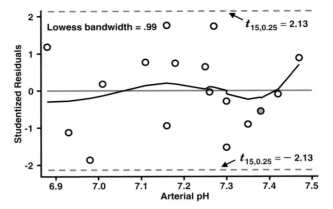

Figure 2.11   Scatterplot of studentized residuals against arterial pH for the linear regression performed in Section 2.9. A lowess regression is fitted to these residuals.

correct, then t_i should have a t distribution with $n - 3$ degrees of freedom. Plotting these residuals against x_i is useful for assessing the homoscedasticity assumption and detecting departures from linearity. Figure 2.11 shows a plot of studentized residuals against pH values for the linear regression performed in Section 2.9. A lowess regression curve of the studentized residuals against pH is also plotted. This curve should be flat and close to zero when the regression is from a large data set in which the linear model is valid. Dashed horizontal lines are drawn at $\pm t_{n-3, 0.25} = \pm t_{15, 0.25} = \pm 2.13$; if the model is correct 95% of the residuals should lie between these dotted lines. This is, in fact, the case and there is no obvious pattern in the distribution of the residuals. The variation of the residuals does not appear to vary with pH and the lowess regression curve is fairly flat and close to zero. Hence, this graph suggests that the linear regression model is appropriate for these data.

It is always a good idea to double check data points with large studentized residuals. They may indicate data errors or some anomaly in the way the experiment was conducted. If the data point is valid but has high influence you may wish to report your findings both with and without this data point included in the analysis.

2.16. Studentized Residual Analysis Using Stata

The following log file and comments illustrate a residual analysis of the ethylene glycol poison data.

```
. * 2.16.Poison.log

. *

. * Perform a residual analysis of the linear regression of plasma glycolate
. * against arterial pH from the poison data set (Brent et al., 1999).

. *

. use C:\WDDtext\2.12.Poison.dta, clear

. format ph %9.1g

. regress glyco ph
```

{Output omitted. See Section 2.12}

```
. predict residual, rstudent                                        {1}

. display invttail(_N-3, .025)                                      {2}
2.1314495

. ksm residual ph, lowess bwidth(.99) gap(2) xlabel(6.9,7.0 to 7.5)

. ksm residual ph, lowess bwidth(.99) gap(2) xlabel(6.9,7.0 to 7.5)  {3}
> ylabel(-2.0 -1 to 2.0) yline(-2.13 0 2.13,.95) symbol(Oi)
```

{Graph omitted. See Figure 2.11}

Comments

1 The *rstudent* option of the *predict* command causes studentized residuals to be derived and stored in the specified variable – in this case *residual*. (Note that the *predict* command applies to the most recent estimation command; *ksm* is also an estimation command. Hence, if we had calculated a lowess regression in between the preceding *predict* and *regress* commands, we would have had to repeat the *regress* command prior to calculating the studentized residuals.)

2 The critical value $t_{n-3,0.25} = t_{15,0.25} = 2.13$. If the linear model is correct 95% of the studentized residuals should lie between ± 2.13.

3 The *ksm* command accepts many of the options of the *graph* command. This command produces a graph that is very similar to Figure 2.11.

2.17. Transforming the x and y Variables

2.17.1. Stabilizing the Variance

Suppose that we regress y against x, and then perform a residual plot as in Section 2.16. If this plot shows evidence of heteroscedasticity we can sometimes rectify the problem by transforming the y variable. If the residual standard deviation appears to be proportional to the expected value $\hat{y}_i$, try using a **logarithmic transformation**. That is, try the model

$$\log[y_i] = \alpha + \beta x_i + \varepsilon_i. \tag{2.27}$$

If the residual variance is proportional to the expected value $\hat{y}_i$, then the **square root transform**

$$\sqrt{y_i} = \alpha + \beta x_i + \varepsilon_i. \tag{2.28}$$

will stabilize the variance. Note, however, that transforming the y variable affects the shape of the curve $\log[\hat{y}[x]]$ as well as the residual standard deviation. Hence, if the relationship between x and y is linear but the residual standard deviation increases with $\hat{y}_i$, then equation (2.27) may stabilize the residual variance but impose an invalid non-linear relationship between $E[y_i]$ and x_i. In this case non-linear regression methods may be needed (Hamilton, 1992; Draper and Smith, 1998).

2.17.2. Correcting for Non-linearity

Figure 2.12 shows four common patterns on non-linearity between x and y variables. If x is positive, then models of the form

$$y_i = \alpha + \beta (x_i)^P + \varepsilon_i, \tag{2.29}$$

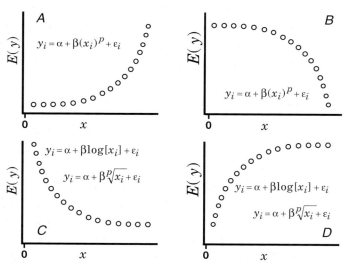

Figure 2.12   Transforms to consider to achieve a linear relationship between $E[y_i]$ and either $\log[x_i]$, $(x_i)^P$ or $\sqrt[p]{x_i}$. We choose a constant $p > 1$ that gives the best linear relationship for the transformed data.

$$y_i = \alpha + \beta \log[x_i] + \varepsilon_i, \text{ or} \qquad (2.30)$$

$$y_i = \alpha + \beta \sqrt[p]{x_i} + \varepsilon_i \qquad (2.31)$$

should be considered for some $p > 1$. Data similar to panels A and B of this figure may be modeled with equation (2.29). Data similar to panels C and D may be modeled with equations (2.30) or (2.31). The best value of p is found empirically. Alternatively, data similar to panels A or C may be modeled with

$$\log[y_i] = \alpha + \beta x_i + \varepsilon_i \qquad (2.32)$$

or

$$\sqrt[p]{y_i} = \alpha + \beta x_i + \varepsilon_i. \qquad (2.33)$$

Data similar to panels B or D may be modeled with

$$y_i^p = \alpha + \beta x_i + \varepsilon_i. \qquad (2.34)$$

These models may correctly model the relationship between x and y but introduce heteroscedasticity in the model errors. In this case non-linear regression methods should be used.

Data transformations can often lead to more appropriate statistical models. In most cases, however, the results of our analyses should be presented in terms of the untransformed data. It is important to bear in mind that the ultimate purpose of statistics in biomedical research is to help clinicians and scientists communicate with each other. For this reason, results should be presented in a way that will be easily understood by readers who do not necessarily have strong backgrounds in biostatistics.

2.17.3. Example: Research Funding and Morbidity for 29 Diseases

Gross et al. (1999) studied the relationship between NIH research funding for 29 different diseases and disability-adjusted person-years of life lost due to these illnesses. Scatter plots of these two variables are shown in the panels of Figure 2.13. Panel A shows the untransformed scatter plot. Funding for AIDS is 3.7 times higher than for any other disease, which makes the structure of the data hard to see. Panel B is similar to panel A except the AIDS data has been deleted and the y-axis has been rescaled. This scatterplot has a concave shape similar to panel D of Figure 2.12, which suggests using a log or power transform (equations 2.30 or 2.31). Panel C of Figure 2.13 shows funding plotted against log disability-adjusted life-years. The resulting scatter plot has a convex shape similar to panel A of Figure 2.12. This suggests using

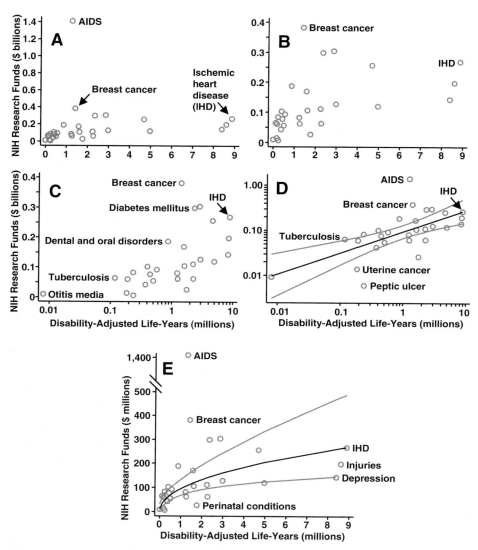

Figure 2.13   Scatter plots of NIH funding against disability-adjusted life-years lost for 29 diseases (Gross et al., 1999). The x- and y-axes of these variables are plotted on either linear or logarithmic scales. The relationship between log funds and log life-years in panel D is reasonably linear.

either a less concave transform of the x-axis or using a log transform of the y-axis. In panel D of Figure 2.13 we plot log funding against log disability. The relationship between these transformed variables is now quite linear. AIDS remains an outlier but is far less discordant with the other diseases than it is in panel A. The linear regression line and associated 95% confidence intervals are shown in this panel. The model for this linear regression is

$$E[\log[y_i] \mid x_i] = \alpha + \beta \log[x_i],$$ (2.35)

where y_i and x_i are the research funds and disability-adjusted life-years lost for the ith disease, respectively. The slope estimate is $\beta = 0.48$, which differs from zero with overwhelming statistical significance. Gross et al. (1999) published a figure that is similar to panel D. Although this figure helps to validate their statistical model, it is not an ideal graphic for displaying the relationship between funding and lost life-years to their audience. This relationship is more easily understood in panel E of Figure 2.13, which uses the untransformed data. The transformed regression line and confidence intervals from panel D are redrawn in this panel. If $\log[\hat{y}_i] = a + b\log[x_i]$ is the estimated regression line for the model specified by equation (2.35) then the predicted funding level for the ith disease is

$$\hat{y}_i = e^a x_i^b.$$ (2.36)

Equation (2.36) is the middle curve in panel E. The 95% confidence intervals for this curve are obtained by taking anti-logs of the confidence intervals in panel D. Panel E shows that funding does increase with increasing loss of life-years but that the rate of increase slows as the number of life-years lost increases. Clearly other factors in addition to numbers of life-years lost affect funding decisions. This is particularly true with respect to AIDS (see Varmus, 1999). Of course, panels D and E display the same information. However, panel D de-emphasizes the magnitude of AIDS funding and overemphasizes the magnitude of the number of disability-adjusted life-years lost to this disease.

2.18. Analyzing Transformed Data with Stata

The following log file illustrates how data may be transformed to obtain data that are appropriate for linear regression.

```
. * 2.18.Funding.log

. *

. * Explore the relationship between NIH research funds and disability-
. * adjusted life-years lost due to the 29 diseases discussed by
. * Gross et al. (1999). Look for transformed values of these variables
. * that are linearly related. Perform a linear regression on these
. * transformed variables. Replot this regression line as a function of
. * the untransformed variables.
```

```
. *
. use C:\WDDtext\2.18.Funding.dta, clear                                    {1}

. format dollars %9.1g

. graph dollars disabil ,xlabel(0, 1 to 9) ylabel(0, 0.2 to 1.4) gap(5)     {2}
```
{Graph omitted. See Figure 2.13, panel A.}
```
. graph dollars disabil if dollars < 1 ,xlabel(0, 1 to 9) ylabel            {3}
> (0, .1 to .4) ytick(.05 .15 .25 .35) gap(3)
```
{Graph omitted. See Figure 2.13, panel B.}
```
. generate logdis = log(disabil)

. label variable logdis "Log Adj. Life-Years"                               {4}

. graph dollars logdis if dollars < 1, xtick(-2.3,-1.61,-1.2,-.92,-.69,     {5}
> -.51,-.36,-.22,-.11,0,.69,1.1,1.39,1.61,1.79,1.95,2.08,2.20,2.3)
> xlabel(-4.61 -2.3 0 2.3) ylabel(0 .1 .2 .3 .4) ytick(.05 .15 .25 .35) gap(3)
```
{Graph omitted. See Figure 2.13, panel C.}
```
. generate logdol = log(dollars)

. label variable logdol "Funding (log $ billions)"

. graph logdol logdis, xtick(-2.3,-1.61,-1.2,-.92,-.69,-.51,-.36,-.22,      {6}
> -.11,0,.69,1.1,1.39,1.61,1.79,1.95,2.08,2.20,2.3) xlabel(-4.61,-2.3 0 2.3)
> ytick(-4.61, -3.91, -3.51, -3.22, -3.00, -2.81, -2.66, -2.53, -2.41, -2.3,
> -1.61,-1.2,-.92,-.69,-.51,-.36,-.22,-.11,0) ylabel(-4.61,-2.3,0) gap(5)
```
{Graph omitted.}
```
. regress logdol logdis                                                     {7}
```

```
  Source |       SS       df       MS              Number of obs =      29
---------+-----------------------------            F( 1,    27) =    18.97
   Model | 14.8027627     1  14.8027627            Prob > F      =   0.0002
Residual | 21.0671978    27   .780266584           R-squared     =   0.4127
---------+-----------------------------            Adj R-squared =   0.3909
   Total | 35.8699605    28   1.28107002           Root MSE      =   .88333
-------------------------------------------------------------------------------
  logdol |     Coef.   Std. Err.       t     P>|t|     [95% Conf. Interval]
---------+---------------------------------------------------------------------
  logdis |   .4767575   .109458     4.356   0.000     .2521682     .7013468   {8}
   _cons |  -2.352205   .1640383   -14.339   0.000    -2.688784    -2.015627
-------------------------------------------------------------------------------
```

```
. predict yhat, xb

. predict stdp, stdp
```

```
. generate ci_u = yhat + invttail(_N-2,.025)*stdp

. generate ci_l = yhat - invttail(_N-2,.025)*stdp

. sort logdis

. graph logdol yhat ci_l ci_u logdis, connect(.111) symbol(Oiii)        {9}
> xlabel(-4.61,-2.3 0 2.3) xtick(-2.3,-1.61,-1.2,-.92,-.69,-.51,-.36,-.22,
> -.11,0,.69,1.1,1.39,1.61,1.79,1.95,2.08,2.20,2.3) ylabel(-4.61,-2.3,0)
> ytick(-4.61,-3.91,-3.51,-3.22,-3.00,-2.81,-2.66,-2.53,-2.41,-2.3,-1.61,
> -1.2,-.92,-.69,-.51,-.36,-.22,-.11,0) gap(5)
```
                                        {Graph omitted. See Figure 2.13, panel D.}
```
. generate yhat2 = exp(yhat)                                           {10}

. generate ci_u2 = exp(ci_u)

. generate ci_l2 = exp(ci_l)

. graph dollars yhat2 ci_u2 ci_l2 disabil, xlabel(0, 1 to 9)          {11}
> ylabel(0, .2 to 1.4) gap(5) connect(.111) symbol(Oiii)
```
                                                              {Graph omitted}
```
. graph dollars yhat2 ci_u2 ci_l2 disabil if dollars < 1, xlabel     {12}
> (0, 1 to 9) ylabel(0,.1, .2,.3, .4,.5) gap(3) connect(.111) symbol(Oiii)
```
                                        {Graph omitted. See Figure 2.13, panel E.}

Comments

1 This data set is from Table 1 of Gross et al. (1999). It contains the annual allocated NIH research funds and disability-adjusted life-years lost for 29 diseases. These two variables are denoted *dollars* and *disabil* in this data set, respectively.

2 This command produces a scatter plot that is similar to panel A of Figure 2.13. In this figure the annotation of individual diseases was added with a graphics editor.

3 AIDS is the only disease receiving more than one billion dollars. Restricting this graph to diseases with less than one billion dollars in funding produces a graph similar to panel B of Figure 2.13. The *ytick* command draws tick marks on the *y*-axis at the indicated values.

4 This label variable command adds "Log Adj. Life-Years" as a label to the *logdis* variable. This label will be used as the axis title in plots that use *logdis* as either the *x*- or *y*-axis.

5 This graph produces a scatter plot that is similar to panel C of Figure 2.13. The *xtick* option draws tick marks on the *x*-axis at $\log[0.1] = -2.3$, $\log[0.2], \log[0.3], \ldots, \log[0.9], \log[1], \log[2], \ldots, \log[9]$ and $\log[10] = 2.3$; *x*-axis labels are placed at $\log[0.01] = -4.61$, $\log[0.1], \log[1]$ and

log[10]. In Figure 2.13, panel C these labels have been replaced by 0.01, 0.1, 1, and 10 using a graphics editor.

6 This command produces a scatter plot of log funding against log life-years lost.

7 This command fits the regression model of equation (2.35).

8 The slope of the regression of log funding against log life-years lost is 0.4768. The P value associated with the null hypothesis that $\beta = 0$ is < 0.0005.

9 This plot is similar to panel D of Figure 2.13.

10 The variable *yhat2* equals the left hand side of equation (2.36); *ci_u2* and *ci_l2* give the upper and lower bounds of the 95% confidence interval for *yhat2*.

11 This graph plots funding against life-years lost. The regression curve and 95% confidence intervals are shown.

12 Deleting AIDS (diseases with dollars ≥ 1) permits using a more narrow range for the y-axis. The resulting graph is similar to panel E of Figure 2.13. In panel E, however, the y-axis is expressed in millions rather than billions and a graphics editor has been used to break the y-axis and add the data for AIDS.

2.19. Testing the Equality of Regression Slopes

Consider the relationship between systolic blood pressure (SBP) and body mass index (BMI) in men and women. Suppose that we have data on samples of n_1 men and n_2 women. Let x_{i1} and y_{i1} be the SBP and BMI for the ith man and let x_{i2} and y_{i2} be similarly defined for the ith woman. Let

$$y_{i1} = \alpha_1 + \beta_1 x_{i1} + \varepsilon_{i1} \text{ and}$$

$$y_{i2} = \alpha_2 + \beta_2 x_{i2} + \varepsilon_{i2}$$

be linear models of the relationship between SBP and BMI in men and women, where ε_{i1} and ε_{i2} are normally distributed error terms with mean 0 and standard deviation σ. It is of interest to know whether the rate at which SBP increases with increasing BMI differs between men and women. That is, we wish to test the null hypothesis that $\beta_1 = \beta_2$. To test these hypothesis we first perform separate linear regressions on the data from the men and women. Let a_1, b_1 and s_1^2 estimate the y-intercept, slope and error variance for the men and let a_2, b_2 and s_2^2 be similarly defined for the women. Let $\hat{y}_{i1} = a_1 + b_1 x_{i1}$ and $\hat{y}_{i2} = a_1 + b_2 x_{i2}$. Then a pooled estimate of the error variance σ^2 is

$$s^2 = \left(\sum_{i=1}^{n_1} (y_{i1} - \hat{y}_{i1})^2 + \sum_{i=1}^{n_2} (y_{i2} - \hat{y}_{i2})^2 \right) / (n_1 + n_2 - 4)$$

$$= \left(s_1^2(n_1 - 2) + s_2^2(n_2 - 2) \right) / (n_1 + n_2 - 4). \qquad (2.37)$$

The variance of the slope difference is

$$\mathrm{var}[b_1 - b_2] = s^2 \left(1 \middle/ \sum_{i=1}^{n_1} (x_{i1} - \bar{x}_1)^2 + 1 \middle/ \sum_{i=1}^{n_2} (x_{i2} - \bar{x}_2)^2 \right). \qquad (2.38)$$

But

$$\mathrm{var}[b_1] = s_1^2 \middle/ \sum_{i=1}^{n_1} (x_{i1} - \bar{x}_1)^2$$

and hence

$$\sum_{i=1}^{n_1} (x_{i1} - \bar{x}_1)^2 = s_1^2 / \mathrm{var}[b_1].$$

This allows us to rewrite equation (2.38) as

$$\mathrm{var}[b_1 - b_2] = s^2 \left(\mathrm{var}[b_1]/s_1^2 + \mathrm{var}[b_2]/s_2^2 \right). \qquad (2.39)$$

Under the null hypothesis that $\beta_1 = \beta_2$,

$$t = (b_1 - b_2)/\sqrt{\mathrm{var}[b_1 - b_2]} \qquad (2.40)$$

has a t distribution with $n_1 + n_2 - 4$ degrees of freedom. A 95% confidence interval for $\beta_1 - \beta_2$ is

$$(b_1 - b_2) \pm t_{n_1+n_2-4,\,0.05} \sqrt{\mathrm{var}[b_1 - b_2]}. \qquad (2.41)$$

2.19.1. Example: The Framingham Heart Study

The Framingham Heart Study (Levy, 1999) has collected cardiovascular risk factor data and long-term follow-up on almost 5000 residents of the town of Framingham, Massachusetts. They have made available a didactic data set from this study that includes baseline systolic blood pressure (SBP) and body mass index (BMI) values on $n_1 = 2047$ men and $n_2 = 2643$ women (see also Section 3.10). Table 2.1 summarizes the results of two separate linear regressions of log[SBP] against log[BMI] in men and women from this data set. The observed rate at which log[SBP] increases with increasing log[BMI] in men is $b_1 = 0.272\,646$ mm Hg per unit of BMI (kg/m^2). This is appreciably less than the corresponding rate of $b_2 = 0.398\,595$ in women.

Table 2.1. Results of linear regressions of log systolic blood pressure against log body mass index in men and women from the Framingham Heart Study (Levy, 1999).

Sex	i	Number of subjects n_i	y intercept a_i	Slope b_i	MSE s_i^2	se$[b_i]$	var$[b_i]$
Men	1	2047	3.988 043	0.272 646	0.018 7788	0.023 2152	0.000 5389
Women	2	2643	3.593 017	0.398 595	0.026 1167	0.018 5464	0.000 3440

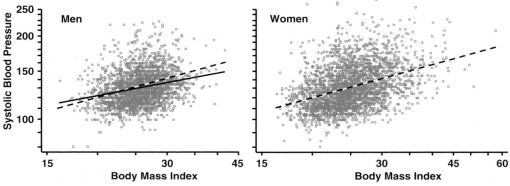

Figure 2.14   Linear regressions of log systolic blood pressure against log body mass index in men and women from the Framingham Heart Study (1999). The regression line for women (dashed line) has been superimposed over the corresponding line for men (solid line).

Figure 2.14 shows scatter plots of log[SBP] vs. log[BMI] in men and women together with lines depicting the expected log[SBP] from these linear regressions. The regression line for women (dashed line) is also superimposed on the scatterplot for men to provide an indication of the magnitude of the slope difference.

Substituting these values into equations (2.37) and (2.39) gives $s^2 = (0.018\,7788 \times (2047 - 2) + 0.026\,1167 \times (2643 - 2))/(2047 + 2643 - 4) = 0.022\,91$ and var$[b_1 - b_2] = 0.022\,91 \times (0.000\,5389/0.018\,7788 + 0.000\,3440/0.026\,1167) = 0.000\,959$. Therefore, a t statistic to test the equality of these slopes is $t = (0.272\,646 - 0.398\,595)/\sqrt{0.000\,959} = -4.07$ with 4686 degrees of freedom. The P value associated with this test is $P = 0.000\,05$. A 95% confidence interval for $\beta_1 - \beta_2$ is $0.272\,646 - 0.398\,595 \pm t_{4686,0.025}\sqrt{0.000\,959} = -0.126 + 1.96 \times 0.0310 = (-0.19, -0.065)$. This test allows us to conclude with great confidence that the difference in slopes between men and women in these regressions is not due to chance variation. Whether this difference is due to an inherent difference between men and women or is due to confounding with other variables remains to be determined. It is worth noting, however, that these differences are clinically appreciable. A man with a BMI of 35 will have an expected SBP of $\exp[3.988 + 0.2726 \times \log[35]] = 142$ mm Hg. The corresponding expected SBP for a woman with this BMI is $\exp[3.593 + 0.3986 \times \log[35]] = 150$ mm Hg.

2.20. Comparing Slope Estimates with Stata

The following log file and comments illustrate how to perform the calculations and draw the graphs from the preceding section using Stata.

```
. * 2.20.Framingham.log
. *
. * Regression of log systolic blood pressure against log body mass
. * index at baseline in men and women from the Framingham Heart Study.
. *
. use C:\WDDtext\2.20.Framingham.dta, clear                           {1}

. generate logsbp = log(sbp)                                          {2}

. generate logbmi = log(bmi)
(9 missing values generated)

. codebook sex                                                        {3}
                                                           {Output omitted}

        tabulation:   Freq.   Numeric   Label
                       2049        1    Men
                       2650        2    Women


. regress logsbp logbmi if sex==1                                     {4}

      Source |       SS       df       MS              Number of obs =    2047
-------------+------------------------------           F(  1,    2045) =  137.93
       Model |  2.5901294      1   2.5901294           Prob > F      =  0.0000
    Residual | 38.4025957   2045   .018778775          R-squared     =  0.0632
-------------+------------------------------           Adj R-squared =  0.0627
       Total | 40.9927251   2046   .020035545          Root MSE      =  .13704
```

```
-----------------------------------------------------------------------
   logsbp|      Coef.    Std. Err.        t    P>|t|     [95% Conf. Interval]
---------+-------------------------------------------------------------
   logbmi|    .272646     .0232152   11.744    0.000      .2271182    .3181739
   _cons|   3.988043     .0754584   52.851    0.000       3.84006    4.136026
-----------------------------------------------------------------------
```

. **predict** *yhatmen, xb*   {5}

(9 missing values generated)

. **regress** *logsbp logbmi if sex==2*   {6}

```
   Source|       SS        df         MS           Number of obs =      2643
---------+ ---------------------------           F( 1,    2641) =    461.90
    Model|  12.0632111        1   12.0632111      Prob > F       =    0.0000
 Residual|  68.9743032     2641   .026116737      R-squared      =    0.1489
---------+ ---------------------------           Adj R-squared =    0.1485
    Total|  81.0375143     2642   .030672791      Root MSE       =    .16161
-----------------------------------------------------------------------
   logsbp|      Coef.    Std. Err.        t    P>|t|     [95% Conf.   Interval]
---------+-------------------------------------------------------------
   logbmi|   .3985947     .0185464   21.492    0.000      .3622278    .4349616
   _cons|   3.593017     .0597887   60.095    0.000      3.475779    3.710254
-----------------------------------------------------------------------
```

. **predict** *yhatwom, xb*

(9 missing values generated)

. **sort** *logbmi*

. **graph** *logsbp yhatwom logbmi if sex==2,* **connect**(.1[-#]) **symbol**(oi)   {7}
> **xlabel**(*2.71,3.4,3.81,4.09*) **xtick**(*3.0,3.22,3.56,3.69,3.91,4.01*)
> **ylabel**(*4.61,5.01,5.30,5.52*) **ytick**(*4.38,4.5,4.7,4.79,4.87,4.94,5.08,5.14,*
> *5.19,5.25,5.35,5.39,5.43,5.48*) **gap**(*4*) **yscale**(*4.382,5.599*)

{Graph omitted. See Figure 2.14, right panel}

. **graph** *logsbp yhatmen yhatwom logbmi if sex==1 ,* **connect**(.11[-#]) **symbol**(oii)
> **xlabel**(*2.71,3.4,3.81,4.09*) **xtick**(*3.0,3.22,3.56,3.69,3.91,4.01*)
> **ylabel**(*4.61,5.01,5.30,5.52*) **ytick**(*4.38,4.5,4.7,4.79,4.87,4.94,5.08,5.14,*
> *5.19,5.25,5.35,5.39,5.43,5.48*) **gap**(*4*) **yscale**(*4.382,5.599*)

{Graph omitted. See Figure 2.14, left panel}

. **generate** *s2 = (0.018778775*2045 + 0.026116737*2641)/(2047 + 2643 - 4)*   {8}

. **generate** *varb_dif = s2*(0.0232152^2/0.018778775 + 0.0185464^2/0.026116737)*   {9}

. **generate** *t = (0.272646 - 0.3985947)/sqrt(varb_dif)*   {10}

```
. generate ci95_lb = (0.272646 - 0.3985947)                          {11}
>                   - invttail(4686,.025)*sqrt(varb_dif)
. generate ci95_ub = (0.272646 - 0.3985947)
>                   + invttail(4686,.025)*sqrt(varb_dif)

. list s2 varb_dif t ci95_lb ci95_ub in 1/1                          {12}
             s2   varb_dif            t    ci95_lb     ci95_ub
  1.   .0229144   .0009594    -4.066185   -.1866736   -.0652238

. display 2*ttail(4686,abs(t))                                       {13}

. 00004857
```

Comment

1 This data set contains long term follow-up on 4699 people from the town of Framingham. In this example, we focus on three variables collected at each patient's baseline exam: *sbp, bmi* and *sex*. The variable *sbp* records systolic blood pressure in mm Hg; *bmi* records body mass index in kg/m^2.

2 An exploratory data analysis (not shown here) indicates that the relationship between log[*sbp*] and log[*bmi*] comes closer to meeting the assumptions of a linear model than does the relationship between *sbp* and *bmi*.

3 There are 2049 men and 2650 women in this data set; *sex* is coded 1 or 2 for men or women, respectively.

4 This regression command is restricted to records where *sex*==*1* is true. That is, to records of men. The statistics from this regression that are also in Table 2.1 are highlighted. Two of the 2049 men in this data set are missing values for either *sbp* or *bmi*, giving a total of 2047 observations in the analysis.

5 The variable *yhatmen* contains the expected value of each man's log[*sbp*] given his body mass index. These expected values are based on the regression of *logsbp* against *logbmi* among men. There are nine subjects with missing values of *logbmi* (two men and seven women). The variable *yhatmen* is missing for these people. Note that this *predict* command defines *yhatmen* for all subjects including women. The command *predict yhatmen if sex==1, xb* would have defined *yhatmen* for men only.

6 This regression of *logsbp* against *logbmi* is restricted to women with non-missing values of *sbp* and *bmi*.

7 This graph is similar to the right panel of Figure 2.14. The axis labels are written in terms of *logsbp* and *logbmi*. In Figure 2.14 these labels have been replaced by the corresponding values of *sbp* and *bmi* using a graphics editor.

In Figure 2.14 we want the x- and y-axes to be drawn to the same scales in order to facilitate comparisons between men and women. By default, the range of the y-axis includes all *ytick* and *ylabel* values plus all values of the y-variable. In panels of Figure 2.14 the range of values of *logsbp* is different for men and women and extends beyond the *ytick* and *ylabel* values. To force the scale of the y-axis to be the same for both men and women we use the *yscale* option, which specifies a minimum range for the y-axis. The y-axes for men and women will be identical as long as this range includes all *logsbp* values for both men and women. The *xscale* option works the same way for the x-axis, but is not needed here since the *xlabel* values span the range of observed *logbmi* values for both men and women.

In Figure 2.14 we distinguish between the regression lines for women and men by using a dashed line for women. Stata allows a wide variety of patterned lines. The desired pattern is specified by symbols placed in brackets following the connect symbol of the *connect* option. For example, in this command the *connect(.l[−#])* option contains two connect symbols: "." and "*l*". These symbols dictate how the first and second variables are to be connected, which in this example are *logsbp* and *yhatwom* (see comment 12 of Section 2.12). The second of these symbols, "*l*", is followed by "*[−#]*", which specifies that a dashed line is to connect the observations of the second variable (*yhatwom*). Hence, the effect of this command is to use a dashed line for the regression of *logsbp* against *logbmi* among women. It is important when using a patterned line that the data be sorted by the x-axis variable prior to the *graph* command. See the Stata Graphics Manual for further details.

8 This command defines *s2* to equal s^2 in equation (2.37); *s2* is set equal to this constant for each record in the database.

9 This command defines *varb_dif* to equal $\mathrm{var}(b_1 - b_2)$ in equation (2.39).

10 This is the t statistic given in equation (2.40).

11 The next two lines calculate the lower and upper bound of the 95% confidence interval given in equation (2.41).

12 This command lists the values of *s2, varb_dif, t, ci95_lb* and *ci95_ub* in the first record of the data file (all the other records contain identical values). Note that these values agree with those given for s^2, $\mathrm{var}[b_1 - b_2]$ and $(b_1 - b_2) \pm t_{n_1+n_2-4,\,0.025}\sqrt{\mathrm{var}(b_1 - b_2)}$ in the example from Section 2.19.1.

13 The function *ttail(df,t)* gives the probability that a t statistic with *df* degrees of freedom is greater than t. The function *abs(t)* gives the absolute value of t. Hence *2*ttail(4686,abs(t))* gives the two-sided P value associated with a t statistic with 4686 degrees of freedom. In this example, $t = -4.07$ giving $P = -0.00005$.

2.21. Additional Reading

Armitage and Berry (1994) and
Pagano and Gauvreau (2000) provide excellent introductions to simple linear regression. The approach to testing the equality of two regression slopes described in Section 2.19 is discussed in greater detail by Armitage and Berry.

Cleveland (1993) discusses lowess regression along with other important graphical techniques for data analysis.

Hamilton (1992) provides a brief introduction to non-linear regression.

Draper and Smith (1998) provide a more thorough and more mathematically advanced discussion of non-linear regression.

Cleveland (1979) is the original reference on lowess regression.

Levy (1999) provides a review of the research findings of the Framingham Heart Study.

Framingham Heart Study (1997) provides the 40 year follow-up data from this landmark study. The didactic data set used in this text is a subset of the 40 year data set that is restricted to patients who were free of coronary heart disease at the time of their baseline exam.

Brent et al. (1999) studied patients with ethylene glycol poisoning. We used data from this study to illustrate simple linear regression.

Gross et al. (1999) studied the relationship between research funding and disability-adjusted life-years lost due to 29 diseases. We used data from this study to illustrate data transformations in linear regression.

2.22. Exercises

Eisenhofer et al. (1999) investigated the use of plasma normetanephrine and metanephrine for detecting pheochromocytoma in patients with von Hippel–Lindau disease and multiple endocrine neoplasia type 2. The *2.ex.vonHippelLindau.dta* data set contains data from this study on 26 patients with von Hippel–Lindau disease and nine patients with multiple endocrine neoplasia. The variables in this data set are

$$disease = \begin{cases} 0: \text{Patient has von Hippel–Lindau disease} \\ 1: \text{Patient has multiple endocrine neoplasia type 2} \end{cases}$$

p_ne = plasma norepinephrine (pg/ml)
$tumorvol$ = tumor volume (ml).

1 Regress plasma norepinephrine against tumor volume. Draw a scatter plot of norepinephrine against tumor volume together with the

estimated linear regression curve. What is the slope estimate for this regression? What proportion of the total variation in norepinephrine levels is explained by this regression?

2 Calculate the studentized residuals for the regression in question 1. Determine the 95% prediction interval for these residuals. Draw a scatter plot of these residuals showing the 95% prediction interval and the expected residual values. Comment on the adequacy of the model for these data.

3 Plot the lowess regression curve for norepinephrine against tumor volume. How does this curve differ from the regression curve in exercise 1?

4 Experiment with different transformations of norepinephrine and tumor volume. Find transformations that provide a good fit to a linear model.

5 Regress the logarithm of norepinephrine against the logarithm of tumor volume. Draw a scatter plot of these variables together with the linear regression line and the 95% confidence intervals for this line. What proportion of the total variation in the logarithm of norepinephrine levels is explained by this regression? How does this compare with your answer to question 1?

6 Using the model from question 5, what is the predicted plasma norepinephrine concentration for a patient with a tumor volume of 100 ml? What is the 95% confidence interval for this concentration? What would be the 95% prediction interval for a new patient with a 100 ml tumor?

7 Calculate the studentized residuals for the regression in question 5. Determine the 95% prediction interval for these residuals. Draw a scatter plot of these residuals showing the 95% prediction interval and the expected residual values. Include the lowess regression curve of these residuals against tumor volume on your graph. Contrast your answer to that for question 2. Which model provides the better fit to the data?

8 Perform separate linear regressions of log norepinephrine against log tumor volume in patients with von Hippel–Lindau disease and in patients with multiple endocrine neoplasia. What are the slope estimates for these two diseases? Give 95% confidence intervals for these slopes. Test the null hypothesis that these two slope estimates are equal. What is the 95% confidence interval for the difference in slopes for these diseases?

The following exercises concern the Framingham Heart Study data set *2.20.Framingham.dta.*

9 Evaluate the relationship between systolic blood pressure (SBP) and body mass index (BMI). Do these variables meet the assumptions of a linear

model? If not, explore different transformations of these two variables that will result in variables that come closer to meeting the linear model assumptions.

10 Replicate the regressions of log[SBP] against log[BMI] for men and women in Section 2.20. What are the predicted SBPs for men and women with a BMI of 40? Do you think that the difference between these two blood pressures is clinically significant?

11 Plot the predicted SBPs in men and women as a function of BMI. Plot the 95% confidence intervals for these predicted values.

The following question is for those who would like to sharpen their intuitive understanding of simple linear regression.

12 When a data point has leverage $h_i = 1$, the regression line always goes through the data point. Can you construct an example where this happens? Enter your example into Stata and confirm that $h_i = 1$ for your designated data point. (Hint: this is not a math question. All you need to remember is that the regression line minimizes the sum of squares of the residuals. By experimenting with different scatter plots, find a set of x values for which the sum of squared residuals is always minimized by having a zero residual at your designated data point.)

Multiple Linear Regression

In simple linear regression we modeled the value of a response variable as a linear function of a single covariate. In multiple linear regression we expand on this approach by using two or more covariates to predict the value of the response variable.

3.1. The Model

It is often useful to predict a patient's response from multiple explanatory variables. The simple linear regression model (equation 2.4) can be generalized to do this as follows. Suppose we have observations on n patients. The **multiple linear regression model** assumes that

$$y_i = \alpha + \beta_1 x_{i1} + \beta_2 x_{i2} + \cdots + \beta_k x_{ik} + \varepsilon_i, \tag{3.1}$$

where

$\alpha, \beta_1, \beta_2, \ldots, \beta_k$ are unknown parameters,
$x_{i1}, x_{i2}, \ldots, x_{ik}$ are the values of known variables measured on the ith patient,
ε_i has a normal distribution with mean 0 and standard deviation σ,
$\varepsilon_1, \varepsilon_2, \ldots, \varepsilon_n$ are mutually independent, and
y_i is the value of the response variable for the ith patient.

We usually assume that the patient's response y_i is causally related to the variables $x_{i1}, x_{i2}, \ldots, x_{ik}$ through the model. These latter variables are called **covariates** or **explanatory variables**; y_i is called the **dependent** or **response variable.** The model parameters are also called **regression coefficients.**

Multiple linear regression is often useful when we wish to improve our ability to predict a response variable and we have several explanatory variables that affect the patient's response.

3.2. Confounding Variables

A **confounding variable** is one of little immediate interest that is correlated with the risk factor and is independently related to the outcome variable of interest. For example, blood pressure and body mass index (BMI) both tend to increase with age. Also, blood pressure and BMI are positively correlated. If we select a stout and lean subject at random from a population, the stout person is likely to be older than the lean subject and this difference in age will account for some of their difference in blood pressure. If we are interested in the effect of BMI *per se* on blood pressure we must adjust for the effect of age on the relationship between these two variables. We say that age confounds the effect of BMI on blood pressure. One way to adjust for age is to compare BMI and blood pressure in a sample of patients who are all the same age. It may, however, be difficult to find such a sample and the relationship between BMI and blood pressure may be different at different ages. Another approach is through multiple linear regression. The interpretation of β_1 in equation (3.1) is that it estimates the rate of change in y_i with x_{i1} among patients with identical values of $x_{i2}, x_{i3}, \ldots, x_{ik}$. To see this more clearly, suppose that we have two covariates x_{i1} and x_{i2}. Let $\alpha = 0, \beta_1 = 1, \beta_2 = 2$ and $\varepsilon_i = 0$ for all i (i.e., $\sigma = 0$). Then equation (3.1) reduces to $y_i = x_{i1} + 2x_{i2}$. Figure 3.1 shows a sample of values that fit this model in which x_{i1} and x_{i2} are positively correlated. Note that the values of y_i increase from 0 to 4 as x_{i2} increases from 0 to 1. Hence, the slope of the simple regression curve of y_i against x_{i2} is 4. However, when x_{i1} is held constant, y_i increases from x_{i1} to $x_{i1} + 2$ as x_{i2} increases from 0 to 1. Hence, the rate at which y_i increases with x_{i2} adjusted for x_{i1} is $\beta_2 = 2$.

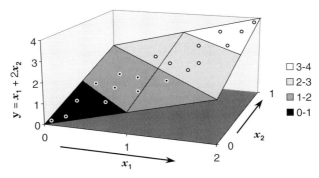

Figure 3.1   This graph shows points on the plane defined by the equation $y = x_1 + 2x_2$. The rate at which y increases with increasing x_2 is 2 when x_1 is held constant and equals 4 when x_2 is not.

3.3. Estimating the Parameters for a Multiple Linear Regression Model

Let $\hat{y}_i = a + b_1 x_{i1} + b_2 x_{i2} + \cdots + b_k x_{ik}$ be an estimate of y_i given x_{i1}, $x_{i2}, \ldots, x_{ik}$. We choose our estimates of $a, b_1, \ldots, b_k$ to be those values that minimize the sum of squared residuals $\sum (y_i - \hat{y}_i)^2$. These values are said to be the **least squares estimates** of $\alpha, \beta_1, \beta_2, \ldots,$ and β_k. This is precisely analogous to what we did in Section 2.6 for simple linear regression, only now there are k covariates instead of 1. When there are just two covariates the observations $\{(x_{i1}, x_{i2}, y_i) : i = 1, \ldots, n\}$ can be thought of as a cloud of points in three dimensions. The estimates $\hat{y}_i = a + b_1 x_{i1} + b_2 x_{i2}$ all lie on a plane that bisects this cloud (see Figure 3.1). The **residual** $y_i - \hat{y}_i$ is the vertical distance between the observation y_i and this plane. We choose the values of a, b_1 and b_2, that give the plane that minimizes the sum of squares of these vertical distances. When the points all lie on the same plane (as in Figure 3.1) the values of a, b_1 and b_2, that define this plane give residuals that are all zero. These values are our least squares estimates of α, β_1 and β_2, since they give a sum of squared residuals that equals zero.

3.4. R^2 Statistic for Multiple Regression Models

As in simple linear regression, the total variation of the dependent variable is measured by the total sum of squares (TSS), which equals $\sum (y_i - \bar{y})^2$. The variation explained by the model, the model sum of squares (MSS), equals $\sum (\hat{y}_i - \bar{y})^2$. The proportion of the variation explained by the model is $R^2 = \text{MSS}/\text{TSS}$. This is the same formula given in Section 2.8 for simple linear regression. This statistic is a useful measure of the explanatory power of the model. It is not, however, the square of a correlation coefficient, as was the case for simple linear regression.

3.5. Expected Response in the Multiple Regression Model

Let $\mathbf{x}_i = (x_{i1}, x_{i2}, \ldots, x_{ik})$ be a compact way of denoting the values of all of the covariates for the ith patient. Then, if the model is true, it can be shown that the expected value of both y_i and $\hat{y}_i$ given her covariates is

$$E[y_i \mid \mathbf{x}_i] = E[\hat{y}_i \mid \mathbf{x}_i] = \alpha + \beta_1 x_{i1} + \beta_2 x_{i2} + \cdots + \beta_k x_{ik}. \tag{3.2}$$

We estimate the expected value of y_i among subjects whose covariate values are identical to those of the ith patient by $\hat{y}_i$. The equation

$$\hat{y}_i = a + b_1 x_{i1} + b_2 x_{i2} + \cdots + b_k x_{ik} \tag{3.3}$$

may be rewritten

$$\hat{y}_i = \bar{y} + b_1(x_{i1} - \bar{x}_1) + b_2(x_{i2} - \bar{x}_2) + \cdots + b_k(x_{ik} - \bar{x}_k). \tag{3.4}$$

Thus $\hat{y}_i = \bar{y}$ when $x_{i1} = \bar{x}_1, x_{i2} = \bar{x}_2, \ldots,$ and $x_{ik} = \bar{x}_k$.

3.6. The Accuracy of Multiple Regression Parameter Estimates

In equation (3.1) the error term ε_i has a variance of σ^2. We estimate this variance by

$$s^2 = \sum (y_i - \hat{y}_i)^2 / (n - k - 1). \tag{3.5}$$

As was the case with simple linear regression, you can think of s^2 as being the average squared residual as long as n is much larger than $k + 1$. It is often called the **mean squared error** (MSE). It can be shown that the expected value of s^2 is σ^2. The standard deviation σ is estimated by s which is called the **root MSE**.

The standard errors of the parameter estimates $a, b_1, b_2, \ldots, b_k$ are estimated by formulas of the form

$$se[b_j] = s / f_j[\{x_{ij} : i = 1, \ldots, n; j = 1, \ldots, k\}], \tag{3.6}$$

where $f_j[\{x_{ij} : i = 1, \ldots, n; j = 1, \ldots, k\}]$ is a complicated function of all of the covariates on all of the patients. Fortunately, we do not need to spell out this formula in detail as all statistical software packages can derive it for us. The important thing to remember about equation (3.6) is that the standard error of b_j increases as s, the standard deviation of the residuals, increases, and decreases as the dispersion of the covariates increases. Equation (3.6) is a generalization of equation (2.13), which gives the standard error of the slope coefficient for the simple linear regression model.

Under the null hypothesis that $\beta_j = 0$,

$$b_j / se[b_j] \tag{3.7}$$

has a t distribution with $n - k - 1$ degrees of freedom. That is, the number of degrees of freedom equals n, the number of patients, minus $k + 1$, the number of parameters in the model. We can use equation (3.7) to test this null hypothesis. A 95% confidence interval for β_j is given by

$$b_j \pm t_{n-k-1, 0.025} \times se[b_j]. \tag{3.8}$$

3.7. Leverage

Many of the concepts and statistics that we introduced for simple linear regression have counterparts in multiple linear regression. One of these is leverage. The **leverage** h_i is a measure of the potential ability of the ith patient to influence the parameter estimates. Patients with high leverage will have an appreciable influence on these estimates if the residual $e_i = y_i - \hat{y}_i$ is large. The formula for h_i is a complex function of the covariates $\{x_{ij} : i = 1, \ldots, n; j = 1, \ldots, k\}$ but does not involve the response values $\{y_i : i = 1, \ldots, n\}$. It can be shown that $1/n \leq h_i \leq 1$. A leverage greater than 0.2 is generally considered to be large. Leverage is easily calculated by any modern statistical software package.

The variance of $\hat{y}_i$ given all of the covariates $\mathbf{x}_i$ for the ith patient is estimated by

$$\text{var}\,[\hat{y}_i \mid \mathbf{x}_i] = s^2 h_i. \tag{3.9}$$

Hence h_i can also be thought of as the variance of $\hat{y}_i$ given $\mathbf{x}_i$ expressed in units of s^2. Note that equation (3.9) is analogous to equation (2.21) for simple linear regression.

3.8. 95% Confidence Interval for $\hat{y}_i$

It can be shown that $(\hat{y}_i - \text{E}[y_i \mid \mathbf{x}_i])/\sqrt{\text{var}[\hat{y}_i \mid \mathbf{x}_i]}$ has a t distribution with $n - k - 1$ degrees of freedom. From equation (3.9) we have that the standard error of $\hat{y}_i$ given this patient's covariates is $s\sqrt{h_i}$. Hence, the 95% confidence interval for $\hat{y}_i$ is

$$\hat{y}_i \pm t_{n-k-1,0.025}(s\sqrt{h_i}). \tag{3.10}$$

3.9. 95% Prediction Intervals

Suppose that a new patient has covariates $x_1, x_2, \ldots, x_k$, which we will denote by $\mathbf{x}$, and leverage h. Let $\hat{y}[\mathbf{x}] = a + b_1 x_1 + b_2 x_2 + \cdots + b_k x_k$ be her estimated expected response given these covariates. Then the estimated variance of her predicted response y is

$$\text{var}\,[y \mid \mathbf{x}] = s^2 (h + 1), \tag{3.11}$$

and a 95% prediction interval for y is

$$\hat{y}[\mathbf{x}] \pm t_{n-k-1,0.025}(s\sqrt{h + 1}). \tag{3.12}$$

Equations (3.9), (3.11), and (3.12) are precisely analogous to equations (2.21), (2.22) and (2.23) for simple linear regression.

3.10. Example: The Framingham Heart Study

The Framingham Heart Study (Levy, 1999) has collected long-term follow-up and cardiovascular risk factor data on almost 5000 residents of the town of Framingham, Massachusetts. Recruitment of patients started in 1948. At the time of the baseline exams there were no effective treatments for hypertension. I have been given permission to use a subset of the 40-year data from this study in this text (Framingham Heart Study, 1997). We will refer to this subset as the Framingham Heart Study didactic data set. It consists of data on 4699 patients who were free of coronary heart disease at their baseline exam. At this exam, the following variables were recorded on each patient. The Stata names for these variables are given in the first column below:

sbp   = systolic blood pressure (SBP) in mm Hg,

dbp   = dyastolic blood pressure (DBP) in mm Hg,

age   = age in years,

scl   = serum cholesterol (SCL) in mg/100ml,

bmi   = body mass index (BMI) = weight/height^2 in kg/m^2,

sex   = gender coded as $\begin{cases} 1: \text{if subject is male} \\ 2: \text{if subject is female,} \end{cases}$

month   = month of year in which baseline exam occurred, and

id   = a patient identification variable (numbered 1 to 4699).

Follow-up information on coronary heart disease is also provided:

followup = the subject's follow-up in days, and

chdfate = $\begin{cases} 1: \text{if the patient develops CHD at the end of follow-up} \\ 0: \text{otherwise.} \end{cases}$

In Section 2.19.1 we showed that the rate at which SBP increased with BMI was greater for women than for men. In this example, we will explore this relationship in greater detail, and will seek to build a multiple linear regression model that adequately explains how SBP is affected by the other variables listed above. Although we usually have hypotheses to test that were postulated in advance of data collection, there is almost always an exploratory component to the modeling of a multivariate data set. It is all too easy to force an inappropriate model on the data. The best way to avoid doing this is to become familiar with your data through a series of analyses of

Table 3.1. Summary of results of three separate simple linear regressions of log systolic blood pressure against log body mass index, age, and log serum cholesterol.

Model	Slope coefficient	t	$P > \lvert t \rvert$	95% confidence interval	R^2
$\log[sbp_i] = \alpha + \beta \times \log[bmi_i]$	0.355	24.7	< 0.0005	0.33–0.38	0.12
$\log[sbp_i] = \alpha + \beta \times age_i$	0.00752	29.6	< 0.0005	0.0070–0.0080	0.16
$\log[sbp_i] = \alpha + \beta \times \log[scl_i]$	0.196	16.3	< 0.0005	0.17–0.22	0.05

increasing complexity and to do residual analyses that will identify individual patients whose data may result in misleading conclusions.

3.10.1. Preliminary Univariate Analyses

We first perform separate simple linear regressions of SBP on each of the continuous covariates: age, BMI, and serum cholesterol. Residual analyses should be performed and the variables should be transformed if appropriate (see Sections 2.15–2.18). These analyses indicate that reasonable linear fits can be obtained by regressing log SBP against log BMI, log SBP against age, and log SBP against log SCL. Table 3.1 summarizes the results of these simple linear regressions. Figure 3.2 shows the corresponding scatter plots and linear regression lines. These univariate regressions show that SBP is related to age and SCL as well as BMI. Although the statistical significance of the slope coefficients is overwhelming, the R^2 statistics are low. Hence, each of these risk factors individually only explain a modest proportion of the total variability in systolic blood pressure. By building a multivariate model of these variables we seek to achieve a better understanding of the relationship between these variables.

Note that the importance of a parameter depends not only on its magnitude but also on the range of the corresponding covariate. For example, the age coefficient is only 0.007 52 as compared to 0.355 and 0.196 for log[BMI] and log[SCL]. However, the range of age is from 30 to 68 as compared to 2.79–4.05 for log[BMI] and 4.74–6.34 for log[SCL]. The large age range increases the variation in log[SBP] that is associated with age. In fact, age explains more of the variation in log[SBP] (has a higher R^2 statistic) than either of the other two covariates.

Changing the units of measurement of a covariate can have a dramatic effect on the size of the slope estimate, but no effect on its biologic meaning. For example, suppose we regressed blood pressure against weight in grams. If we converted weight from grams to kilograms we would increase the magnitude of the slope parameter by 1000 and decrease the range of observed

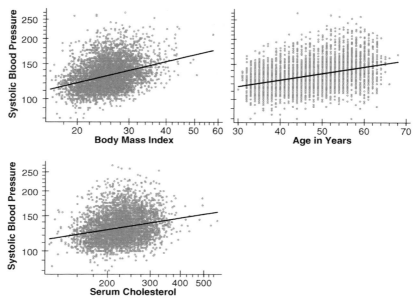

Figure 3.2   Simple linear regressions of log systolic blood pressure against log body mass index, age and log serum cholesterol. These data are from the Framingham Heart Study (Levy, 1999). All measurements were taken at each subject's baseline exam.

weights by 1000. The appearance of the plotted regression line and the statistical significance of the regression analysis would be unchanged.

3.11. Scatterplot Matrix Graphs

Another useful exploratory graphic is the scatter plot matrix, which consists of all possible 2 × 2 scatter plots of the specified variables. Such graphs can be effective at showing the interrelationships between multiple variables observed on a sample of patients. Figure 3.3 shows such a plot for log[SBP], log[BMI], age and log[SCL] from the Framingham Heart Study. The graph is restricted to women recruited in January to reduce the number of data points and allow individual patient values to be discernible. A non-linear regression line is fitted to each scatter plot by connecting median bands with cubic splines. The details of this technique are not of great importance. It is similar to lowess regression in that it attempts to fit a regression line to the data without making any model assumptions, and it is reasonably resistant to outliers. Although it does not always give as satisfactory a fit as lowess regression it is much faster to compute. Like lowess regression, a parameter may be specified to control the degree of smoothing of the curve.

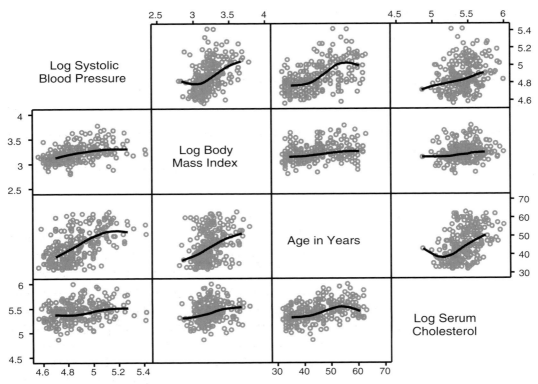

Figure 3.3   Matrix scatter plots of data from women recruited into the Framingham Heart Study during one month. This graph shows all possible 2×2 scatter plots of the specified variables. A non-linear regression curve is fitted to each scatter plot.

3.11.1. Producing Scatterplot Matrix Graphs with Stata

The following log file and comments illustrate how to produce a scatterplot matrix graph with Stata.

```
. * 3.11.1.Framingham.log

. *

. * Plot a scatterplot matrix of log(sbp), log(bmi), age and log(scl) for

. * women from the Framingham Heart Study who were recruited in January.

. *

. use C:\WDDtext\2.20.Framingham.dta, clear

. generate logsbp = log(sbp)

. label variable logsbp "Log Systolic Blood Pressure"

. generate logbmi = log(bmi)
(9 missing values generated)
```

```
. label variable logbmi "Log Body Mass Index"

. generate logscl = log(scl)
(33 missing values generated)

. label variable logscl "Log Serum Cholesterol"

. set textsize 120                                                    {1}

. graph logsbp logbmi age logscl if month == 1 & sex == 2, matrix label symbol(o)  {2}
> connect(s) band(4)
```

{Graph omitted. See Figure 3.3}

Comments

1 This command sets text on subsequent graphs to be 20% larger than the default value; *set textsize 80* would make subsequent text 20% smaller.

2 The *matrix* option generates a matrix scatterplot for *logsbp, logbmi, age* and *logscl*. The *if* clause restricts the graph to women (*sex* == 2) who entered the study in January (*month* == 1). The *label* option adds axis labels to the graphic at evenly spaced intervals; *band*(4) specifies that a non-linear regression line is to be fitted to each scatterplot. The number in parenthesis indicates the degree of smoothing, with lower values indicating greater smoothing; *connect*(*s*) indicates that the regression lines should be smooth.

3.12. Modeling Interaction in Multiple Linear Regression

3.12.1. The Framingham Example

Let $\mathbf{x}_i = (logbmi_i, age_i, logscl_i, sex_i)$ denote the covariates for log[BMI], age, log[SCL] and sex for the ith patient. Let $logsbp_i$ denote his or her log[SBP]. The first model that comes to mind for regressing log[SBP] against these covariates is

$$E[logsbp_i \mid \mathbf{x}_i] = \alpha + \beta_1 \times logbmi_i + \beta_2 \times age_i + \beta_3 \times logscl_i + \beta_4 \times sex_i.$$

$$(3.13)$$

A potential weakness of this model is that it implies that the effects of the covariates on $logsbp_i$ are additive. To understand what this means consider the following. Suppose we look at patients with identical values of age_i and $logscl_i$. Then for these patients $\alpha + \beta_2 \times age_i + \beta_3 \times logscl_i$ will equal a constant and model (3.13) implies that

$$E[logsbp_i \mid \mathbf{x}_i] = \text{constant} + \beta_1 \times logbmi_i + \beta_4 \qquad (3.14)$$

for men, and

$$E[logsbp_i \mid \mathbf{x}_i] = \text{constant} + \beta_1 \times logbmi_i + 2\beta_4 \qquad (3.15)$$

for women (recall that the covariate sex_i takes the values 1 and 2 for men and women, respectively). Subtracting equation (3.14) from equation (3.15) gives that the difference in expected log[SBP] for men and women with identical BMIs is β_4. Hence, the β_4 parameter allows men and women with the same BMI to have different expected log[SBP]s. However, the slope of the $logsbp_i$ vs. $logbmi_i$ relationship for both men and women is β_1. Our analysis in Section 2.19.1 indicated, however, that this slope is higher for women than for men. This is an example of what we call **interaction**, in which the effect of one covariate on the dependent variable is influenced by the value of a second covariate. Models such as (3.13) are said to be **additive** in that the joint effect of any two covariates equals the sum of the individual effects of these parameters. Figure 3.4 illustrates the difference between additive and interactive models. In the additive model, the regression lines for, say, men and women are parallel; in the model with interaction they diverge.

We need a more complex model to deal with interaction. In the Framingham example let

$$woman_i = sex_i - 1.$$

Then

$$woman_i = \begin{cases} 1: \text{if } i^{\text{th}} \text{ subject is female} \\ 0: \text{if } i^{\text{th}} \text{ subject is male.} \end{cases}$$

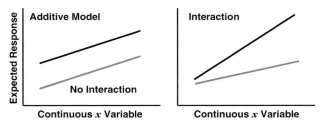

Figure 3.4   Effect of a dichotomous and a continuous covariate on expected patient response. On the left the dichotomous variable (black and gray lines) does not interact with the continuous variable (*x*-axis) giving parallel regression lines. On the right the two variables interact and the effect of the dichotomous variable is much greater for large values of *x* than for small values.

Consider the model

$$E[logsbp_i \mid \mathbf{x}_i] = \alpha + \beta_1 \times logbmi_i + \beta_2 \times woman_i$$

$$+ \beta_3 \times logbmi_i \times woman_i. \tag{3.16}$$

In this and subsequent models, $\mathbf{x}_i$ represents the values of all of the model's covariates for the ith patient, in this case $logbmi_i$ and $woman_i$. Model (3.16) reduces to

$$E[logsbpi_i \mid \mathbf{x}_i] = \alpha + \beta_1 \times logbmi_i$$

for men and

$$E[logsbpi_i \mid \mathbf{x}_i] = \alpha + (\beta_1 + \beta_3) \times logbmi_i + \beta_2$$

for women. Hence, the regression slopes for men and women are β_1 and $\beta_1 + \beta_3$, respectively. The parameter β_3 is the difference in slopes between men and women.

3.13. Multiple Regression Modeling of the Framingham Data

In Section 2.19.1 we showed that there was a significant difference between the slopes of the simple linear regressions of log[SBP] against log[BMI] in men and women. A reasonable approach to multiple regression modeling of these data is to regress log[SBP] against log[BMI], sex, age, log[SCL] and the interaction of sex with log[BMI], age and log[SCL]. That is, we consider the model

$$E[\log[sbp_i] \mid \mathbf{x}_i] = \alpha + \beta_1 \times \log[bmi_i] + \beta_2 \times age_i + \beta_3 \times \log[scl_i]$$

$$+ \beta_4 \times woman_i + \beta_5 \times woman_i \times \log[bmi_i]$$

$$+ \beta_6 \times woman_i \times age_i + \beta_7 \times woman_i \times \log[scl_i]. \tag{3.17}$$

The estimates of the regression coefficients from model (3.17) are given in Table 3.2. The covariate associated with each coefficient is given in the left most column of this table. The P values correspond to the test of the null hypothesis that the true values of these parameters are zero. The R^2 value for this model is 0.2550, which is about twice the R^2 from the simple linear regression of log[sbp] against log[bmi]. Hence, model (3.17) explains 25.5% of the variation in log[SBP]. We seek the simplest model that satisfactorily explains the data. The estimate of coefficient β_7 is very small and has a non-significant P value of 0.70. This P value is larger than any of the other parameter P values in the model. Hence, the $woman_i \times \log(scl_i)$ interaction

Table 3.2. Parameter estimates from models (3.17), (3.18), and (3.19) for analyzing the Framingham Heart Study baseline data (Levy, 1999).

Covariate	Model (3.17)			Model (3.18)			Model (3.19)		
	Parameter	Parameter estimate	P Value	Parameter	Parameter estimate	P Value	Parameter	Parameter estimate	P Value
1	α	3.5494	< 0.0005	α	3.5726	< 0.0005	α	3.5374	< 0.0005
$\log[bmi_i]$	β_1	0.2498	< 0.0005	β_1	0.2509	< 0.0005	β_1	0.2626	< 0.0005
age_i	β_2	0.0035	< 0.0005	β_2	0.0035	< 0.0005	β_2	0.0035	< 0.0005
$\log[scl_i]$	β_3	0.0651	< 0.0005	β_3	0.0601	< 0.0005	β_3	0.0596	< 0.0005
$woman_i$	β_4	-0.2292	0.11	β_4	-0.2715	0.004	β_4	-0.2165	< 0.0005
$woman_i \times \log[bmi_i]$	β_5	0.0189	0.52	β_5	0.0176	0.55			
$woman_i \times age_i$	β_6	0.0049	< 0.0005	β_6	0.0048	< 0.0005	β_5	0.0049	< 0.0005
$woman_i \times \log[scl_i]$	β_7	-0.0090	0.70						

term is not contributing much to our ability to predict log[SBP]. Dropping this interaction term from the model gives

$$E[\log[sbp_i] \mid \mathbf{x}_i] = \alpha + \beta_1 \times \log[bmi_i] + \beta_2 \times age_i + \beta_3 \times \log[scl_i] + \beta_4$$
$$\times woman_i + \beta_5 \times woman_i \times \log[bmi_i] + \beta_6 \times woman_i \times age_i. \qquad (3.18)$$

Model (3.18) gives parameter estimates for α, log[BMI], age, log[SCL] and sex that are very similar to those of model (3.17). The R^2 is unchanged, indicating that we have not lost any explanatory power by dropping the $woman_i \times \log[scl_i]$ interaction term. Dropping ineffectual terms from the model not only clarifies the relationship between the response variable and the covariates, but also increases the statistical power of our analyses.

In model (3.18) the $woman_i \times \log[bmi_i]$ interaction term is small and non-significant. Dropping this term gives

$$E[\log[sbp_i] \mid \mathbf{x}_i] = \alpha + \beta_1 \times \log[bmi_i] + \beta_2 \times age_i + \beta_3 \times \log[scl_i] + \beta_4$$
$$\times woman_i + \beta_5 \times woman_i \times age_i. \qquad (3.19)$$

This deletion has little effect on the remaining coefficient estimates, all of which are now highly statistically significant. The R^2 statistic is 0.2549, which is virtually unchanged from the previous two models. All of the remaining terms in the model remain highly significant and should not be dropped.

3.14. Intuitive Understanding of a Multiple Regression Model

3.14.1. The Framingham Example

When we did simple linear regressions of log[SBP] against log[BMI] for men and women we obtained slope estimates of 0.273 and 0.399 for men and women, respectively. The multiple regression model (3.19) gives a single slope estimate of 0.2626 for both sexes, but finds that the effect of increasing age on log[SBP] is twice as large in women than men. That is, for women this slope is $\beta_2 + \beta_5 = 0.0035 + 0.0049 = 0.0084$ while for men it is $\beta_2 = 0.0035$. How reasonable is our model? In Section 3.2 we said that the parameter for a covariate in a multiple regression model measures the slope of the relationship between the response variable and this covariate when all other covariates are held constant. One way to increase our intuitive understanding of the model is to plot separate simple linear regressions of SBP against BMI in groups of patients who are homogeneous with respect to the other variables in the model. Figure 3.5 shows linear regressions of log[SBP] against log[BMI] in subgroups defined by sex and 10-year age groups. These regressions are restricted to subjects whose log[SCL] lies in the inter-quartile range for this variable, which is from 5.28 to 5.42. The vertical and horizontal lines show the mean log[BMI] and log[SBP] in each panel. The black regression lines plot the simple linear regression of log[SBP] against log[BMI] for the patients in each panel. The thick gray lines are drawn through each panel's joint mean value for log[SBP] and log[BMI] and have slope 0.263 (the estimated parameter for log[BMI] from model (3.19)). A dashed line is also drawn through the joint mean values in the panels for women and has slope 0.399. This is the slope of the simple linear regression of log[SBP] against log[BMI] restricted to women (see Section 2.19.1). Note that the slopes of the black and gray lines are almost identical in all of the panels except for women aged 30–40 and 40–50. For women aged 30–40 the black simple regression slope for this panel is less than both the gray multiple regression slope and the dashed simple regression slope for all women. The gray multiple regression slope comes much closer to the simple regression slope for this panel than does the dashed simple regression line for all women. For women aged 40–50 the simple regression slope exceeds the multiple regression slope and comes close to the dashed line for all women. However, by and large, this figure supports the finding that there is little variation in the rate at which SBP increases with BMI among people of the same sex and similar age and SCL.

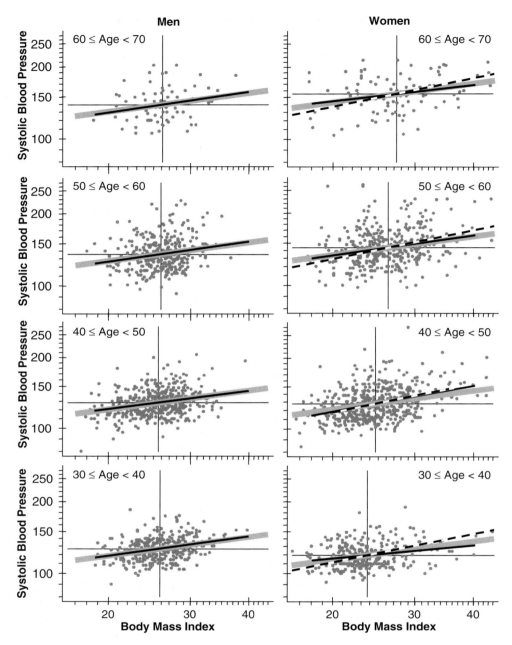

Figure 3.5   The black sloping lines in these panels are simple linear regressions of log systolic blood pressure (SBP) against log body mass index (BMI) in men and women of similar age and serum cholesterol (SCL) levels from the Framingham Heart Study. The thick gray lines have the slope of the log[BMI] parameter in the multiple linear regression model (3.19). The dashed lines have the slope of the simple linear regression of log[SBP] against log[BMI] among women in this study. This graph confirms the finding of model (3.19) that the relationship between log[SBP] and log[BMI] is similar among men and women of similar age and SCL levels (see text).

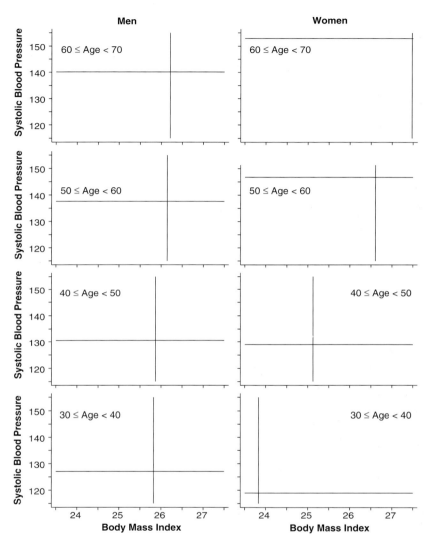

Figure 3.6   The mean systolic blood pressure and body mass index of patients from the Framingham Heart Study are indicated by horizontal and vertical lines in panels defined by age and sex. This figure illustrates the marked interaction between gender, body mass index, and age on systolic blood pressure.

The interrelationship between SBP, sex, BMI and age is better illustrated in Figure 3.6. In this figure SBP and BMI are drawn on a linear scale. In each panel the vertical and horizontal lines mark the mean SBP and BMI for all subjects with the gender and age range specified for the panel. In their thirties men, on average, are fatter than women and have higher systolic blood pressures. The average increase in BMI with increasing age among men, however, is modest. In contrast, the mean BMI increases in women from 23.8 in their thirties to 27.5 in their sixties. This corresponds to an average increase in weight of 9.5 kg (21 lb) for a woman 160 cm (5 ft 3 in) tall. Moreover, SBP increases much faster with age for women than men, and by their sixties, women have a higher mean SBP than their male counterparts. Thus, Figure 3.6 is consistent with our analysis model (3.19), which found that there is a pronounced interaction of sex and age on log[SBP] but no evidence of interaction between sex and log[BMI] on log[SBP].

A factor that should be considered in interpreting Figures 3.5 and 3.6. is that these figures do not take differential mortality rates between men and women into account. Hence, the comparatively modest BMI of men in their sixties is, in part, influenced by the fact that some of the fatter members of their birth cohort died before age 60. We will discuss how to analyze mortality data in the Chapters 6 and 7.

3.15. Calculating 95% Confidence and Prediction Intervals

Suppose we have a new female patient who is 60 years old, has a body mass index of 40 kg/m^2 and serum cholesterol of 400 mg/100ml. The parameter estimates from model (3.19) are $\alpha = 3.5374$, $\beta_1 = 0.2626$, $\beta_2 = 0.003\,517$, $\beta_3 = 0.059\,59$, $\beta_4 = -0.2165$, and $\beta_5 = 0.004\,862$. Substituting these values into equation (3.19) gives that her expected log systolic blood pressure (SBP) under this model is $\hat{y} = 3.5374 + 0.2626 \times \log[40] + 0.003\,517 \times 60 + 0.059\,59 \times \log[400] - 0.2165 \times 1 + 0.004862 \times 1 \times 60 = 5.15$. Thus, our estimate of her SBP is $e^{5.15} = 172$ mm Hg. For these data and this model, the root MSE is $s = 0.1393$. For this specific patient the leverage is $h = 0.003\,901$ (s and h, together with the parameter estimates are calculated for us by our regression software package). Hence, from equation (3.10) we have that a 95% confidence interval for $\hat{y}$ is $5.15 \pm 1.96 \times 0.1393 \times \sqrt{0.003\,901} = (5.132, 5.167)$. Substituting into equation (3.12) gives that a 95% prediction interval for $\hat{y}$ for this patient is $5.15 \pm 1.96 \times 0.1393 \times \sqrt{0.003\,901 + 1} = (4.876, 5.423)$. Hence, we can predict with 95% confidence that her SBP will lie between $e^{4.876} = 131$ and $e^{5.423} = 227$ mm Hg.

3.16. Multiple Linear Regression with Stata

The *3.11.1.Framingham.log* file continues as follows and illustrates how to perform the analyses discussed in Sections 3.13, 3.14 and 3.15.

```
. *
. * Use multiple regression models to analyze the effects of log(sbp),
. * log(bmi), age and log(scl) on log(sbp)
. *
. generate woman = sex -1

. generate wo_lbmi = woman * logbmi
(9 missing values generated)

. generate wo_age = woman * age

. generate wo_lscl = woman * logscl
(33 missing values generated)

. regress logsbp logbmi age logscl woman wo_lbmi wo_age wo_lscl          {1}
                                              {Output omitted. See Table 3.2}
. regress logsbp logbmi age logscl woman wo_lbmi wo_age                  {2}
                                              {Output omitted. See Table 3.2}
. regress logsbp logbmi age logscl woman wo_age                         {3}
```

```
  Source |       SS       df       MS              Number of obs =    4658
---------+------------------------------           F( 5,  4652) = 318.33
   Model | 30.8663845        5  6.1732769          Prob > F      = 0.0000
Residual | 90.2160593     4652 .019392962          R-squared     = 0.2549    {4}
---------+------------------------------           Adj R-squared = 0.2541
   Total | 121.082444     4657 .026000095          Root MSE      = .13926
```

```
--------------------------------------------------------------------------
  logsbp |    Coef.  Std. Err.    t    P>|t|     [95% Conf. Interval]       {5}
---------+----------------------------------------------------------------

  logbmi |  .262647  .0137549 19.095  0.000    .2356808    .2896131
     age | .0035167  .0003644  9.650  0.000    .0028023    0042311          {6}
  logscl | .0595923  .0114423  5.208  0.000    .0371599    .0820247
   woman | -.2165261 .0233469 -9.274  0.000   -.2622971   -.1707551
  wo_age | .0048624  .0004988  9.749  0.000    .0038846    .0058403
   _cons | 3.537356  .0740649 47.760  0.000    3.392153    3.682558         {7}
--------------------------------------------------------------------------
```

```
. *
. * Calculate 95% confidence and prediction intervals for a 60 year-old woman
. * with a SCL of 400 and a BMI of 40.
. *
.edit                                                                      {8}
```

```
- preserve
- set obs 4700
- replace scl = 400 in 4700
- replace age = 60 in 4700
- replace bmi = 40 in 4700
- replace woman = 1 in 4700
- replace id = 9999 in 4700

. replace logbmi = log(bmi) if id == 9999                                  {9}
(1 real change made)

. replace logscl = log(scl) if id == 9999
(1 real change made)

. replace wo_age = woman*age if id == 9999
(1 real change made)

. predict yhat,xb                                                          {10}
(41 missing values generated)

. predict h, leverage                                                      {11}
(41 missing values generated)

. predict std_yhat, stdp                                                   {12}
(41 missing values generated)

. predict std_f, stdf                                                      {13}
(41 missing values generated)

. generate cil_yhat = yhat - invt(4658-5-1,.95)*std_yhat                   {14}
(41 missing values generated)

. generate ciu_yhat = yhat + invt(4658-5-1,.95)*std_yhat
(41 missing values generated)

. generate cil_f = yhat - invt(4658-5-1,.95)*std_f                         {15}
(41 missing values generated)

. generate ciu_f  = yhat + invt(4658-5-1,.95)*std_f
(41 missing values generated)

. generate cil_sbpf = exp(cil_f)                                           {16}
(41 missing values generated)

. generate ciu_sbpf = exp(ciu_f)
(41 missing values generated)

. list bmi age scl woman logbmi logscl yhat h std_yhat std_f cil_yhat      {17}
> ciu_yhat cil_f ciu_f cil_sbpf ciu_sbpf if id==9999
```

```
Observation 4700

        bmi            40         age            60         scl           400
      woman             1      logbmi      3.688879      logscl      5.991465
       yhat      5.149496           h       .003901    std_yhat      .0086978
      std_f        .13953    cil_yhat      5.132444    ciu_yhat      5.166547
      cil_f      4.875951       ciu_f       5.42304    cil_sbpf      131.0987
   ciu_sbpf      226.5669

. display invt(4652,.95)

1.960474
```

Comments

1 This command regresses *logsbp* against the other covariates given in the command line. It evaluates model (3.17).

2 This command evaluates model (3.18).

3 This command evaluates model (3.19).

4 The output from the regress command for multiple linear regression is similar to that for simple linear regression that was discussed in Section 2.12. The R^2 statistic = MSS/TSS = 30.866/121.08 = 0.2549. The mean squared error (MSE) is $s^2 = 0.019\ 392\ 962$, which we defined in equation (3.5). Taking the square root of this variance estimate gives the Root MSE = s = 0.139 26.

5 For each covariate in the model, this table gives the estimate of the associated regression coefficient, the standard error of this estimate, the t statistic for testing the null hypothesis that the true value of the parameter equals zero, the P value that corresponds to this t statistic, and the 95% confidence interval for the coefficient estimate. The coefficient estimates in the second column of this table are also given in Table 3.2 in the second column on the right.

6 Note that although the age parameter estimate is small it is almost ten times larger that its associated standard error. Hence this estimate differs from zero with high statistical significance. The large range of the age of study subjects means that the influence of age on *logsbp* will be appreciable even though this coefficient is small.

7 The estimate of the constant coefficient α is 3.537 356.

8 Use the Stata editor to create a new record with covariates *scl*, *age*, *bmi* and *women* equal to 400, 60, 40 and 1 respectively. For subsequent manipulation set *id* equal to 9999 (or any other identification number that has not already been assigned).

9 The *replace* command redefines those values of an existing variable for which the *if* command qualifier is true. In this command, *logbmi* is only calculated for the new patient with $id = 9999$. This and the following two statements defines the covariates *logbmi*, *logscl* and *wo_age* for this patient.

10 The variable *yhat* is set equal to $\hat{y}_i$ for each record in memory. That is, *yhat* equals the estimated expected value of *logsbp* for each patient. This includes the new record that we have just created. Note that the regression parameter estimates are unaffected by this new record since it was created after the *regress* command was given.

11 The *leverage* option of the *predict* command creates a new variable called *h* that equals the leverage for each patient. Note that *h* is defined for our new patient even though no value of *logsbp* is given. This is because the leverage is a function of the covariates and does not involve the response variable.

12 The *stdp* option sets *std_yhat* equal to the standard error of *yhat*, which equals $s\sqrt{h_i}$.

13 The *stdf* option sets *std_f* equal to the standard deviation of *logsbp* given the patient's covariates. That is, $std\_f = s\sqrt{h_i + 1}$.

14 This command and the next define *cil_yhat* and *ciu_yhat* to be the lower and upper bounds of the 95% confidence interval for *yhat*, respectively. This interval is given by equation (3.10). Note that there are 4658 patients in our regression and there are 5 covariates in our model. Hence the number of degrees of freedom equals $4658 - 5 - 1 = 4652$.

15 This command and the next define *cil_sbpf* and *ciu_sbpf* to be the lower and upper bounds of the 95% prediction interval for *logsbp* given the patient's covariates. This interval is given by equation (3.12).

16 This command and the next define the 95% prediction interval for the SBP of a new patient having the specified covariates. We exponentiate the prediction interval given by equation (3.12) to obtain the interval for SBP as opposed to log[SBP].

17 This command lists the covariates and calculated values for the new patient only (that is, for records for which $id = 9999$ is true). The highlighted values in the output were also calculated by hand in Section 3.15.

3.17. Automatic Methods of Model Selection

In Section 3.13 we illustrated how to fit a multiple regression model by hand. When a large number of covariates are available, it can be useful to use an automatic model selection program for this task. There are four approaches to automatic model selection that are commonly used.

3.17.1. Forward Selection using Stata

The **forward selection** algorithm involves the following steps:

(i) Fit all possible simple linear models of the response variable against each separate covariate. Select the covariate with the lowest *P* value and include it in the models of the subsequent steps.

(ii) Fit all possible models with the covariate(s) selected in the preceding step(s) plus one other of the remaining covariates. Select the new co-variate that has the lowest *P* value and add it to all subsequent models.

(iii) Repeat step (ii) to add additional variables, one variable at a time. Continue this process until either none of the remaining covariates has a *P* value less than some threshold or until all of the covariates have been selected.

This algorithm is best understood by working through an example. We do this with the Framingham data using Stata. The *3.11.1.Framingham.log* file continues as follows.

```
. *
. * Repeat the preceding analysis using an automatic forward
. * selection algorithm
. *
.drop if id == 9999                                              {1}
(1 observation deleted)

. sw regress logsbp logbmi age logscl woman wo_lbmi wo_age wo_lscl,   {2}
> forward pe(.1)
                        begin with empty model
p = 0.0000  < 0.1000  adding   age                              {3}
p = 0.0000  < 0.1000  adding   logbmi                           {4}
p = 0.0000  < 0.1000  adding   logscl                           {5}
p = 0.0005  < 0.1000  adding   wo_age
p = 0.0000  < 0.1000  adding   woman                            {6}
```

{Output omitted. See Section 3.16}

Comments

1 This *drop* command deletes all records for which *id* == 9999 is true. In this instance the new patient added in Section 3.16 is deleted.

2 The *sw* prefix specifies that an automatic model selection algorithm is to be used to fit a multiple regression model (*sw* stands for stepwise);

regress specifies a linear regression model. The response variable is *logsbp*. The covariates to be considered for inclusion in the model are *logbmi*, *age*, *logscl*, *woman*, *wo_lbmi*, *wo_age* and *wo_lscl*. The *forward* option specifies that a forward selection method is to be used; *pe*(.1) sets the significance threshold for entering covariates into the model to be 0.1 (*pe* stands for *P* value for entry). At each step new variables will only be considered for entry into the model if their *P* value after adjustment for previously entered variables is < 0.1. Recall that earlier in the *3.11.1. Framingham.log* file we defined *logbmi* = log[*bmi$_i$*], *logscl* = log[*scl*], *wolbmi* = *woman* × log[*bmi*], *woage* = *woman* × *age*, and *wolscl* = *woman* × log[*scl*].

The choice of the significance threshold is up to the user. The idea is that we wish to include covariates that may have a real effect on the response variable while excluding those that most likely do not. We could set this value to 0.05, in which case only statistically significant covariates would be included. However, this would prevent us from considering variables that might be important, particularly in combination with other risk factors. A threshold of 0.1 is often used as a reasonable compromise.

3   In the first step the program considers the following simple regression models.

$$E[\log[sbp_i] \mid \mathbf{x}_i] = \alpha + \beta_1 \times \log[bmi_i]$$
$$E[\log[sbp_i] \mid \mathbf{x}_i] = \alpha + \beta_1 \times age_i$$
$$E[\log[sbp_i] \mid \mathbf{x}_i] = \alpha + \beta_1 \times \log[scl_i]$$
$$E[\log[sbp_i] \mid \mathbf{x}_i] = \alpha + \beta_1 \times woman_i$$
$$E[\log[sbp_i] \mid \mathbf{x}_i] = \alpha + \beta_1 \times woman_i \times \log[bmi_i]$$
$$E[\log[sbp_i] \mid \mathbf{x}_i] = \alpha + \beta_1 \times woman_i \times age_i$$
$$E[\log[sbp_i] \mid \mathbf{x}_i] = \alpha + \beta_1 \times woman_i \times \log[scl_i]$$

Of these models, the one with age has the most significant slope parameter. The *P* value associated with this parameter is < 0.000 05, which is also < 0.1. Therefore, we select *age* for inclusion in our final model and go on to step 2.

4   In step 2 we consider the following models.

$$E[\log[sbp_i] \mid \mathbf{x}_i] = \alpha + \beta_1 \times age_i + \beta_2 \times \log[bmi_i]$$
$$E[\log[sbp_i] \mid \mathbf{x}_i] = \alpha + \beta_1 \times age_i + \beta_2 \times \log[scl_i]$$
$$E[\log[sbp_i] \mid \mathbf{x}_i] = \alpha + \beta_1 \times age_i + \beta_2 \times woman_i$$
$$E[\log[sbp_i] \mid \mathbf{x}_i] = \alpha + \beta_1 \times age_i + \beta_2 \times woman_i \times \log[bmi_i]$$
$$E[\log[sbp_i] \mid \mathbf{x}_i] = \alpha + \beta_1 \times age_i + \beta_2 \times woman_i \times age_i$$
$$E[\log[sbp_i] \mid \mathbf{x}_i] = \alpha + \beta_1 \times age_i + \beta_2 \times woman_i \times \log[scl_i]$$

The most significant new term in these models is $\log[bmi_i]$, which is selected.

5 In step 3 the evaluated models all contain the term $\alpha + \beta_1 \times age_i + \beta_2 \times \log[bmi_i]$. The new covariates that are considered are $\log[scl_i]$, $woman_i$ and the three interaction terms involving $\log[bmi_i]$, age_i and $\log[scl_i]$. The most significant of these covariates is $\log[scl_i]$, which is included in the model.

6 This process is continued until at the end of step 5 we have model (3.19). In step 6 we consider adding the remaining terms $woman_i \times \log[bmi_i]$ and $woman_i \times \log[scl_i]$. However, neither of these covariates have a P value < 0.1. For this reason we stop and use (3.19) as our final model. The remaining output is identical to that given in Section 3.16 for this model.

It should also be noted that any stepwise regression analysis is restricted to those patients who have non-missing values for all of the covariates considered for the model. If the final model does not contain all of the considered covariates, it is possible that some patients with complete data for the final model will have been excluded because they were missing values for rejected covariates. When this happens it is a good idea to rerun your final model as a conventional regression analysis in order not to exclude these patients.

3.17.2. Backward Selection

The **backward selection** algorithm is similar to the forward method except that we start with all the variables and eliminate the variable with the least significance. The data are refitted with the remaining variables and the process is repeated until all remaining variables have a P value below some threshold.

The Stata command to use backward selection for our Framingham example is

```
sw regress logsbp logbmi age logscl woman wo_lbmi wo_age wo_lscl, pr(.1)
```

Here $pr(.1)$ means that the program will consider variables for removal from the model if their associated P value is ≥ 0.1. If you run this command in this example you will get the same answer as with forward selection, which is reassuring. In general, however, there is no guarantee that this will happen. The logic behind the choice of the removal threshold is the same as for the entry threshold. We wish to discard variables that most likely are unimportant while keeping those that may have a meaningful effect on the response variable.

3.17.3. Forward Stepwise Selection

The **forward stepwise selection** algorithm is like the forward method except that at each step, previously selected variables whose P value has risen above some threshold are dropped from the model. Suppose that x_1 is the best single predictor of the response variable y and is chosen in step 1. Suppose that x_2 and x_3 are chosen next and together predict y better than x_1. Then it may make sense to keep x_2 and x_3 and drop x_1 from the model.

In the Stata *sw* command this is done with the options *forward pe(.1) pr(.2)*, which would consider new variables for entry with $P < 0.1$ and previously selected variables for removal with $P \geq 0.2$. In other words the most significant covariate is entered into the model as long as the associated P value is < 0.1. Once selected it is kept in the model as long as its associated P value is < 0.2.

3.17.4. Backward Stepwise Selection

Backward stepwise selection is similar to the backward selection in that we start with all of the covariates in the model and then delete variables with high P values. It differs from backward selection in that at each step variables that have been previously deleted are also considered for reentry if their associated P value has dropped to a sufficiently low level. In the Stata *sw* command, backward stepwise selection is specified with the *pe* and *pr* options. For example, *pe(.1) pr(.2)*, would consider variables for removal from the model if their P values are ≥ 0.2, and would reconsider previously deleted variables for reentry if $P < 0.1$.

3.17.5. Pros and Cons of Automated Model Selection

Automatic selection methods are fast and easy to use. If you use them, it is a good idea to use more than one method to see if you come up with the same model. If, say, the forward and backward methods produce the same model then you have some evidence that the selected model is not an artifact of the selection procedure. A disadvantage of these methods is that covariates are entered or discarded without regard to the biologic interpretation of the model. For example, it is possible to include an interaction term but exclude one or both of the individual covariates that define this interaction. This may make the model difficult to interpret. Fitting models by hand is sometimes worth the effort.

3.18. Collinearity

Multiple linear regression can lead to inaccurate models if two or more of the covariates are highly correlated. To understand this situation, consider predicting a person's height from the lengths of their arms. A simple linear regression of height against either left or right arm length will show that both variables are excellent predictors of height. If, however, we include both arm lengths in the model we will either fail to get unique estimates of the model parameters, or the confidence intervals for these parameters will be very wide. This is because the arm lengths of most people are almost identical, and the multiple regression model seeks to measure the predictive value of the left arm length above and beyond that of the right, and vice versa. That is, the model measures the height versus left arm length slope among people whose right arm lengths are identical. This slope can only be estimated if there is variation in left arm lengths among people with identical right arm lengths. Since this variation is small or non-existent, the model is unable to estimate the separate effects of both left and right arm lengths on height.

This problem is called **collinearity**, and occurs whenever two covariate are highly correlated. When this happens you should avoid putting both variables in the model. Collinearity will also occur when there is a linear relationship between three or more of the covariates. This situation is harder to detect than that of a pair of highly correlated variables. You should be aware, however, that you may have a collinearity problem if adding a covariate to a model results in a large increase in the standard error estimates for two or more of the model parameters. When there is an exact linear relationship between two or more of the covariates, the minimum least squares estimates of the parameters are not uniquely defined. In this situation, Stata will drop one of these covariates from the model. Other software packages may abort the analysis.

3.19. Residual Analyses

Residual analyses in multiple linear regression are analogous to those for simple linear regression discussed in Section 2.15. Recall that the residual for the ith patient is $e_i = y_i - \hat{y}_i$. The variance of e_i is given by $s^2(1 - h_i)$, where s^2 is our estimate of σ^2 defined by equation (3.5). Dividing e_i by its standard deviation gives the **standardized residual**

$$z_i = e_i/(s\sqrt{1 - h_i}). \tag{3.20}$$

When the influence h_i is large, the magnitude of e_i will be reduced by the observation's ability to pull the expected response $\hat{y}_i$ towards y_i. In order to avoid missing large outliers with high influence we calculate the **studentized residual**

$$t_i = e_i/(s_{(i)}\sqrt{1 - h_i}), \tag{3.21}$$

where $s_{(i)}$ is the estimate of σ obtained from equation (3.5) with the ith case deleted (t_i is also called the **jackknifed residual**). If the multiple linear model is correct, then t_i will have a t distribution with $n - k - 2$ degrees of freedom. It is often helpful to plot the studentized residuals against the expected value of the response variable as a graphical check of the model's adequacy. Figure 3.7 shows such a plot for model (3.19) of the Framingham data. A lowess regression of the studentized residuals against the expected SBP is also included in this graph. If our model fitted perfectly, the lowess regression line would be flat and very close to zero. The studentized residuals would be symmetric about zero, with 95% of them lying between $\pm t_{n-k-2,0.25} = \pm t_{4658-5-2,0.25} = \pm 1.96$. In this example, the residuals are slightly skewed in a positive direction; 94.2% of the residuals lie between ± 1.96. The regression line is very close to zero except for low values of the expected log[SBP]. Hence, Figure 3.7 indicates that model (3.19) fits the

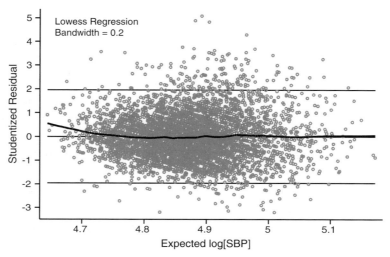

Figure 3.7   Scatter plot of studentized residuals vs. expected log[SBP] for model (3.19) of the Framingham Heart Study data. The thick black line is a lowess regression of the studentized residual against the expected log[SBP]. This plot indicates that model (3.19) provides a good, although not perfect, fit to these data.

data quite well, although not perfectly. The very large sample size, however, should keep the mild departure from normality of our residuals from adversely affecting our conclusions.

It is always a good idea to double-check observations with unusually large studentized residuals. These residuals may be due to coding errors, to anomalies in the way that the experiment was performed or the data was collected, or to unusual attributes of the patient that may require comment when the study is written up for publication.

3.20. Influence

We do not want our conclusions to be unduly influenced by any individual unusual patient. For this reason, it is important to know what effect individual subjects have on our parameter estimates. An observation can be very influential if it has both high leverage and a large studentized residual.

3.20.1. $\Delta\hat{\beta}$ Influence Statistic

The $\Delta\hat{\beta}$ **influence statistic** estimates the change in the value of a parameter due to the deletion of a single patient from the analysis. This change is expressed in terms of the parameter's standard error. Specifically, the influence of the ith patient on the jth parameter is estimated by

$$\Delta\hat{\beta}_{ij} = (b_j - b_{j(i)})/\text{se}[b_{j(i)}], \tag{3.22}$$

where b_j is the least squares estimate of β_j in equation (3.1), $b_{j(i)}$ is the corresponding estimate of β_j with the ith patient deleted from the analysis, and $\text{se}[b_{j(i)}]$ is an estimate of the standard error of $b_{j(i)}$; this estimate differs slightly from the usual one given with multiple linear regression output in order to reduce the computation time needed to compute $\Delta\hat{\beta}_{ij}$ for every patient in the analysis (Hamilton, 1992). A value of $|\Delta\hat{\beta}_{ij}|$ that is greater than one identifies a single observation that shifts the jth parameter estimate by more than a standard error. Large values of $\Delta\hat{\beta}_{ij}$ indicate that either special consideration is warranted for the jth patient or we have built a model that is too complex for our data. Simplifying the regression model will often lead to more robust, although possibly more modest, inferences about our data.

When considering the influence of an individual data point on a specific parameter, it is important to consider the magnitude of the parameter's standard error as well as the magnitude of the $\Delta\hat{\beta}$ statistic. If the standard error is small and the data point does not change the significance of the parameter, then it may be best to leave the data point in the analysis. On the other hand, if the standard error is large and the individual data point changes a small and non-significant parameter estimate into a large and significant one, then we may wish to either drop the data point from the analysis or choose a simpler model that is less affected by individual outliers. Of course any time we delete a data point from a published analysis we must make it clear what we have done and why.

3.20.2. Cook's Distance

Another measure of influence is **Cook's distance:**

$$D_i = \frac{z_i^2 h_i}{(k+1)(1-h_i)}, \tag{3.23}$$

which measures the influence of the ith patient on all of the regression coefficients taken together (Cook, 1977). Note that the magnitude of D_i increases as both the standardized residual z_i and the leverage h_i increase. Values of D_i that are greater than one identify influential patients. Hamilton (1992) recommends examining patients whose Cook's distance is greater than $4/n$. This statistic can be useful in models with many parameters in that it provides a single measure of influence for each patient. Its major disadvantage is that it is not as easily interpreted as the $\Delta\hat{\beta}$ statistic.

3.20.3. The Framingham Example

The entire Framingham data set is too large for any individual patient to have substantial influence over the parameters of model (3.19). To illustrate an analysis of influence, we look at 50 patients from this study. Applying this model to these patients gives an estimate of the log[BMI] coefficient of $b_1 = 0.1659$. Figure 3.8 shows a scatterplot of $\Delta\hat{\beta}_{i1}$ against the studentized residuals t_i for these data. If the model is correct, 95% of these residuals should have a t distribution with $50 - 5 - 2 = 43$ degrees of freedom and lie between $\pm t_{43,0.05} = \pm 2.02$. There are three (6%) of these residuals that lie outside these bounds. Although this number is consistent with our model, patient 49 has a very large residual, with $t_{49} = 4.46$. (Under our model assumptions, we would only expect to see a residual of this size less than once in every 20 000 patients.) For this patient, $h_{49} = 0.155$ and $\Delta\hat{\beta}_{49,1} = -1.42$. Hence, this patient's very large residual and moderate leverage deflects b_1, the log[BMI] coefficient estimate, by 1.42 standard errors. In contrast, for patient 48 we have $t_{48} = 2.58$, $h_{48} = 0.066$ and

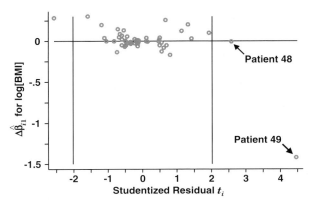

Figure 3.8   Scatterplot of $\Delta\hat{\beta}_{i1}$ versus t_i for 50 Framingham Heart Study patients using model (3.19). Patient 49 has an enormous studentized residual that has great influence on the log[BMI] parameter. The other patients have little influence on this parameter. Patient 48 has a large residual but virtually no influence due to the low leverage of this observation.

$\Delta\hat{\beta}_{48,1} = -0.006$. Thus, even though this patient has a large residual, his small leverage results in a trivial influence on the the log[BMI] coefficient. If we exclude patient 49 and apply model (3.19) to the remaining patients, we get an estimate of this coefficient of $b_{1(49)} = 0.3675$ with standard error 0.1489. Note that $(b_1 - b_{1(49)})/0.1489 = (0.1659 - 0.3675)/0.1489 = -1.354$, which agrees with $\Delta\hat{\beta}_{49,1}$ to two significant figures. Deleting this single patient raises the estimate of β_1 by 122%.

The standardized residual for patient 49 is 3.730, and the Cook's distance is

$$D_{49} = \frac{3.730^2 \times 0.1545}{(5+1)(1-0.1545)} = 0.424.$$

This value, while less than one, is substantially greater than $4/n = 0.08$. Had we only investigated patients with $D_i > 1$ we would have missed this very influential patient.

Of course, we can always look for influential patients by visually scanning scatterplots of the response variable and each individual covariate (see Figure 2.10). In multivariate analyses, however, it is advisable to look also at the influence statistics discussed above. This is because it is possible for the combined effects of a patient's multiple covariates to have a substantial influence on the parameter estimates without appearing to be an influential outlier on any particular 2×2 scatterplot.

3.21. Residual and Influence Analyses Using Stata

The *3.11.1.Framingham.log* file continues as follows and illustrates how to perform the residual and influence analyses discussed in Section 3.20.3. The output explicitly mentioned in these discussions is highlighted below.

```
. *

. * Draw a scatterplot of studentized residuals against the estimated
. * expected value of logsbp together with the corresponding lowess
. * regression curve.
. *

. predict t, rstudent                                                {1}
(41 missing values generated)
. ksm t yhat, lowess generate(t_hat) bwidth(.2)
```
                                                        {Graph omitted}
```
. label variable yhat "Expected log[SBP]"

. label variable t "Studentized Residual"

. sort yhat

. graph t t_hat yhat, symbol(oi) connect(.l) yline(-1.96,0,1.96)
> ylabel(-3,-2 to 5) xlabel(4.7,4.8 to 5.1) gap(2)
```
                                        {Graph omitted. See Figure 3.7}
```
. generate out = t > 1.96 | t < -1.96                                {2}

. tabulate out                                                       {3}
```

```
     out | Freq.    Percent      Cum.
-------- +---------------------------
       0 |  4425      94.17      94.17
       1 |   274       5.83     100.00
-------- +---------------------------
   Total |  4699     100.00
```

```
. *

. * Perform an influence analysis on patients 2000 through 2050
. *

. keep if id >= 2000 & id <= 2050
(4648 observations deleted)

. regress logsbp logbmi age logscl woman wo_age                      {4}
```

```
  Source |       SS       df       MS                Number of obs =      50
---------+------------------------------              F( 5,  44)    =    2.49
   Model | .381164541     5   .076232908              Prob > F      = 0.0456
Residual | 1.34904491     44  .030660112              R-squared     = 0.2203
---------+------------------------------              Adj R-squared = 0.1317
   Total | 1.73020945     49  .035310397              Root MSE      =  .1751
```

```
----------------------------------------------------------------------------
  logsbp |    Coef.    Std. Err.      t     P>|t|   [ 95% Conf. Interval]
-------- +------------------------------------------------------------------
  logbmi |  .1659182   .1696326    0.978   0.333   -.1759538    .5077902
     age | -.0006515   .0048509   -0.134   0.894   -.0104278    .0091249
   logscl |  .0983239   .1321621    0.744   0.461   -.1680314    .3646791
   woman | -.4856951   .294151    -1.651   0.106   -1.078517    .1071272
  wo_age |  .0116644   .0063781    1.829   0.074   -.0011899    .0245187
   _cons |  3.816949   .9136773    4.178   0.000    1.975553    5.658344
----------------------------------------------------------------------------
```

. **drop** *t h*   {5}
. **predict** *h*, **leverage**
(1 missing value generated)

. **predict** *z*, **rstandard**   {6}
(1 missing value generated)

. **predict** *t*, **rstudent**
(1 missing value generated)

. **predict** *deltab1*, **dfbeta(***logbmi***)**   {7}
(1 missing value generated)

. **predict** *cook*, *cooksd*   {8}
(1 missing value generated)

. **display invttail(***43,.025***)**
2.0166922

. **label variable** *deltab1* **"Delta Beta for log[BMI]"**

. **graph** *deltab1 t*, **xline(***-2.017, 2.017***) yline(***0***) xlabel(***-2,-1 to 4***)**
> **xtick(***-2.5,-1.5 to 4.5***) ylabel(***-1.5,-1,-.5,0***) symbol(***O***)**
> **gap(***3***)**

{Graph omitted. See Figure 3.8}

. **sort** *t*

. **list** *id h z t deltab1 cook* **in** *-3/-1*   {9}

```
          id          h          z          t      deltab1        cook
49.     2048    .0655644   2.429988   2.581686    -.0063142     .069052
50.     2049    .1545165   3.730179   4.459472    -1.420916    .4238165
51.     2046          .          .          .            .            .
```

. regress *logsbp logbmi age logscl woman wo_age if id ~= 2049*   {10}

```
  Source |       SS      df       MS              Number of obs =      49
---------+------------------------------          F( 5,   43)   =    3.13
   Model | .336072673      5  .067214535          Prob > F      = 0.0169
Residual | .922432819     43  .021451926          R-squared     = 0.2670
---------+------------------------------          Adj R-squared = 0.1818
   Total | 1.25850549     48  .026218864          Root MSE      = .14646

-----------------------------------------------------------------------
  logsbp |    Coef.   Std. Err.       t    P>|t|   [ 95% Conf. Interval]
---------+-------------------------------------------------------------
  logbmi |  .3675337   .1489199    2.468   0.018    .0672082    .6678592
     age | -.0006212   .0040576   -0.153   0.879   -.0088042    .0075617
  logscl |  .0843428    .110593    0.763   0.450   -.1386894    .3073749
   woman | -.3053762   .2493465   -1.225   0.227   -.8082314     .197479
  wo_age |  .0072062   .0054279    1.328   0.191   -.0037403    .0181527
   _cons |  3.244073   .7749778    4.186   0.000    1.681181    4.806965
-----------------------------------------------------------------------
```

. **display** *(.1659182 -.3675337)/.1489199*   {11}
-1.353852

Comments

1 The *rstudent* option of the *predict* command defines t to equal the studentized residual for each patient.

2 The variable *out* is a logical variable that equals 1 when "$t > 1.96 \mid t < -1.96$" is true and equals 0 otherwise. In other words, *out* equals 1 if either $t > 1.96$ or $t < -1.96$, and equals 0 if $-1.96 \le t \le 1.96$.

3 The tabulate command lists the distinct values taken by *out*, together with the frequency, percentage and cumulative percentage of these values. Note that 94.2% of the studentized residuals lie between ± 1.96 (see Section 3.19).

4 Apply model (3.19) to patients with *id* numbers between 2000 and 2050. Note that one patient in this range has a missing serum cholesterol and is excluded from this analysis. Thus, 50 patients are included in this linear regression.

5 The drop command deletes the t and h variables from memory. We do this because we wish to redefine these variables as being the studentized residual and leverage from the preceding linear regression

6 The *rstandard* option defines z to equal the standardized residuals for each patient.

7 The *dfbeta*(*logbmi*) option defines *deltab1* to equal the $\Delta\hat{\beta}$ influence statistic for the *logbmi* parameter.

8 The *cooksd* option defines *cook* to equal Cook's distance for each patient.

9 The "*in* −3/−1" command qualifier restricts this listing to the last three records in the file. As the previous command sorted the file by t, the records with the three largest values of t are listed. Stata sorts missing values after non-missing ones. The last record in the file is for patient 2046. This is the patient with the missing serum cholesterol who was excluded from the regression analysis; t is missing for this patient. The two patients with the largest studentized residuals are patients 2048 and 2049 who have residuals $t = 2.58$ and $t = 4.46$, respectively. These patients are referred to as patients 48 and 49 in Section 3.20.3, respectively.

10 Repeat the regression excluding patient 2049. Note the large change in the *logbmi* coefficient that results from deleting this patient (see Section 3.20.3).

11 The difference in the *logbmi* coefficient estimates that result from including or excluding patient 2049 is −1.35 standard errors.

3.22. Additional Reading

Armitage and Berry (1994), and

Pagano and Gauvreau (2000) provide good introductions to multiple linear regression.

Hamilton (1992) and

Cook and Weisberg (1999) are more advanced texts that emphasize a graphical approach to multiple linear regression. Hamilton (1992) provides a brief introduction to non-linear regression.

Draper and Smith (1998) is a classic reference on multiple linear regression.

Cook (1977) is the original reference on Cook's distance.

Levy (1999) reviews the findings of the Framingham Heart Study.

3.23. Exercises

1 Linear regression was applied to a large data set having age and weight as covariates. The estimated coefficients for these two variables and their standard errors are as follows:

Covariate	Estimated coefficient	Estimated standard error
Age	1.43	0.46
Weight	25.9	31.0

Can we reject the null hypothesis that the associated parameter equals zero for either of these variables? Can we infer anything about the biologic significance of these variables from the magnitudes of the estimated coefficients? Justify your answers.

The following questions concern the study by Gross et al. (1999) about the relationship between funding by the National Institutes of Health and the burden of 29 diseases. The data from Table 1 of this study are given in a Stata data file called *3.ex.Funding.dta* on the *www.mc.vanderbilt. edu/prevmed/wddtext.htm* web page. The variable names and definitions in this file are

disease   = condition or disease,
id   = a numeric disease identification number,
dollars   = thousands of dollars of NIH research funds per year,
incid   = disease incidence rate per 1000,
preval   = disease prevalence rate per 1000,
hospdays = thousands of hospital-days,
mort   = disease mortality rate per 1000,
yrslost   = thousands of life-years lost,
disabil   = thousands of disability-adjusted life-years lost.

2 Explore the relationship between *dollars* and the other covariates listed above. Fit a model that you feel best captures this relationship.

3 Perform a forward stepwise linear regression of log[*dollars*] against the following potential covariates: log[*incid*], log[*preval*], log[*hospdays*], log[*mort*], log[*yrslost*] and log[*disabil*]. Use thresholds for entry and removal of covariates into or from the model of 0.1 and 0.2, respectively. Which covariates are selected by this procedure?

4 Repeat question 3 only now using a backward stepwise model selection procedure. Use the same thresholds for entry and removal. Do you get the same model as in question 3?

5 Regress log[*dollars*] against the same covariates chosen by the stepwise procedure in question 4. Do you get the same parameter estimates? If not, why not?

6 Regress log[*dollars*] against log[*hospdays*], log[*mort*], log[*yrslost*] and

log[*disabil*]. Calculate the expected log[*dollars*] and studentized residuals for this regression. What bounds should contain 95% of the studentized residuals under this model? Draw a scatterplot of these residuals against expected log[*dollars*]. On the graph draw the lowess regression curve of the residuals against the expected values. Draw horizontal lines at zero and the 95% bounds for the studentized residuals. What does this graph tell you about the quality of the fit of this model to these data?

7 In the model from question 6, calculate the $\Delta\hat{\beta}$ influence statistic for log[*mort*]. List the values of this statistic together with the disease name, studentized residual and leverage for all diseases for which the absolute value of this $\Delta\hat{\beta}$ statistic is greater than 0.5. Which disease has the largest influence on the log[*mort*] parameter estimate? How many standard errors does this data point shift the log[*mort*] parameter estimate? How big is its studentized residual?

8 Draw scatterplots of log[*dollars*] against the other covariates in the model from question 6. Identify the disease in these plots that had the most influence on log[*mort*] in question 7. Does it appear to be particularly influential in any of these scatterplots?

9 Repeat the regression from question 6 excluding the observation on perinatal conditions. Compare your coefficient estimates with those from question 6. What is the change in the estimate of the coefficient for log[*mort*] that results from deleting this disease? Express this difference as a percentage change and as a difference in standard errors.

10 Perform influence analyses on the other covariates in the model from question 6. Are there any observations that you feel should be dropped from the analysis? Do you think that a simpler model might be more appropriate for these data?

11 Regress log[*dollars*] against log[*disabil*] and log[*hospdays*]. What is the estimated expected amount of research funds budgeted for a disease that causes a million hospital-days a year and the loss of a million disability-adjusted life-years? Calculate a 95% confidence interval for this expected value. Calculate a 95% prediction interval for the funding that would be provided for a new disease that causes a million hospital-days a year and the loss of a million disability-adjusted life-years.

12 In question 11, suppose that we increase the number of disability-adjusted life-years lost by two million while keeping the number of hospital-days constant. What will happen to the estimated expected number of research funds spent on this disease under this model?

13 Perform an influence analysis on the model from question 11. Is this analysis more reassuring than the one that you performed in question 10? Justify your answer.

4

Simple Logistic Regression

In simple linear regression we fit a straight line to a scatterplot of two continuous variables that are measured on study subjects. Often, however, the
response variable of interest has dichotomous outcomes such as survival or
death. We wish to be able to predict the probability of a patient's death given
the value of an explanatory variable for the patient. Using linear regression
to estimate the probability of death is usually unsatisfactory since it can
result in probability estimates that are either greater than one (certainty)
or less than zero (impossibility). Logistic regression provides a simple and
plausible way to estimate such probabilities.

4.1. Example: APACHE Score and Mortality in Patients with Sepsis

Figure 4.1 shows 30-day mortality in a sample of septic patients as a function
of their baseline APACHE scores (see Section 1.2.1). Patients are coded as 1
or 0 depending on whether they are dead or alive at 30 days, respectively. We
wish to predict death from baseline APACHE score in these patients. Note
that all patients with an APACHE score of less than 17 survived, while all
but one patient with a score greater than 27 died. Mortal outcome varied
for patients with scores between 17 and 27.

4.2. Sigmoidal Family of Logistic Regression Curves

Let $\pi[x]$ be the probability that a patient with score x will die. In logistic
regression we fit probability functions of the form

$$\pi[x] = \exp[\alpha + \beta x]/(1 + \exp[\alpha + \beta x]), \tag{4.1}$$

where α and β are unknown parameters that we will estimate from the data.
Equation (4.1) is the **logistic probability function.** This equation describes
a family of sigmoidal curves, four examples of which are given in Figure 4.2.
For now, assume that $\beta > 0$. For negative values of x, $\exp[\alpha + \beta x]$ is very
close to zero when x is small (i.e. when $-x$ is large). Hence $\pi[x]$ approaches
$0/(1 + 0) = 0$ as x gets small. For positive values of x, $\exp[\alpha + \beta x]$ is very

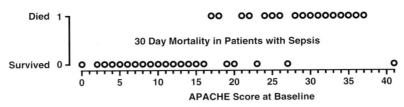

Figure 4.1   Scatter plot showing mortal outcome by baseline APACHE Score for 30 patients admitted to an intensive care unit with sepsis.

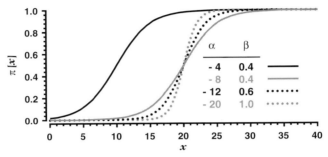

Figure 4.2   Four examples of logistic regression curves given by equation 4.1. The two solid curves have the same value of the β parameter, which gives identical slopes. The different values of the α parameter shifts the gray curve 10 units to the right. The slopes of these curves increase as β gets larger.

large when x is big and hence $\pi[x] = a\_big\_number/(1 + a\_big\_number)$ approaches 1 as x gets large. The magnitude of β controls how quickly $\pi[x]$ rises from 0 to 1. When $x = -\alpha/\beta$, $\alpha + \beta x = 0$, $e^0 = 1$, and hence $\pi[x] = 1/(1 + 1) = 0.5$. Thus, for given β, α controls where the 50% survival point is located. In Figure 4.2, the solid black curve reaches $\pi[x] = 0.5$ when $x = -\alpha/\beta = 4/0.4 = 10$. The solid gray curve has the same slope as the black curve but is shifted 10 units to the right. The solid gray curve and the dotted curves all reach their midpoint at $x = -\alpha/\beta = 20$. The slopes of the dotted curves are greater than that of the solid gray curve because of their larger value of β. It can be shown that the slope of a logistic regression curve when $\pi[x] = 0.5$ equals $\beta/4$.

We wish to choose the best curve to fit data such as that shown in Figure 4.1. Suppose that there is a sharp survival threshold with deaths occurring only in those patients whose x value is above this threshold. Then we would want to fit a regression curve with a large value of β that will give a rapid transition between estimated probabilities of death of 0 and 1. On the other hand, if the observed mortality increases gradually with increasing

x then we would want a curve with a much smaller value of β that will predict a more gradual rise in the probability of death.

4.3. The Log Odds of Death Given a Logistic Probability Function

Equation (4.1) gives that the probability of death under a logistic probability function is $\pi[x] = \exp[\alpha + \beta x]/(1 + \exp[\alpha + \beta x])$. Hence, the probability of survival is

$$1 - \pi[x] = \frac{1 + \exp[\alpha + \beta x] - \exp[\alpha + \beta x]}{1 + \exp[\alpha + \beta x]} = \frac{1}{1 + \exp[\alpha + \beta x]}.$$

The **odds** of death is

$$\pi[x]/(1 - \pi[x]) = \exp[\alpha + \beta x], \tag{4.2}$$

and the **log odds** of death equals

$$\log\left[\frac{\pi[x]}{1 - \pi[x]}\right] = \alpha + \beta x. \tag{4.3}$$

For any number π between 0 and 1 the **logit function** is defined by

$$\text{logit}[\pi] = \log[\pi/(1 - \pi)].$$

In the sepsis example let

$$d_i = \begin{cases} 1: \text{if the } i^{\text{th}} \text{ patient dies} \\ 0: \text{if the } i^{\text{th}} \text{ patient lives, and} \end{cases}$$

x_i equal the APACHE score of the ith patient.

Then we can rewrite equation (4.3) as

$$\text{logit}[\pi[x_i]] = \alpha + \beta x_i. \tag{4.4}$$

In simple linear regression we modeled a continuous response variable as a linear function of a covariate (see equation 2.4). In simple logistic regression we will model the logit of the probability of survival as a linear function of a covariate.

4.4. The Binomial Distribution

Suppose that m people are at risk of death during some interval and that d of these people die. Let each patient have probability π of dying during the interval, and let the fate of each patient be independent of the fates of all the others. Then d has a **binomial distribution** with parameters m and π. The mean of this distribution is $m\pi$, and its standard error is $\sqrt{m\pi(1-\pi)}$.

The probability of observing d deaths among these m patients is

$$\Pr[d \text{ deaths}] = \frac{m!}{(m-d)!d!}\,\pi^d(1-\pi)^{(m-d)} \quad : d = 0, 1, \ldots, m. \quad (4.5)$$

Equation (4.5) is an example of a **probability distribution** for a discrete random variable, which gives the probability of each possible outcome.

The mean of any random variable x is also equal to its expected value and is written $E[x]$. Also, if x is a random variable and k is a constant then $E[kx] = kE[x]$. Hence

$E[d] = \pi m$ and $E[d/m] = \pi$.

For example, if we have $m = 100$ patients whose individual probability of death is $\pi = 1/2$ then the expected number of deaths is $E[d] = 0.5 \times 100 = 50$. That is, we would expect that one half of the patients will die. Of course, the actual number of deaths may vary considerably from 50 although the probability of observing a number of deaths that is greatly different from this value is small. Figure 4.3 shows the probability distribution for the number of deaths observed in $m = 12$ patients with an individual probability of death of $\pi = 0.25$. In this example the expected number of deaths is three. The probability of observing three deaths is 0.258, which is higher than the probability of any other outcome. The probability of observing nine or more deaths is very small.

A special case of the binomial distribution occurs when we have a single patient who either does, or does not, die. In this case $m = 1$, and we observe either $d = 0$ or $d = 1$ deaths with probability $1 - \pi$ and π, respectively. The expected value of d is $E[d] = m\pi = \pi$. The random variable d is said to have a **Bernoulli distribution** when $m = 1$.

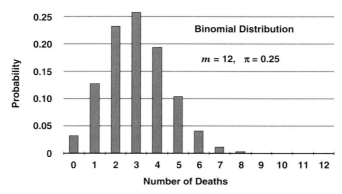

Figure 4.3   Binomial probability distribution resulting from observing 12 patients with an individual probability of death of 0.25.

4.5. Simple Logistic Regression Model

Suppose we have an unbiased sample of n patients from a target population. Let

$$d_i = \begin{cases} 1: \text{if the } i^{\text{th}} \text{ patient suffers some event of interest} \\ 0: \text{otherwise, and} \end{cases}$$

x_i be a continuous covariate observed on the ith patient.

The **simple logistic regression model** assumes that d_i has a Bernoulli distribution with

$$\text{E}[d_i \mid x_i] = \pi[x_i] = \exp[\alpha + \beta x_i]/(1 + \exp[\alpha + \beta x_i]), \qquad (4.6)$$

where α and β are unknown parameters associated with the target population. Equivalently, we can rewrite the logistic regression model using equation (4.4) as

$$\text{logit}[\text{E}[d_i \mid x_i]] = \alpha + \beta x_i. \qquad (4.7)$$

4.6. Generalized Linear Model

Logistic regression is an example of a **generalized linear model**. These models are defined by three attributes: the distribution of the model's random component, its linear predictor, and its link function. For logistic regression these are defined as follows:

1. The **random component** of the model is d_i, the patient's fate. In simple logistic regression, d_i has a Bernoulli distribution with expected value $\text{E}[d_i \mid x_i]$. (In Section 4.14 we will generalize this definition to allow d_i to have any binomial distribution.)
2. The **linear predictor** of the model is $\alpha + \beta x_i$.
3. The **link function** describes a functional relationship between the expected value of the random component and the linear predictor. Logistic regression uses the logit link function $\text{logit}[\text{E}[d_i \mid x_i]] = \alpha + \beta x_i$.

4.7. Contrast Between Logistic and Linear Regression

Not surprisingly, linear regression is another example of a generalized linear model. In linear regression, the expected value of y_i given x_i is

$$\text{E}[y_i \mid x_i] = \alpha + \beta x_i \text{ for } i = 1, 2, \dots, n.$$

The random component of the model, y_i, has a normal distribution with mean $\alpha + \beta x_i$ and standard deviation σ. The linear predictor is $\alpha + \beta x_i$, and the link function is the identity function $I[x] = x$. That is, $I[E[y_i \mid x_i]] = E[y_i \mid x_i] = \alpha + \beta x_i$. The generalized linear model is useful in that it provides a common approach to fitting several important models in biostatistics and epidemiology.

4.8. Maximum Likelihood Estimation

We have yet to discuss how to choose the best logistic regression model to fit a specific data set. In linear regression we used the method of least squares to estimate regression coefficients. That is, we chose those estimates of α and β that minimized the sum of the squared residuals. This approach does not work well in logistic regression, or for the entire family of generalized linear models. Instead we use another approach called **maximum likelihood estimation**. The easiest way to explain this approach is through a simple example.

Suppose that we observe an unbiased sample of 50 AIDS patients, and that five of these patients die in one year. We wish to estimate π, the annual probability of death for these patients. We assume that the number of observed deaths has a binomial distribution obtained from $m = 50$ patients with probability of death π for each patient. Let $L[\pi \mid d = 5] = (50!/45! \times 5!)\pi^5(1 - \pi)^{45}$ be the probability of the observed outcome (five deaths) given different values of π. $L[\pi \mid d = 5]$ is called a **likelihood function** and is plotted in Figure 4.4.

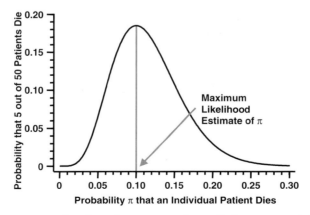

Figure 4.4   Suppose that five of 50 AIDS patients die in a year and that these deaths have a binomial distribution. Let π be the probability that an individual patient dies in a given year. Then the likelihood function $L[\pi \mid d = 5]$ for this observation gives the probability of the observed outcome ($d = 5$ deaths) under different hypothesized values of π.

The **maximum likelihood estimate** of π is the value of π that assigns the greatest probability to the observed outcome. In this example the maximum likelihood estimate, denoted $\hat{\pi}$, equals $d/m = 0.1$. This is a plausible estimate in that, if the observed mortality rate is 10%, our best guess of the true mortality rate is also 10%. Note that if $\pi = \hat{\pi} = 0.1$ then $\mathrm{E}[d] = 50\pi = 5 = d$. Thus, in this example, the maximum likelihood estimate of π is also the value that sets the expected number of deaths equal to the observed number of deaths.

In general, maximum likelihood estimates do not have simple closed solutions, but must be solved iteratively using numerical methods. This, however, is not a serious drawback given ubiquitous and powerful desktop computers.

A likelihood function looks deceptively like a probability density function. It is important to realize that they are quite different. A probability density function uses fixed values of the model parameters and indicates the probability of different outcomes under this model. A likelihood function holds the observed outcome fixed and shows the probability of this outcome for the different possible values of the parameters.

4.8.1. Variance of Maximum Likelihood Parameter Estimates

It can be shown that when a maximum likelihood estimate is based on large number of patients, its variance is approximately equal to $-1/C$, where C is the curvature of the logarithm of the likelihood function at $\hat{\pi}$. (In mathematical jargon, the curvature of a function is its second derivative. A function that bends downward has a negative curvature. The more sharply it bends the greater the absolute value of its curvature.) An intuitive explanation of this result is as follows. If the likelihood function reaches a sharp peak at $\hat{\pi}$ that falls away rapidly as π moves away from $\hat{\pi}$, then the curvature C at $\hat{\pi}$ will have high magnitude and $-1/C$ will be low. This means that the data are consistent with only a small range of π and hence $\hat{\pi}$ is likely to be close to π. Thus, in a repeated sequence of similar experiments there will be little variation in $\hat{\pi}$ from experiment to experiment giving a low variance for this statistic. On the other hand, if the likelihood function drops slowly on both sides of $\hat{\pi}$ then $|C|$ will be small and $-1/C$ will be large. The data will be consistent with a wide range of π and a repeated sequence of similar experiments will produce a wide variation in the values of $\hat{\pi}$. Hence, the variance of $\hat{\pi}$ will be large.

In the AIDS example from Section 4.8, C can be shown to equal $-m/(\hat{\pi}(1 - \hat{\pi}))$. Hence, the approximate variance of $\hat{\pi}$ is

$$\text{var}[\hat{\pi}] = -1/C = \hat{\pi}(1 - \hat{\pi})/m. \tag{4.8}$$

The true variance of $\hat{\pi}$ is $\pi(1 - \pi)/m$, and equation (4.8) converges to this true value as m becomes large. Substituting $\hat{\pi} = 0.1$ and $m = 50$ into equation (4.8) gives that the variance of $\hat{\pi}$ is approximately $0.1 \times 0.9/50 = 0.0018$. The corresponding standard error is $\text{se}[\hat{\pi}] = \sqrt{0.0018} = 0.0424$.

4.9. Statistical Tests and Confidence Intervals

In this section we briefly introduce three fundamental types of statistical tests, which we will use in this and later chapters: likelihood ratio tests, score tests and Wald tests. Each of these tests involves a statistic whose distribution is approximately normal or chi-squared. The accuracy of these approximations increases with increasing study sample size. We will illustrate these tests using the AIDS example from Section 4.8.

4.9.1. Likelihood Ratio Tests

Suppose that we wish to test the null hypothesis that $\pi = \pi_0$. Let $L[\pi]$ denote the likelihood function for π given the observed data. We look at the **likelihood ratio** $L[\pi_0]/L[\hat{\pi}]$. If this ratio is small then we would be much more likely to have observed the data that was actually obtained if the true value of π was $\hat{\pi}$ rather than π_0. Hence, small values of $L[\pi_0]/L[\hat{\pi}]$ provide evidence that $\pi \neq \pi_0$. Moreover, it can be shown that if the null hypothesis is true, then

$$\chi^2 = -2 \log[L[\pi_0]/L[\hat{\pi}]] \tag{4.9}$$

has an approximately chi-squared distribution with one degree of freedom. Equation (4.9) is an example of a **likelihood ratio test**. The P value associated with this test is the probability that a chi-squared distribution with one degree of freedom exceeds the value of this test statistic.

In our AIDS example, the likelihood ratio is

$$L[\pi_0]/L[\hat{\pi}] = \left(\pi_0^5(1 - \pi_0)^{45}\right)/(\hat{\pi}^5(1 - \hat{\pi})^{45}).$$

Suppose that we wished to test the null hypothesis that $\pi_0 = 0.2$. Now since $\hat{\pi} = 0.1$, equation (4.9) gives us that

$$\chi^2 = -2 \log[(0.2^5 \times 0.8^{45})/(0.1^5 \times 0.9^{45})] = 3.67.$$

The probability that a chi-squared distribution with one degree of freedom exceeds 3.67 is $P = 0.055$.

4.9.2. Quadratic Approximations to the Log Likelihood Ratio Function

Consider quadratic equations of the form $f[x] = -a(x - b)^2$, where $a \geq 0$. Note that all equations of this form achieve a maximum value of 0 at $x = b$. Suppose that $g[x]$ is any smooth function that has negative curvature at x_0. Then it can be shown that there is a unique equation of the form $f[x] = -a(x - b)^2$ such that f and g have the same slope and curvature at x_0. Let

$$q[\pi] = \log[L[\pi]/L[\hat{\pi}]] \tag{4.10}$$

equal the logarithm of the likelihood ratio at π relative to $\hat{\pi}$. Suppose that we wish to test the null hypothesis that $\pi = \pi_0$. Then the likelihood ratio test is given by $-2q[\pi_0]$ (see equation (4.9)). In many practical situations, equation (4.10) is difficult to calculate. For this reason $q[\pi]$ is often approximated by a quadratic equation. The maximum value of $q[\pi]$ is $q[\hat{\pi}] = \log[L[\hat{\pi}]/L[\hat{\pi}]] = 0$. We will consider approximating $q[\pi]$ by quadratic equations that also have a maximum value of 0. Let

> $f_s[\pi]$ be the quadratic equation that has the same slope and curvature as $q[\pi]$ at π_0 and achieves a maximum value of 0,
> $f_w[\pi]$ be the quadratic equation that has the same slope and curvature as $q[\pi]$ at $\hat{\pi}$ and achieves a maximum value of 0.

Tests that approximate $q[\pi]$ by $f_s[\pi]$ are called score tests. Tests that approximate $q[\pi]$ by $f_w[\pi]$ are called Wald tests. We will introduce these two types of tests in the next two sections.

4.9.3. Score Tests

Suppose we again wish to test the null hypothesis that $\pi = \pi_0$. If the null hypothesis is true then it can be shown that

$$\chi^2 = -2 f_s[\pi_0] \tag{4.11}$$

has an approximately chi-squared distribution with one degree of freedom. Equation (4.11) is an example of a **score test**. Score tests are identical to likelihood ratio tests except that a likelihood ratio test is based on the true log likelihood ratio function $q[\pi]$ while a score test approximates $q[\pi]$ by $f_s[\pi]$.

In the AIDS example,

$$\hat{\pi} = 0.1 \text{ and } q[\pi] = \log((\pi/0.1)^5((1 - \pi)/0.9)^{45}).$$

It can be shown that

$q[\pi]$ has slope $\dfrac{5}{\pi} - \dfrac{45}{1 - \pi}$ and curvature $-\dfrac{5}{\pi^2} - \dfrac{45}{(1 - \pi)^2}$.

We wish to test the null hypothesis that $\pi_0 = 0.2$. The slope and curvature of $q[\pi]$ at $\pi = 0.2$ are -31.25 and -195.3125, respectively. It can be shown that $f_s[\pi] = -97.656\,25(\pi - 0.04)^2$ also has this slope and curvature at $\pi = 0.2$. Therefore, if the true value of $\pi = 0.2$ then $-2 f_s[0.2] = 2 \times 97.656\,25(0.2 - 0.04)^2 = 5$ has an approximately chi-squared distribution with one degree of freedom. The P value associated with this score statistic is $P = 0.025$, which is lower than the corresponding likelihood ratio test.

4.9.4. Wald Tests and Confidence Intervals

If the null hypothesis that $\pi = \pi_0$ is true, then

$$\chi^2 = -2 f_w [\pi_0] \tag{4.12}$$

also has an approximately chi-squared distribution with one degree of freedom. Equation (4.12) is an example of a **Wald Test.** It is identical to the likelihood ratio test except that a likelihood ratio test is based on the true log likelihood ratio function $q[\pi]$, while a Wald test approximates $q[\pi]$ by $f_w[\pi]$. In Section 4.8.1 we said that the variance of a maximum likelihood estimate can be approximated by $\text{var}[\hat{\pi}] = -1/C$. It can be shown that

$$-2 f_w[\pi_0] = (\pi_0 - \hat{\pi})^2/\text{var}[\hat{\pi}]. \tag{4.13}$$

The standard error of $\hat{\pi}$ is approximated by $\text{se}[\hat{\pi}] = \sqrt{-1/C}$. Recall that a chi-squared statistic with one degree of freedom equals the square of a standard normal random variable. Hence, an equivalent way of performing a Wald test is to calculate

$$z = (\hat{\pi} - \pi_0)/\text{se}[\hat{\pi}], \tag{4.14}$$

which has an approximately standard normal distribution. An approximate 95% confidence interval for π is given by

$$\hat{\pi} \pm 1.96 \text{se}[\hat{\pi}]. \tag{4.15}$$

Equations (4.15) is known as a **Wald confidence interval.**

In the AIDS example, $\hat{\pi} = 0.1$ and $\text{se}[\hat{\pi}] = 0.0424$. Consider the null hypothesis that $\pi_0 = 0.2$. Equation (4.14) gives that $z = (0.1 - 0.2)/0.0424 =$

-2.36. The probability that a z statistic is less than -2.36 or greater than 2.36 is $P = 0.018$. The 95% confidence interval for π is $0.1 \pm 1.96 \times 0.0424 = (0.017, 0.183)$.

4.9.5. Which Test Should You Use?

The three tests outlined above all generalize to more complicated situations. Given a sufficiently large sample size all of these methods are equivalent. However, likelihood ratio tests and score tests are more accurate than Wald tests for most problems that are encountered in practice. For this reason, you should use a likelihood ratio or score test whenever they are available. The likelihood ratio test has the property that it is unaffected by transformations of the parameter of interest and is preferred over the score test for this reason. The Wald test is much easier to calculate than the other two, which are often not given by statistical software packages. It is common practice to use Wald tests when they are the only ones that can be easily calculated.

Wide divergence between these three tests can result when the log likelihood function is poorly approximated by a quadratic curve. In this case it is desirable to transform the parameter is such a way as to give the log likelihood function a more quadratic shape.

In this text, the most important example of a score test is the logrank test, which is discussed in Chapter 6. In Chapters 5, 7 and 9 we will look at changes in model deviance as a means of selecting the best model for our data. Tests based on these changes in deviance are an important example of likelihood ratio tests. All of the confidence intervals in this text that are derived from logistic regression, survival or Poisson regression models are Wald intervals. Tests of statistical significance in these models that are derived directly from the parameter estimates are Wald tests.

4.10. Sepsis Example

Let us use logistic regression to model the relationship between mortal risk and APACHE score in the example from Section 4.1. Let $d_i = 1$ if the ith patient dies within 30 days, and let $d_i = 0$ otherwise. Let x_i be the ith patient's APACHE score at baseline. Applying the logistic regression model (4.7) to these data we obtain maximum likelihood parameter estimates of $\hat{\alpha} = -4.3478$ and $\hat{\beta} = 0.201\,24$. Inserting these estimates into equation (4.6) gives the estimated probability of death associated with each APACHE

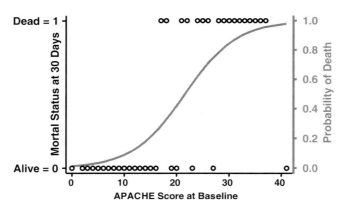

Figure 4.5   The gray curve in this figure shows the estimated probability of death within 30 days for septic patients with the indicated APACHE score at baseline. This curve is obtained by applying a logistic regression model to the observed mortal outcomes of 38 septic patients.

score. For example, the estimated probability of death associated with an APACHE score of 16 is

$$\hat{\pi}[16] = \exp[\hat{\alpha} + \hat{\beta} \times 16]/(1 + \exp[\hat{\alpha} + \hat{\beta} \times 16])$$

$$= \exp[-4.3478 + 0.201\,24 \times 16]/(1 + \exp[-4.3478$$

$$+ 0.201\,24 \times 16])$$

$$= 0.2445.$$

Figure 4.5 shows a plot of this probability of death as a function of baseline APACHE score.

4.11. Logistic Regression with Stata

The following log file and comments illustrates how to fit a logistic regression model to the sepsis data set given in Figure 4.1.

```
. * 4.11.Sepsis.log
. *
. * Simple logistic regression of mortal status at 30 days (fate) against
. * baseline APACHE score (apache) in a random sample of septic patients
. *
. use C:\WDDtext\4.11.Sepsis.dta, clear
. summarize fate apache                                              {1}
```

```
Variable  |    Obs      Mean   Std. Dev.      Min        Max
----------+-----------------------------------------------------
    fate  |    38    .4473684    .5038966       0          1
  apache  |    38    19.55263    11.30343       0         41
```

. **glm fate apache, family(binomial) link(logit)**   {2}

                                                    {Output omitted}

```
Variance function:   V(u)   =   u*(1-u)          [Bernoulli]
Link function    :   g(u)   =   ln(u/1-u))       [Logit]
```

                                                    {Output omitted}

```
----------------------------------------------------------------
    fate  |     Coef.   Std. Err.      z   P>|z|   [95% Conf. Interval]
----------+-----------------------------------------------------------
  apache  |   .2012365   .0608998   3.304  0.001   .0818752   .3205979   {3}
   _cons  |  -4.347807   1.371609  -3.170  0.002  -7.036111  -1.659503
----------------------------------------------------------------
```

. **predict logodds, xb**   {4}

. **generate prob = exp(logodds)/(1 + exp(logodds))**   {5}

. **list apache fate logodds prob in 1/3**

```
       apache   fate    logodds      prob
  1.       16   Alive  -1.128022   .2445263
  2.       25   Dead    .6831066   .6644317
  3.       19   Alive  -.5243126   .3718444
```

. **set textsize 120**

. **sort apache**

. **graph fate prob apache, connect(.1) symbol(Oi) xlabel(0,10,20,30,40)**
> **ylabel(0,1) gap(3) r1title(Probability of Death) rlabel(0,.2,.4,.6,.8,1)** {7}

                                          {Graph omitted. See Figure 4.5}

Comments

1 This data set contains 38 observations. The variable *fate* equals 1 for patients who die within 30 days; *fate* equals 0 otherwise. Baseline APACHE
   scores range from 0 to 41.

2 This *glm* command regresses *fate* against *apache* using a generalized linear
   model. The *family* and *link* options specify that the random component
   of the model is binomial and the link function is logit. In other words, a
   logistic model is to be used. Stata has two commands that can perform

logistic regression: *glm*, which can analyze any generalized linear model, and *logistic*, which can only be used for logistic regression. We will introduce the *logistic* command in Section 4.13.1.

3 The maximum likelihood parameter estimates are $\hat{\alpha} = -4.3478$ and $\hat{\beta} = 0.201\,24$.

4 The *xb* option of this *predict* command specifies that the linear predictor will be estimated for each patient and stored in a variable named *logodds*. Recall that *predict* is a post estimation command whose meaning is determined by the latest estimation command, which in this example is *glm*.

5 This command defines *prob* to equal the estimated probability that a patient will die. It is calculated using equation (4.6).

6 The first patient has an APACHE score of 16. Hence, the estimated linear predictor for this patient is $logodds = \hat{\alpha} + \hat{\beta}x_i = \_cons + apache \times 16 = -4.3478 + 0.201\,24 \times 16 = -1.128$. The second patient has $APACHE = 25$ giving $logodds = -4.3478 + 0.201\,24 \times 25 = 0.683$. For the first patient, $prob = \exp[logodds]/(1 + \exp[logodds]) = 0.2445$, which agrees with our calculation from Section 4.10.

7 This graph command produces a graph that is similar to Figure 4.5. The *r1title* and *rlabel* options provide a title and axis labels for a vertical axis on the right of the graph.

4.12. Odds Ratios and the Logistic Regression Model

The log odds of death for patients with APACHE scores of x and $x + 1$ are

$$logit[\pi[x]] = \alpha + \beta x \qquad (4.16)$$

and

$$logit[\pi[x+1]] = \alpha + \beta(x+1) = \alpha + \beta x + \beta \qquad (4.17)$$

respectively. Subtracting equation (4.16) from equation (4.17) gives

$$
\begin{aligned}
\beta &= logit[\pi[x+1]] - logit[\pi[x]] \\
&= \log\left[\frac{\pi[x+1]}{1 - \pi[x+1]}\right] - \log\left[\frac{\pi[x]}{1 - \pi[x]}\right] \\
&= \log\left[\frac{\pi[x+1]/[1 - \pi[x+1]]}{\pi[x]/[1 - \pi[x]]}\right].
\end{aligned}
$$

Hence $\exp[\beta]$ is the odds ratio for death associated with a unit increase in x. A property of logistic regression is that this ratio remains constant for all values of x.

4.13. 95% Confidence Interval for the Odds Ratio Associated with a Unit Increase in *x*

Let $s_{\hat{\beta}}$ denote the estimated standard error of $\hat{\beta}$ from the logistic regression model. Now $\hat{\beta}$ has an approximately normal distribution. Therefore, a 95% confidence interval for β is estimated by $\hat{\beta} \pm 1.96 s_{\hat{\beta}}$, and a 95% confidence interval for the odds ratio associated with a unit increase in x is

$$(\exp[\hat{\beta} - 1.96 s_{\hat{\beta}}], \exp[\hat{\beta} + 1.96 s_{\hat{\beta}}]). \tag{4.18}$$

In the sepsis example in Section 4.10, the parameter estimate for *apache* (that is, β) was 0.201 24 with a standard error of $s_{\hat{\beta}} = 0.060\ 90$. Hence, the 95% confidence interval for β is $0.201\ 24 \pm z_{0.025} \times 0.060\ 90 = 0.201\ 24 \pm 1.96 \times 0.060\ 90 = (0.0819, 0.3206)$. The odds ratio for death associated with a unit rise in APACHE score is $\exp[0.2012] = 1.223$ with a 95% confidence interval of $(\exp[0.0819], \exp[0.3206]) = (1.085, 1.378)$.

4.13.1. Calculating this Odds Ratio with Stata

Stata can perform these calculations automatically. The following log file and comments illustrates how to do this using the *logistic* command:

```
. * 4.13.1.Sepsis.log
. *
. * Calculate the odds ratio associated with a unit rise in APACHE score
. *
. use C:\WDDtext\4.11.Sepsis.dta, clear
. logistic fate apache                                                    {1}

Logit estimates                              Number of obs   =        38
                                             LR chi2(1)      =     22.35
                                             Prob > chi2     =    0.0000
Log likelihood = -14.956085                  Pseudo R2       =    0.4276

-----------------------------------------------------------------------------
    fate |  Odds Ratio   Std. Err.     z     P>|z|   [95% Conf.  Interval]
---------+-------------------------------------------------------------------
  apache |    1.222914    .0744759   3.304   0.001    1.085319   1.377953    {2}
-----------------------------------------------------------------------------
```

Comments

1 Regress *fate* against *apache* using logistic regression. This command performs the same calculations as the *glm* command given in Section 4.11.

However, the output is somewhat different. Also, there are some useful post estimation commands that are available after running *logistic* that are not available after running *glm*.

2 The number under the *Odds Ratio* heading is the exponentiated coefficient estimate for *apache*. As indicated above, this is the odds ratio associated with a unit rise in APACHE score. The 95% confidence interval for this odds ratio is identical to that calculated above.

4.14. Logistic Regression with Grouped Response Data

The number of patients under study often exceeds the number of distinct covariates. For example, in the Ibuprofen in Sepsis Study there were 38 distinct baseline APACHE scores observed on 454 patients (Bernard et al., 1997). Suppose that $\{x_i : i = 1, \ldots, n\}$ denote the distinct values of a covariate, and there are m_i patients who have the identical covariate value x_i. Let d_i be the number of deaths in these m_i patients and let $\pi[x_i]$ be the probability that any one of them will die. Then d_i has a binomial distribution with mean $m_i \pi[x_i]$, and hence $E[d_i \mid x_i]/m_i = \pi[x_i]$. Thus, the logistic model becomes

$$\text{logit}[E[d_i \mid x_i]/m_i] = \alpha + \beta x_i, \tag{4.19}$$

or equivalently

$$E[d_i/m_i \mid x_i] = \pi[x_i] = \exp[\alpha + \beta x_i]/(1 + \exp[\alpha + \beta x_i]). \tag{4.20}$$

In equation (4.19) d_i is the random component of the model, which has a binomial distribution. If i indexes patients rather than distinct values of the covariate then $m_i = 1$ for all i and equation (4.19) reduces to equation (4.7).

4.15. 95% Confidence Interval for $\pi[x]$

Let $\sigma_{\hat{\alpha}}^2$ and $\sigma_{\hat{\beta}}^2$ denote the variance of $\hat{\alpha}$ and $\hat{\beta}$, and let $\sigma_{\hat{\alpha}\hat{\beta}}$ denote the covariance between $\hat{\alpha}$ and $\hat{\beta}$. Then it can be shown that the standard error of $\hat{\alpha} + \hat{\beta}x$ is

$$\text{se}[\hat{\alpha} + \hat{\beta}x] = \sqrt{\sigma_{\hat{\alpha}}^2 + 2x\sigma_{\hat{\alpha}\hat{\beta}} + x^2\sigma_{\hat{\beta}}^2}. \tag{4.21}$$

Any logistic regression software that calculates the maximum likelihood estimates of α and β can also provide estimates of $\sigma_{\hat{\alpha}}^2, \sigma_{\hat{\beta}}^2$ and $\sigma_{\hat{\alpha}\hat{\beta}}$. We substitute these estimates into equation (4.21) to obtain an estimate of the standard error of $\hat{\alpha} + \hat{\beta}x$. This allows us to estimate the 95% confidence interval for $\alpha + \beta x$ to be $\hat{\alpha} + \hat{\beta} x \pm 1.96 \times \mathrm{se}[\hat{\alpha} + \hat{\beta} x]$. Hence, a 95% confidence interval for $\pi[x]$ is $(\hat{\pi}_L[x], \hat{\pi}_U[x])$, where

$$\hat{\pi}_L[x] = \frac{\exp[\hat{\alpha} + \hat{\beta} x - 1.96 \times \mathrm{se}[\hat{\alpha} + \hat{\beta} x]]}{1 + \exp[\hat{\alpha} + \hat{\beta} x - 1.96 \times \mathrm{se}[\hat{\alpha} + \hat{\beta} x]]} \tag{4.22}$$

and

$$\hat{\pi}_U[x] = \frac{\exp[\hat{\alpha} + \hat{\beta} x + 1.96 \times \mathrm{se}[\hat{\alpha} + \hat{\beta} x]]}{1 + \exp[\hat{\alpha} + \hat{\beta} x + 1.96 \times \mathrm{se}[\hat{\alpha} + \hat{\beta} x]]}. \tag{4.23}$$

4.16. 95% Confidence Intervals for Proportions

It is useful to be able to estimate a 95% confidence interval for the proportion d_i/m_i. Let d be the number of deaths observed in m patients. Let

$p \quad = d/m$ be the observed proportion of deaths,
$q \quad = 1 - p$, and
$z_{\alpha/2} =$ the critical value such that $100(\alpha/2)\%$ of observations from standard normal distribution exceed $z_{\alpha/2}$.

Then Fleiss (1981) gives a $100(1-\alpha)\%$ confidence interval for p, which is (P_L, P_U), where

$$P_L = \frac{\left(2mp + z_{\alpha/2}^2 - 1\right) - z_{\alpha/2}\sqrt{z_{\alpha/2}^2 - (2 + 1/m) + 4p(mq + 1)}}{2\left(m + z_{\alpha/2}^2\right)} \tag{4.24}$$

and

$$P_U = \frac{\left(2mp + z_{\alpha/2}^2 + 1\right) + z_{\alpha/2}\sqrt{z_{\alpha/2}^2 + (2 - 1/m) + 4p(mq - 1)}}{2\left(m + z_{\alpha/2}^2\right)}. \tag{4.25}$$

For a 95% confidence interval $\alpha = 0.05$ and $z_{\alpha/2} = 1.96$ in equations (4.24) and (4.25). These equations are valid as long as $0 < d < $ m. Although simpler formulas exist that work well when p is, say, between 0.3 and 0.7, equations (4.24) and (4.25) are recommended when p is close to either 0 or 1.

4.17. Example: The Ibuprofen in Sepsis Trial

The Ibuprofen and Sepsis Trial contained 454 patients with known baseline APACHE scores. The 30-day mortality data for these patients is summarized in Table 4.1. Let x_i denote the distinct APACHE scores observed in this study. Let m_i be the number of patients with baseline score x_i and let d_i be the number of patients with this score who died within 30 days. Applying the logistic regression model (4.19) to these data yields parameter estimates

Table 4.1. Survival data from the Ibuprofen in Sepsis Study. The number of patients enrolled with the indicated baseline APACHE score is given together with the number of subjects who died within 30 days of entry into the study (Bernard et al., 1997).

Baseline APACHE score	Number of patients	Number of deaths	Baseline APACHE score	Number of patients	Number of deaths
0	1	0	20	13	6
2	1	0	21	17	9
3	4	1	22	14	12
4	11	0	23	13	7
5	9	3	24	11	8
6	14	3	25	12	8
7	12	4	26	6	2
8	22	5	27	7	5
9	33	3	28	3	1
10	19	6	29	7	4
11	31	5	30	5	4
12	17	5	31	3	3
13	32	13	32	3	3
14	25	7	33	1	1
15	18	7	34	1	1
16	24	8	35	1	1
17	27	8	36	1	1
18	19	13	37	1	1
19	15	7	41	1	0

$\hat{\alpha} = -2.290\,327$ and $\hat{\beta} = 0.115\,627$. The estimated variance of $\hat{\alpha}$ and $\hat{\beta}$ is $s_{\hat{\alpha}}^2 = 0.076\,468$ and $s_{\hat{\beta}}^2 = 0.000\,256$, respectively. The estimated covariance between $\hat{\alpha}$ and $\hat{\beta}$ is $s_{\hat{\alpha}\hat{\beta}} = -0.004\,103$. Substituting these values into equations (4.20) through (4.25) provides estimates of the probability of death given a baseline score of x, 95% confidence intervals for these estimates, and 95% confidence intervals for the observed proportion of deaths at any given score. For example, patients with a baseline score of 20 will have a linear predictor of $\hat{\alpha} + \hat{\beta} \times 20 = 0.0222$. Substituting this value into equation (4.20) gives $\hat{\pi}[20] = \exp[0.0222]/(1 + \exp[0.0222]) = 0.506$. Equation (4.21) gives us that

$$se[\hat{\alpha} + \hat{\beta} \times 20] = \sqrt{0.076\,468 - 2 \times 20 \times 0.004\,103 + 20^2 \times 0.000\,256}$$
$$= 0.1214.$$

Substituting into equations (4.22) and (4.23) gives

$$\hat{\pi}_L[20] = \exp[0.0222 - 1.96 \times 0.1214]/(1 + \exp[0.0222$$

$$- 1.96 \times 0.1214]) = 0.446,$$

and

$$\hat{\pi}_U[20] = \exp[0.0222 + 1.96 \times 0.1214]/(1 + \exp[0.0222$$

$$+ 1.96 \times 0.1214]) = 0.565.$$

Hence a 95% confidence interval for $\pi(20)$ is (0.446, 0.565).

There are $m = 13$ patients with an APACHE score of 20; $d = 6$ of these subjects died. Hence the observed proportions of dying and surviving patients with this score are $p = 6/13$ and $q = 7/13$, respectively. Substituting these values into equations (4.24) and (4.25) gives

$$P_L = \frac{\left(2 \times 13 \times \frac{6}{13} + 1.96^2 - 1\right) - 1.96\sqrt{1.96^2 - \left(2 + \frac{1}{13}\right) + 4 \times \frac{6}{13}\left(13 \times \frac{7}{13} + 1\right)}}{2\left(13 + 1.96^2\right)} = 0.204$$

and

$$P_U = \frac{\left(2 \times 13 \times \frac{6}{13} + 1.96^2 + 1\right) + 1.96\sqrt{1.96^2 + \left(2 - \frac{1}{13}\right) + 4 \times \frac{6}{13}\left(13 \times \frac{7}{13} - 1\right)}}{2\left(13 + 1.96^2\right)} = 0.739$$

as the bounds of the 95% confidence interval for the true proportion of deaths among people with an APACHE score of 20. Note that the difference between $(\hat{\pi}_L(20), \hat{\pi}_U(20))$ and (P_L, P_U) is that the former is based on all 454 patients and the logistic regression model while the latter is based solely on the 13 patients with APACHE scores of 20.

We can perform calculations similar to those given above to generate Figure 4.6. The black dots in this figure give the observed mortality for each APACHE score. The error bars give 95% confidence intervals for the observed mortality at each score using equations (4.24) and (4.25). Confidence intervals for scores associated with 100% survival or 100% mortality are not given. The solid gray line gives the logistic regression curve using equation (4.20). This curve depicts the expected 30-day mortality as a function of the baseline APACHE score. The dashed lines give the 95% confidence intervals for the regression curve using equations (4.22) and (4.23). These intervals are analogous to the confidence intervals for the linear regression line described in Section 2.10. Note that the expected mortality curve lies within all of the 95% confidence intervals for the observed proportion of deaths at each score. This indicates that the logistic regression model fits the

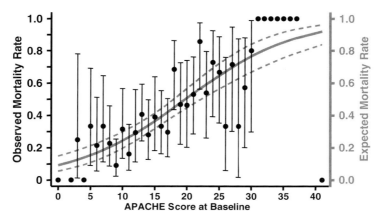

Figure 4.6   Observed and expected 30-day mortality by APACHE score in patients from the Ibuprofen in Sepsis Study (Bernard et al., 1997). The solid gray line gives the expected mortality based on a logistic regression model. The dashed lines give the 95% confidence region for this regression line. The black dots give the observed mortality for each APACHE score. The error bars give 95% confidence intervals for the observed mortality at each score.

data quite well. The width of the 95% confidence intervals for the regression curve depends on the number of patients studied, on the distance along the x-axis from the central mass of observations and on the proximity of the regression curve to either zero or one. Figure 4.7 shows a histogram of the number of study subjects by baseline APACHE score. This figure shows that the distribution of scores is skewed. The interquartile range is 10–20. Note that the width of the confidence interval at a score of 30 in Figure 4.6 is considerably greater than it is at a score of 15. This reflects the fact that 30 is further from the central mass of observations than is 15, and that as a consequence the accuracy of our estimate of $\pi[30]$ is less than that of $\pi[15]$. For very large values of the x variable, however, we know that $\pi[x]$ converges to one. Hence, $\hat{\pi}_L[x]$ and $\hat{\pi}_U[x]$ must also converge to one. In Figure 4.6 the confidence intervals have started to narrow for this reason for scores of 40 or more. We can think of the 95% confidence intervals for the regression line as defining the region that most likely contains the true regression line given that the logistic regression model is, in fact, correct.

4.18. Logistic Regression with Grouped Data using Stata

The following log file and comments illustrates how to use Stata to perform the calculations from the preceding section.

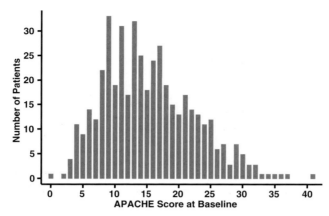

Figure 4.7   Histogram of baseline APACHE scores for patients from the Ibuprofen in Sepsis Study. This distribution is skewed to the right, with few patients having
scores greater than 30. The estimate of the expected mortality rate in Figure 4.6
is most accurate over the range of scores that were most common in this study.

```
. * 4.18.Sepsis.log
. *
. * Simple logistic regression of mortality against APACHE score
. * in the Ibuprofen in Sepsis Study. Each record of 4.18.Sepsis.dta
. * gives the number of patients and number of deaths among subjects
. * with a specified APACHE score. These variables are named patients
. * deaths and apache, respectively.
. *
. use C:\WDDtext\4.18.Sepsis.dta, clear
. *
. * Calculate 95% confidence intervals for observed mortality rates
. *
. generate p = deaths/patients
. generate m = patients
. generate q = 1-p
. generate c = 1.96
```

. generate $ci95lb = (2*m*p+c^2-1-c*sqrt(c^2-(2+1/m)+4*p*(m*q+1)))/(2*(m+c^2))$ $\{1\}$
> if $d \sim=0$ & $d\sim= m$

(11 missing values generated)

. generate $ci95ub = (2*m*p+c^2+1+c*sqrt(c^2+(2-1/m)+4*p*(m*q-1)))/(2*(m+c^2))$ $\{2\}$
> if $d \sim=0$ & $d \sim= m$

```
(11 missing values generated)

. *

. * Regress deaths against APACHE score

. *

. glm deaths apache, family(binomial patients) link(logit)          {3}
                                                        {output omitted}

Generalized linear models                  No. of obs    =    38
                                                        {output omitted}

Variance function: V(u)   =   u*(1-u/patients)      [Binomial]
Link function     : g(u)   =   ln(u/(patients-u))    [Logit]
                                                        {output omitted}

------------------------------------------------------------------------
   deaths |    Coef.    Std. Err.     z      P>|z|     [95% Conf. Interval]
----------+-------------------------------------------------------------
   apache |   .1156272   .0159997   7.227    0.000    .0842684    .146986   {4}
    _cons |  -2.290327   .2765283  -8.282    0.000   -2.832313  -1.748342
------------------------------------------------------------------------

. vce                                                               {5}

          |   apache     _cons
----------+------------------
   apache |   .000256
    _cons |  -.004103    .076468

. predict logodds, xb                                               {6}

. generate e_prob = exp(logodds)/(1+exp(logodds))                   {7}

. label variable e_prob "Expected Mortality Rate"

. *

. * Calculate 95% confidence region for e_prob

. *

. predict stderr, stdp                                              {8}

. generate lodds_lb = logodds - 1.96*stderr

. generate lodds_ub = logodds + 1.96*stderr

. generate prob_lb = exp(lodds_lb)/(1+exp(lodds_lb))                {9}

. generate prob_ub = exp(lodds_ub)/(1+exp(lodds_ub))

. label variable p "Observed Mortality Rate"
```

```
. set textsize 120

. list p e_prob prob_lb prob_ub ci95lb ci95ub apache if apache == 20          {10}

           p      e_prob     prob_lb     prob_ub      ci95lb     ci95ub     apache
20.   .4615385    .505554    .4462291    .564723    .2040146     .7388         20

. graph p e_prob prob_lb prob_ub ci95lb ci95ub apache, symbol(Oiiiii)          {11}
> connect(.ll[-#]l[-#]II) gap(3) xlabel(0 5 to 40) ylabel(0 .2 to 1.0)
> ytick(.1 .2 to .9) rltitle(Expected Mortality Rate) rlabel(0,.2,.4,.6,.8,1.0)
```
                                                    {Graph omitted. See Figure 4.6}
```
. graph apache [freq=patients], bin(42) freq gap(3) lltitle(Number of Patients)
> xlabel(0, 5 to 40) ylabel(0, 5 to 30)                                        {12}
```
                                                    {Graph omitted. See Figure 4.7}

Comments

1 Calculate the lower bound for a 95% confidence interval for the observed proportion of deaths using equation (4.24). This bound is not calculated if all or none of the patients survive.

2 Calculate the corresponding upper bound using equation (4.25).

3 The *family* and *link* option of this *glm* command specify a binomial random component and a logit link function. The *family(binomial patients)* option indicates that each observation describes the outcomes of multiple patients with the same value of *apache*; *patients* records the number of subjects with each *apache* value; *deaths* records the number of deaths observed among these subjects. In other words, we are fitting a logistic regression model using equation (4.20) with $d_i = deaths$, $m_i = patients$ and $x_i = apache$.

4 The estimated regression coefficients for *apache* and the constant term _cons are $\hat{\beta} = 0.115\ 627$ and $\hat{\alpha} = -2.290\ 327$, respectively.

5 The *vce* command prints the variance–covariance matrix for the estimated regression coefficients. This is a triangular array of numbers that gives estimates of the variance of each coefficient estimate and the covariance of each pair of coefficient estimates. In this example there are only two coefficients. The estimated variance of the *apache* and _cons coefficient estimates are $s_{\hat{\beta}}^2 = 0.000\ 256$ and $s_{\hat{\alpha}}^2 = 0.076\ 468$, respectively. The covariance between these estimates is $s_{\hat{\alpha}\hat{\beta}} = -0.004\ 103$. Note that the square roots of $s_{\hat{\beta}}^2$ and $s_{\hat{\alpha}}^2$ equal 0.1600 and 0.2765, which are the standard errors of $\hat{\beta}$ and $\hat{\alpha}$ given in the output from the *glm* command. We do not usually need to output the variance–covariance matrix in

Stata because the *predict* and *lincom* post estimation commands can usually derive all of the statistics that are of interest. We output these terms here in order to corroborate the hand calculations performed in Section 4.17. We will introduce the *lincom* command in Section 5.20. The variance–covariance matrix is further discussed in Section 5.17.

6 This command sets *logodds* equal to the linear predictor $\hat{\alpha} + \hat{\beta} \times$ *apache*.

7 The variable *e_prob* equals $\hat{\pi}[apache]$, the estimated probability of death for patients with the indicated APACHE score.

8 The *stdp* option of this *predict* command sets *stderr* equal to the standard error of the linear predictor.

9 This generate command defines *prob_lb* to equal $\hat{\pi}_L[x]$ as defined by equation (4.22). The next command sets *prob_ub* to equal $\hat{\pi}_U[x]$.

10 This list command outputs the values of variables calculated above for the record with an APACHE score of 20. Note that these values agree with the estimates that we calculated by hand in Section 4.17.

11 The graph produced by this command is similar to Figure 4.6. The two "I"s in the *connect* option specify that the last two *y*-variables, *ci95lb* and *ci95ub*, are to be connected by error bars. The 95% confidence region for *e_prob* = $\hat{\pi}[apache]$ are drawn with dashed lines that are specified by the "l[−#]" code in the *connect* option.

12 This histogram is similar to Figure 4.7. The *freq* option specifies that the *y*-axis will be the number of subjects; *l1title* specifies the title of the *y*-axis.

4.19. Simple 2×2 Case-Control Studies

4.19.1. Example: The Ille-et-Vilaine Study of Esophageal Cancer and Alcohol

Tuyns et al. (1977) conducted a case-control study of alcohol, tobacco and esophageal cancer in men from the Ille-et-Vilaine district of Brittany. Breslow and Day (1980) subsequently published these data. The cases in this study were 200 esophageal cancer patients who had been diagnosed at a district hospital between January 1972 and April 1974. The controls were 775 men who were drawn from local electoral lists. Study subjects were interviewed concerning their consumption of alcohol and tobacco as well as other dietary risk factors. Table 4.2 shows these subjects divided by whether they were moderate or heavy drinkers.

Table 4.2. Cases and controls from the Ille-et-Vilaine study of esophageal cancer, grouped by level of daily alcohol consumption. Subjects were considered heavy drinkers if their daily consumption was $\geq$ 80 grams (Breslow and Day, 1980).

Esophageal	Daily alcohol consumption		
cancer	$\geq$ 80g	< 80g	Total
Yes (cases)	$d_1 = 96$	$c_1 = 104$	$m_1 = 200$
No (controls)	$d_0 = 109$	$c_0 = 666$	$m_0 = 775$
Total	$n_1 = 205$	$n_0 = 770$	$N = 975$

4.19.2. Review of Classical Case-Control Theory

Let π_0 and π_1 denote the prevalence of heavy drinking among controls and cases in the Ille-et-Vilaine case-control study, respectively. That is, π_i is the probability that a control ($i = 0$) or a case ($i = 1$) is a heavy drinker. Then the **odds** that a control patient is a heavy drinker is $\pi_0/(1 - \pi_0)$, and the odds that a case is a heavy drinker is $\pi_1/(1 - \pi_1)$. The **odds ratio** for heavy drinking among cases relative to controls is

$$\psi = (\pi_1/(1 - \pi_1))/(\pi_0/(1 - \pi_0)). \tag{4.26}$$

Let m_0 and m_1 denote the number of controls and cases, respectively. Let d_0 and d_1 denote the number of controls and cases who are heavy drinkers. Let c_0 and c_1 denote the number of controls and cases who are moderate or non-drinkers. (Note that $m_i = c_i + d_i$ for $i = 0$ or 1.) Then the observed prevalence of heavy drinkers is $d_0/m_0 = 109/775$ for controls and $d_1/m_1 = 96/200$ for cases. The observed prevalence of moderate or non-drinkers is $c_0/m_0 = 666/775$ for controls and $c_1/m_1 = 104/200$ for cases. **The observed odds** that a case or control will be a heavy drinker is

$$(d_i/m_i)/(c_i/m_i) = d_i/c_i$$

$= 109/666$ and $96/104$ for controls and cases, respectively. The **observed odds ratio** for heavy drinking in cases relative to controls is

$$\hat{\psi} = \frac{d_1/c_1}{d_0/c_0} = \frac{96/104}{109/666} = 5.64.$$

If the cases and controls are representative samples from their respective underlying populations then:

1 $\hat{\psi}$ is an appropriate estimate of the true odds ratio ψ for heavy drinking in cases relative to controls in the underlying population.

2 This true odds ratio also equals the true odds ratio for esophageal cancer in heavy drinkers relative to moderate drinkers.

3 If, in addition, the disease under study is rare (as is the case for esophageal cancer) then $\hat{\psi}$ also estimates the relative risk of esophageal cancer in heavy drinkers relative to moderate drinkers.

It is the second of the three facts listed above that makes case-control studies worth doing. We really are not particularly interested in the odds ratio for heavy drinking among cases relative to controls. However, we are very interested in the relative risk of esophageal cancer in heavy drinkers compared to moderate drinkers. It is, perhaps, somewhat surprising that we can estimate this relative risk from the prevalence of heavy drinking among cases and controls. Note that we are unable to estimate the incidence of cancer in either heavy drinkers or moderate drinkers. See Hennekens and Buring (1987) for an introduction to case-control studies. A more mathematical explanation of this relationship is given in Breslow and Day (1980).

4.19.3. 95% Confidence Interval for the Odds Ratio: Woolf's Method

An estimate of the standard error of the log odds ratio is

$$se_{\log(\hat{\psi})} = \sqrt{\frac{1}{d_0} + \frac{1}{c_0} + \frac{1}{d_1} + \frac{1}{c_1}}, \tag{4.27}$$

and the distribution of $\log(\hat{\psi})$ is approximately normal. Hence, if we let

$$\hat{\psi}_L = \hat{\psi} \exp\left[-1.96 se_{\log(\hat{\psi})}\right] \tag{4.28}$$

and

$$\hat{\psi}_U = \hat{\psi} \exp\left[1.96 se_{\log(\hat{\psi})}\right], \tag{4.29}$$

then $(\hat{\psi}_L, \hat{\psi}_U)$ is a 95% confidence interval for ψ (Woolf, 1955). In the esophageal cancer and alcohol analysis

$$se_{\log(\hat{\psi})} = \sqrt{\frac{1}{109} + \frac{1}{666} + \frac{1}{96} + \frac{1}{104}} = 0.1752.$$

Therefore, Woolf's estimate of the 95% confidence interval for the odds ratio is $(\hat{\psi}_L, \hat{\psi}_U) = (5.64 \exp[-1.96 \times 0.1752], 5.64 \exp[+1.96 \times 0.1752]) = (4.00, 7.95)$.

4.19.4. Test of the Null Hypothesis that the Odds Ratio Equals One

If there is no association between exposure and disease then the odds ratio ψ will equal one. Let n_j be the number of study subjects who are

$(j = 1)$ or are not $(j = 0)$ heavy drinkers and let $N = n_0 + n_1 = m_0 + m_1$ be the total number of cases and controls. Under the null hypothesis that $\psi = 1$, the expected value and variance of d_1 are

$E[d_1 \mid \psi = 1] = n_1 m_1 / N$ and

$\text{var}[d_1 \mid \psi = 1] = m_0 m_1 n_0 n_1 / N^3.$

Hence,

$$\chi_1^2 = (|d_1 - E[d_{1j} \mid \psi = 1]| - 0.5)^2 / \text{var}[d_1 \mid \psi = 1] \tag{4.30}$$

has a χ^2 distribution with one degree of freedom. In the Ille-et-Vilaine study

$E[d_1 \mid \psi = 1] = 205 \times 200/975 = 42.051$ and

$\text{var}[d_1 \mid \psi = 1] = 775 \times 200 \times 770 \times 205/975^3 = 26.397.$

Therefore, $\chi_1^2 = (|96 - 42.051| - 0.5)^2/(26.397) = 108.22$. The P value associated with this statistic is $< 10^{-24}$, providing overwhelming evidence that the observed association between heavy drinking and esophageal cancer is not due to chance.

In equation (4.30) the constant 0.5 that is subtracted from the numerator is known as Yates' continuity correction (Yates, 1934). It adjusts for the fact that we are approximating a discrete distribution with a continuous normal distribution. There is an ancient controversy among statisticians as to whether such corrections are appropriate (Dupont and Plummer, 1999). Mantel and Greenhouse (1968), Fleiss (1981), Breslow and Day (1980) and many others use this correction in calculating this statistic. However, Grizzle (1967) and others, including the statisticians at Stata, do not. This leads to a minor discrepancy between output from Stata and other statistical software. Without the continuity correction the χ^2 statistic equals 110.26.

4.19.5. Test of the Null Hypothesis that Two Proportions are Equal

We also need to be able to test the null hypothesis that two proportions are equal. For example, we might wish to test the hypothesis that the proportion of heavy drinkers among cases and controls are the same. It is important to realize that this hypothesis, $H_0 : \pi_0 = \pi_1$, is true if and only if $\psi = 1$. Hence equation (4.30) may also be used to test this null hypothesis.

4.20. Logistic Regression Models for 2×2 Contingency Tables

Consider the logistic regression model

$$\text{logit}[E[d_i \mid x_i]/m_i] = \alpha + \beta x_i : i = 0, 1, \tag{4.31}$$

where $x_0 = 0$, $x_1 = 1$ and $E[d_i \mid x_i]/m_i = \pi_i$ is the probability of being a heavy drinker for controls ($i = 0$) or cases ($i = 1$). Then (4.31) can be rewritten as

$$\text{logit}\,[\pi_i] = \log\,[\pi_i/(1 - \pi_i)] = \alpha + \beta x_i. \tag{4.32}$$

Hence,

$$\log[\pi_1/(1 - \pi_1)] = \alpha + \beta x_1 = \alpha + \beta \text{ and} \tag{4.33}$$

$$\log\,[\pi_0/(1 - \pi_0)] = \alpha + \beta x_0 = \alpha.$$

Subtracting these two equations gives

$$\log[\pi_1/(1 - \pi_1)] - \log[\pi_0/(1 - \pi_0)] = \beta, \text{ and hence}$$

$$\log\left[\frac{\pi_1/(1 - \pi_1)}{\pi_0/(1 - \pi_0)}\right] = \log(\psi) = \beta. \tag{4.34}$$

Thus, the true odds ratio ψ equals e^β. We will use logistic regression to derive an estimate $\hat\beta$ of β. We then can estimate the odds ratio by $\hat\psi = e^{\hat\beta}$.

In the esophageal cancer and alcohol study $\hat\beta = 1.730$ and $\hat\psi = e^{1.730} = 5.64$. This is identical to the classical odds ratio estimate obtained in Section 4.19.2. The reader may wonder why we would go to the trouble of calculating $\hat\psi$ with logistic regression when the simple classical estimate gives the same answer. The answer is that we will be able to generalize logistic regression to adjust for multiple covariates; classical methods are much more limited in their ability to adjust for confounding variables or effect modifiers.

4.20.1. Nuisance Parameters

In equation (4.31) α is called a **nuisance parameter**. This is one that is required by the model but is not used to calculate interesting statistics.

4.20.2. 95% Confidence Interval for the Odds Ratio: Logistic Regression

Logistic regression also provides an estimate of the standard error of $\hat\beta$. We use this estimate to approximate the 95% confidence interval for the odds ratio in exactly the same way as for Woolf's confidence interval. That is,

$$(\hat\psi_L, \hat\psi_U) = (\exp[\hat\beta - 1.96 s_{\hat\beta}], \exp[\hat\beta + 1.96 s_{\hat\beta}]). \tag{4.35}$$

4.21. Creating a Stata Data File

Up until now we have used previously created data sets in our Stata examples. We next wish to analyze the data in Table 4.2. As this is a very small table, it provides a good opportunity to explain how to create a new Stata data set. We do this in the following example.

```
. * 4.21.EsophagealCa.log
. *
. * Create a Stata data set from the Ille-et-Vilaine data on esophageal
. * cancer and alcohol given in Table 4.2.
. *
. edit                                                              {1}

. list                                                              {2}

        var1      var2      var3
  1.       0         0       666
  2.       1         0       104
  3.       0         1       109
  4.       1         1        96

. rename var1 cancer                                                {3}

. rename var2 alcohol

. rename var3 patients

. label define yesno 0 "No" 1 "Yes"                                 {4}

. label values cancer yesno                                         {5}

. label define dose 0 "< 80g" 1 ">= 80g"

. label values alcohol dose

. list                                                              {6}

        cancer    alcohol   patients
  1.        No      < 80g        666
  2.       Yes      < 80g        104
  3.        No     >= 80g        109
  4.       Yes     >= 80g         96

. save C:\WDDtext\4.21.EsophagealCa.dta, replace                    {7}
```

Comments

1 Open the Stata Editor window. Enter three rows of values as shown in Figure 4.8. Then, exit the edit window by clicking the "×" in the upper

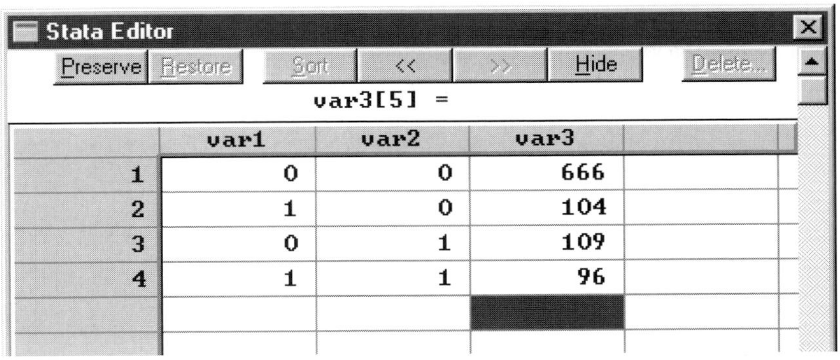

Figure 4.8

This figure shows the Stata Editor window after the data from Table 4.2 has been entered by hand.

right hand corner of the window. This creates three variables with the default names *var1*, *var2* and *var3*. There are four observations corresponding to the four cells in Table 4.2. The variable *var1* classifies the study subjects as either controls ($var1 = 0$) or cases ($var1 = 1$). Similarly, *var2* classifies subjects as either moderate ($var2 = 0$) or heavy ($var2 = 1$) drinkers. The variable *var3* gives the number of subjects in each of the four possible disease–exposure groups.

2 This *list* command shows the values that we have just entered. Without arguments, this command shows all observations on all variables.

3 This *rename* command changes the name of the first variable from *var1* to *cancer*. The Stata *Getting Started* manual also explains how to do this in the Stata Editor window.

4 The *cancer* variable takes the values 0 for controls and 1 for cases. It is often useful to associate labels with the numeric values of such classification variables. To do this we first define a value label called *yesno* that links 0 with "No" and 1 with "Yes".

5 We then use the *label values* command to link the variable *cancer* with the values label *yesno*. Multiple variables can be assigned to the same values label.

6 The *list* command now gives the value labels of the *cancer* and *alcohol* variables instead of their numeric values. The numeric values are still available for use in analysis commands.

7 This *save* command saves the data set that we have created in the *C:\WDDtext* folder with the name *4.21.EsophagealCa.dta*. If a file with the same name already exists in this folder, the *replace* option will replace the old file with the new version.

4.22. Analyzing Case-Control Data with Stata

The Ille-et-Vilaine data set introduced in Section 4.19 may be analyzed as follows:

```
. * 4.22.EsophagealCa.log
. *
. * Logistic regression analysis of 2x2 case-control data from
. * the Ille-et-Vilaine study of esophageal cancer and alcohol.
. *
. use C:\WDDtext\4.22.EsophagealCa.dta, clear
. cc cancer alcohol [freq=patients], woolf                                  {1}
```

```
                   | alcohol                           Proportion
                   | Exposed  Unexposed |   Total          Exposed
   ----------------+-------------------+----------------------------------
           Cases |     96        104  |    200            0.4800
        Controls |    109        666  |    775            0.1406
   ----------------+-------------------+----------------------------------
           Total |    205        770  |    975            0.2103
                   | Point estimate    |        [95% Conf. Interval]
                   +-------------------+----------------------------------
      Odds ratio |     5.640085      |  4.000589         7.951467  (Woolf){2}
   Attr. frac. ex. |    .8226977      |  .7500368         .8742371  (Woolf)
   Attr. frac. pop |    .3948949      |
                   +----------------------------------------------------------
                          chi2(1) = 110.26 Pr>chi2 = 0.0000              {3}
```

```
. logistic alcohol cancer [freq=patients]                                   {4}

  Logit estimates                          Number of obs    =      975
                                            LR chi2(1)       =    96.43
                                            Prob > chi2      =   0.0000
  Log likelihood = -453.2224                Pseudo R2        =   0.0962

  ---------------------------------------------------------------------------
  alcohol |  Odds Ratio    Std. Err.    z     P>|z|    [95% Conf. Interval]
  ---------+-----------------------------------------------------------------
   cancer |   5.640085    .9883491   9.872   0.000    4.000589   7.951467    {5}
  ---------------------------------------------------------------------------
```

Comments

1 This *cc* command performs a classical case-control analysis of the data in the 2×2 table defined by *cancer* and *alcohol*. The command qualifier [*freq = patients*] gives the number of patients who have the specified

values of *cancer* and *alcohol*. The *woolf* option specifies that the 95% confidence interval for the odds ratio is to be calculated using Woolf's method.

An alternative way of performing the same analysis would have been to create a data set with one record per patient. This would have given

666 records with *cancer* = 0 and *alcohol* = 0,

104 records with *cancer* = 1 and *alcohol* = 0,

109 records with *cancer* = 0 and *alcohol* = 1, and

96 records with *cancer* = 1 and *alcohol* = 1.

Then the command

```
cc cancer alcohol, woolf
```

would have given exactly the same results as those shown above.

2 The estimated odds ratio is $\hat{\psi} = 5.64$. Woolf's 95% confidence interval for $\hat{\psi}$ is (4.00, 7.95). These statistics agree with our hand calculations in Sections 4.19.2 and 4.19.3.

3 The test of the null hypothesis that $\psi = 1$ gives an uncorrected χ^2 statistic of 110.26. The *P* value associated with this statistic is (much) less than 0.000 05.

4 Regress *alcohol* against *cancer* using logistic regression. This command fits equation (4.31) to the data. We would also have got the same result if we had regressed *cancer* against *alcohol*.

5 The estimate of the odds ratio and its 95% confidence interval are identical to those obtained from the classical analysis. Recall that the logistic command outputs $\hat{\psi} = \exp[\hat{\beta}]$ rather than the parameter estimate $\hat{\beta}$ itself.

4.23. Regressing Disease Against Exposure

The simplest explanation of simple logistic regression is the one given above. Unfortunately, it does not generalize to multiple logistic regression where we are considering several risk factors at once. In order to make the next chapter easier to understand, let us return to simple logistic regression one more time.

Suppose we have a population who either are or are not exposed to some risk factor. Let π'_j denote the true probability of disease in exposed ($j = 1$) and unexposed ($j = 0$) people. We conduct a case-control study in which we select a representative sample of diseased (case) and healthy (control) subjects from the target population. That is, the selection is done in such a way that the probability that an individual is selected is unaffected by her exposure status. Let

n_j be the number of study subjects who are ($j = 1$) or are not ($j = 0$) exposed,

d_j be the number of cases who are ($j = 1$) or are not ($j = 0$) exposed,

$x_j = j$ denote exposure status, and

π_j be the probability that a study subject is a case given that she is ($j = 1$) or is not ($j = 0$) exposed.

Consider the logistic regression model

$$\text{logit}[E[d_j \mid x_j]/n_j] = \alpha + \beta x_j \quad : j = 0, 1. \tag{4.36}$$

This is a legitimate logistic regression model with $E[d_j \mid x_j]/n_j = \pi_j$. It can be shown, however, that equation (4.36) can be rewritten as

$$\text{logit}[\pi'_j] = \alpha' + \beta x_j \quad : j = 0, 1, \tag{4.37}$$

where α' is a different constant. But, by exactly the same argument that we used to derived equation (4.34) from equation (4.31), we can deduce from equation (4.37) that

$$\log\left[\frac{\pi'_1/(1 - \pi'_1)}{\pi'_0/(1 - \pi'_0)}\right] = \log(\psi) = \beta. \tag{4.38}$$

Hence, β also equals the log odds ratio for disease in exposed vs. unexposed members of the target population, and $\hat{\beta}$ from equation (4.36) estimates this log odds ratio. Thus, in building logistic regression models it makes sense to regress disease against exposure even though we have no estimate of the probability of disease in the underlying population.

In the next chapter we will not always distinguish between terms like π_j and π'_j. It is less awkward to talk about the probability of developing cancer given a set of covariates than to talk about the probability that a study subject with given covariates is also a case. This lack of precision is harmless as long as you remember that in a case-control study we cannot estimate the probability of disease given a patient's exposure status. Moreover, when estimates of π_j are used in formulas for odds ratios, they provide valid odds ratio estimates for the underlying population.

4.24. Additional Reading

McCullagh and Nelder (1989) is a standard, if rather mathematical, reference on Generalized Linear Models.

Breslow and Day (1980) is somewhat easier to read, although it is targeted at an audience with a solid statistical background. They provide an informative contrast between classical methods for case-control studies and logistic regression. This text also has an excellent and extensive discussion of the Ille-et-Vilaine data set that may be read in conjunction with the discussion in this and the next chapter. They provide the complete Ille-et-Vilaine data set in an appendix.

Fleiss (1981) provides a useful discussion of the analysis of rates and proportions.

Hennekens and Buring (1987) provide a good introduction to case-control studies.

Rothman and Greenland (1998) is a more advanced epidemiology text with a worthwhile discussion of case-control studies. This text also has a good discussion of likelihood ratio tests, score tests, and Wald tests.

Clayton and Hills (1993) provide an excellent discussion of the difference between likelihood ratio, score, and Wald tests that includes some helpful graphs.

Wald (1943) is the original reference on Wald tests and confidence intervals.

Yates (1934) is the original reference on the continuity correction for the chi-squared statistic for 2×2 tables.

Dupont and Plummer (1999) provide a brief review of the controversy surrounding continuity corrections in the statistical literature. They also provide a Stata program that calculates Yates' corrected chi-squared statistic for 2×2 tables.

Tuyns et al. (1977) studied the effect of alcohol and tobacco on the risk of esophageal cancer among men from the Ille-et-Vilaine district of France. We used their data to illustrate classical methods of analyzing case control studies as well as logistic regression.

4.25. Exercises

The following questions relate to the *4.ex.Sepsis.dta* data set from my web site, which you should download onto your computer. This data set contains information on patients from the Ibuprofen in Sepsis trial. Variables in this file include:

$$
treat = \begin{cases} 0: \text{if patient received placebo} \\ 1: \text{if patient received ibuprofen,} \end{cases}
$$

$$
death30d = \begin{cases} 0: \text{if patient was alive 30 days after entry into the study} \\ 1: \text{if patient was dead 30 days after entry,} \end{cases}
$$

$$
race = \begin{cases} 0: \text{if patient is white} \\ 1: \text{if patient is black,} \end{cases}
$$

apache = baseline APACHE score, and
id   = patient identification number.

1 Use logistic regression to estimate the probability of death in treated black patients as a function of baseline APACHE score. Do a similar regression for black patients on placebo. Plot these two curves on a single graph. How would you interpret these curves?

2 What is the odds ratio associated with a unit rise in APACHE score in untreated black patients? Give a 95% confidence interval for this odds ratio.

3 What is the estimated expected mortality for a black control patient with a baseline APACHE score of 10? Give the 95% confidence interval for this expected mortality. How many black control patients had a baseline APACHE score of 15 or less? What proportion of these patients died? Give a 95% confidence interval for this proportion.

5

Multiple Logistic Regression

Simple logistic regression generalizes to multiple logistic regression in the same way that simple linear regression generalizes to multiple linear regression. We regress a dichotomous response variable, such as survival, against several covariates. This allows us to either adjust for confounding variables or account for covariates that have a synergistic effect on the response variable. We can add interaction terms to our model in exactly the same way as in linear regression.

Before discussing multiple logistic regression we will first describe a traditional method for adjusting an odds ratio estimate for a confounding variable.

5.1. Mantel–Haenszel Estimate of an Age-Adjusted Odds Ratio

In Section 4.19.1 we introduced the Ille-et-Vilaine study of esophageal cancer and alcohol (Breslow and Day, 1980). Table 5.1 shows these data stratified by ten-year age groups. It is clear from this table that the incidence of esophageal cancer increases dramatically with age. There is also some evidence that the prevalence of heavy drinking also increases with age; the prevalence of heavy drinking among controls increases from 7.8% for men aged 25–30 to 17.3% for men aged 45–54. Thus, age may confound the alcohol–cancer relationship, and it makes sense to calculate an age-adjusted odds ratio for the effect of heavy drinking on esophageal cancer. Mantel and Haenszel (1959) proposed the following method for adjusting an odds ratio in the presence of a confounding variable.

Suppose that study subjects are subdivided into a number of strata by a confounding variable. Let

c_{ij} = the number of controls in the jth stratum who are ($i = 1$), or are not ($i = 0$), exposed (i.e. who are, or are not, heavy drinkers),

d_{ij} = the number of cases in the jth stratum who are ($i = 1$), or are not ($i = 0$), exposed,

$m_{0j} = c_{0j} + c_{1j}$ = the number of controls in the jth stratum,

Table 5.1. Ille-et-Vilaine data on alcohol consumption and esophageal cancer stratified by age (Breslow and Day, 1980).

Age	Cancer	Daily alcohol consumption ≥ 80g	<80g	Total	% ≥ 80g	Odds ratio $\hat{\psi}_j$
25–34	Yes	1	0	1	100.00%	.
	No	9	106	115	7.83%	
	Total	10	106	116	8.62%	
35–44	Yes	4	5	9	44.44%	5.046
	No	26	164	190	13.68%	
	Total	30	169	199	15.08%	
45–54	Yes	25	21	46	54.35%	5.665
	No	29	138	167	17.37%	
	Total	54	159	213	25.35%	
55–64	Yes	42	34	76	55.26%	6.359
	No	27	139	166	16.27%	
	Total	69	173	242	28.51%	
65–74	Yes	19	36	55	34.55%	2.580
	No	18	88	106	16.98%	
	Total	37	124	161	22.98%	
≥ 75	Yes	5	8	13	38.46%	.
	No	0	31	31	0.00%	
	Total	5	39	44	11.36%	
All ages	Yes	96	104	200	48.00%	5.64
	No	109	666	775	14.06%	
	Total	205	770	975	21.03%	

$m_{1j} = d_{0j} + d_{1j}$ = the number of cases in the jth stratum,

$n_{ij} = d_{ij} + c_{ij}$ = the number of subjects in the jth stratum who are ($i = 1$), or are not ($i = 0$), exposed,

$N_j = n_{0j} + n_{1j} = m_{0j} + m_{1j}$ = the number of subjects in the jth stratum,

$\hat{\psi}_j$ = the estimated odds ratio for members of the jth stratum,

$w_j = d_{0j}c_{1j}/N_j$, and

$W = \sum w_j$.

Then the Mantel–Haenszel estimate of the common odds ratio within these strata is

$$\hat{\psi}_{mh} = \sum \left(d_{1j}c_{0j}/N_j \right) / W. \tag{5.1}$$

If $\hat{\psi}_j$ is estimable for all strata, then equation (5.1) can be rewritten

$$\hat{\psi}_{mh} = \sum \hat{\psi}_j w_j / W. \tag{5.2}$$

This implies that $\hat{\psi}_{mh}$ is a weighted average of the odds ratio estimates within each strata. The weight w_j is approximately equal to the inverse of the variance of $\hat{\psi}_j$ when ψ is near one. Thus, equation (5.2) gives the greatest weight to those odds ratio estimates that are estimated with the greatest precision.

In the Ille-et-Vilaine data given in Table 5.1 there are six age strata. We apply equation (5.1) to these data to calculate the age-adjusted odds ratio for esophageal cancer in heavy drinkers compared to moderate drinkers. For example, in Strata 2 we have $w_2 = d_{02}c_{12}/N_2 = 5 \times 26/199 = 0.653$ and $d_{12}c_{02}/N_2 = 4 \times 164/199 = 3.296$. Performing similar calculations for the other strata and summing gives the $W = 11.331$ and $\hat{\psi}_{mh} = 5.158$. The unadjusted odds ratio for this table is 5.640 (see Section 4.19.2). Thus there is a suggestion that age may have a mild confounding effect on this odds ratio.

5.2. Mantel–Haenszel χ^2 Statistic for Multiple 2 × 2 Tables

Under the null hypothesis that the common odds ratio $\psi = 1$, the expected value of d_{1j} is

$$E[d_{1j} \mid \psi = 1] = n_{1j}m_{1j}/N_j \tag{5.3}$$

and the variance of d_{1j} is

$$\text{var}[d_{1j} \mid \psi = 1] = \frac{m_{0j}m_{1j}n_{0j}n_{1j}}{N_j^2(N_j - 1)}. \tag{5.4}$$

The Mantel–Haenszel test statistic for this null hypothesis is

$$\chi_1^2 = \left(\left| \sum d_{1j} - \sum E[d_{1j} \mid \psi = 1] \right| - 0.5 \right)^2 \bigg/ \sum \text{var}[d_{1j} \mid \psi = 1], \tag{5.5}$$

which has a χ^2 distribution with one degree of freedom (Mantel and Haenszel, 1959). In the Ille-et-Vilaine study $\sum d_{1j} = 96$, $\sum E[d_{1j} \mid \psi = 1] = 48.891$ and $\sum \text{var}[d_{1j} \mid \psi = 1] = 26.106$. Therefore $\chi_1^2 = (|96 - 48.891| - 0.5)^2/(26.106) = 83.21$. The P value associated with this statistic is $< 10^{19}$, providing overwhelming evidence that the observed association between heavy drinking and esophageal cancer is not due to chance.

In equation (5.5), the constant 0.5 that is subtracted from the numerator is a continuity correction that adjusts for the fact that we are approximating a discrete distribution with a continuous normal distribution (see Section 4.19.4). Without the continuity correction the χ^2 statistic equals 85.01.

5.3. 95% Confidence Interval for the Age-Adjusted Odds Ratio

Let $P_j = (d_{1j} + c_{0j})/N_j,$

$Q_j = (c_{1j} + d_{0j})/N_j,$

$R_j = d_{1j}c_{0j}/N_j,$ and

$S_j = c_{1j}d_{0j}/N_j.$

Then Robins et al. (1986) estimated the standard error of the log of $\hat{\psi}_{mh}$ to be

$$\text{se}[\log \hat{\psi}_{mh}] = \sqrt{\frac{\sum P_j R_j}{2(\sum R_j)^2} + \frac{\sum (P_j S_j + Q_j R_j)}{2 \sum R_j \sum S_j} + \frac{\sum Q_j S_j}{2(\sum S_j)^2}}. \quad (5.6)$$

Hence, a 95% confidence interval for the common within-stratum odds ratio ψ is

$$(\hat{\psi}_{mh} \exp[-1.96 \, \text{se}[\log \hat{\psi}_{mh}]], \, \hat{\psi}_{mh} \exp[1.96 \, \text{se}[\log \hat{\psi}_{mh}]]). \quad (5.7)$$

In the Ille-et-Vilaine study,

$$\sum R_j = 58.439, \sum S_j = 11.331, \sum P_j R_j = 43.848,$$

$$\sum (P_j S_j + Q_j R_j) = 22.843, \sum Q_j S_j = 3.079, \text{ and } \hat{\psi}_{mh} = 5.158.$$

Therefore,

$$\text{se}(\log \hat{\psi}_{mh}) = \sqrt{\frac{43.848}{2 \, (58.439)^2} + \frac{22.843}{2 \times 58.439 \times 11.331} + \frac{3.079}{2 \, (11.331)^2}}$$

$$= 0.189,$$

and a 95% confidence interval for the age-adjusted odds ratio ψ is $(5.158 \exp[-1.96 \times 0.189], 5.158 \exp[1.96 \times 0.189]) = (3.56, 7.47)$.

5.4. Breslow and Day's Test for Homogeneity

The derivation of the Mantel–Haenszel odds ratio assumes that there is a single true odds ratio for subjects from each stratum. Breslow and Day

Table 5.2. Observed and fitted values for the fifth stratum of the Ille-et-Vilaine data set. The fitted values are chosen so that the resulting odds ratio equals $\hat{\psi}_{mh} = 5.158$, and the total number of cases and controls and heavy and moderate drinkers equal the observed totals for this stratum. These calculations are needed for Breslow and Day's test for homogeneity of the common odds ratio (Breslow and Day, 1980).

Esophageal cancer	Daily alcohol consumption		Total
	$\geq 80g$	$<80g$	
Observed values			
Yes	$d_{15} = 19$	$d_{05} = 36$	$m_{15} = 55$
No	$c_{15} = 18$	$c_{05} = 88$	$m_{05} = 106$
Total	$n_{15} = 37$	$n_{05} = 124$	$N_5 = 161$
Fitted values			
Yes	$d_{15}[\hat{\psi}_{mh}] = 23.557$	$d_{05}[\hat{\psi}_{mh}] = 31.443$	$m_{15} = 55$
No	$c_{15}[\hat{\psi}_{mh}] = 13.443$	$c_{05}[\hat{\psi}_{mh}] = 92.557$	$m_{05} = 106$
Total	$n_{15} = 37$	$n_{05} = 124$	$N_5 = 161$

(1980) proposed the following test of this assumption. First, we find fitted values $c_{ij}[\hat{\psi}_{mh}]$ and $d_{ij}[\hat{\psi}_{mh}]$ for the jth stratum that give $\hat{\psi}_{mh}$ as the within-stratum odds ratio and which add up to the actual number of cases and controls and exposed and unexposed subjects for this stratum. For example, the top and bottom halves of Table 5.2 show the actual and fitted values for the fifth age stratum from the Ille-et-Vilaine study. Note that the fitted values have been chosen so that $(d_{15}[\hat{\psi}_{mh}]/d_{05}[\hat{\psi}_{mh}])/(c_{15}[\hat{\psi}_{mh}]/c_{05}[\hat{\psi}_{mh}]) = (23.557/31.443)/(13.443/92.557) = \hat{\psi}_{mh} = 5.158$ and the column and row totals for the fitted and observed values are identical. The fitted value $d_{1j}[\hat{\psi}_{mh}]$ is obtained by solving for x in the equation

$$\hat{\psi}_{mh} = \frac{(x/(m_{1j} - x))}{(n_{1j} - x)/(n_{0j} - m_{1j} + x)}. \tag{5.8}$$

We then set

$$c_{1j}[\hat{\psi}_{mh}] = n_{1j} - x, \; d_{0j}[\hat{\psi}_{mh}] = m_{1j} - x, \text{ and } c_{0j}[\hat{\psi}_{mh}] = n_{0j} - m_{1j} + x.$$

There is a unique solution to equation (5.8) for which $c_{ij}[\hat{\psi}_{mh}]$ and $d_{ij}[\hat{\psi}_{mh}]$ are non-negative.

The variance of d_{1j} given $\psi = \hat{\psi}_{mh}$ is

$$
\text{var}[d_{1j} \mid \hat{\psi}_{mh}] = \left(\frac{1}{c_{0j}[\hat{\psi}_{mh}]} + \frac{1}{d_{0j}[\hat{\psi}_{mh}]} + \frac{1}{c_{1j}[\hat{\psi}_{mh}]} + \frac{1}{d_{1j}[\hat{\psi}_{mh}]} \right)^{-1}.
$$

$$(5.9)$$

For example, in the fifth stratum

$$
\text{var}[d_{15} \mid \hat{\psi}_{mh} = 5.158] = \left(\frac{1}{92.557} + \frac{1}{31.443} + \frac{1}{13.443} + \frac{1}{23.557} \right)^{-1}
$$

$$
= 6.272.
$$

Let J be the number of strata. Then if the null hypothesis that $\psi_j = \psi$ for all strata is true, and the total study size is large relative to the number of strata,

$$
\chi^2_{J-1} = \sum \frac{(d_{1j} - d_{1j}[\hat{\psi}_{mh}])^2}{\text{var}[d_{1j} \mid \hat{\psi}_{mh}]} \tag{5.10}
$$

has a χ^2 distribution with $J-1$ degrees of freedom. This sum is performed over all strata. We reject the null hypothesis when χ^2_{J-1} is too large. For example, in the fifth stratum of the Ille-et-Vilaine study

$$
\frac{(d_{15} - d_{15}[\hat{\psi}_{mh}])^2}{\text{var}[d_{15} \mid \hat{\psi}_{mh}]} = \frac{(19 - 23.557)^2}{6.272} = 3.31.
$$

Summing this term with analogous terms from the other strata gives $\chi^2_5 = 9.32$. As there are six strata, $J = 5$. The probability that a χ^2 statistic with five degrees of freedom exceeds 9.32 is $P = 0.097$. Hence, although we cannot reject the null hypothesis of equal odds ratios across these strata, there is some evidence to suggest that the odds ratio may vary with age. In Table 5.1 these odds ratios are fairly similar for all strata except for age 65–74, where the odds ratio drops to 2.6. This may be due to chance, or perhaps, to a hardy survivor effect. You must use your judgment in deciding whether it is reasonable to report a single-age adjusted odds ratio in your own work.

5.5. Calculating the Mantel–Haenszel Odds Ratio using Stata

The *5.5.EsophagealCa.dta* data file contains the complete Ille-et-Vilaine data set published by Breslow and Day (1980). The following log file and comments illustrate how to use Stata to perform the calculations given above.

```
. * 5.5.EsophagealCa.log
. *
. * Calculate the Mantel-Haenszel age-adjusted odds ratio from
. * the Ille-et-Vilaine study of esophageal cancer and alcohol.
. *
. use C:\WDDtext\5.5.EsophagealCa.dta, clear
```

```
. table cancer heavy [freq=patients]                                {1}
------------+----------------------
            |     Heavy Alcohol
Esophagea   |      Consumption
l Cancer    |    <80 gm   >= 80 gm
------------+----------------------
        No  |      666        109
        Yes |      104         96
------------+----------------------
```

```
. table cancer heavy [freq=patients], by(age)                       {2}
------------+----------------------
Age         |
(years)     |
and         |     Heavy Alcohol
Esophagea   |      Consumption
l Cancer    |    <80 gm   >= 80 gm
------------+----------------------
25-34       |
        No  |      106          9
        Yes |                   1
------------+----------------------
35-44       |
        No  |      164         26
        Yes |        5          4
------------+----------------------
45-54       |
        No  |      138         29
        Yes |       21         25
------------+----------------------
55-64       |
        No  |      139         27
        Yes |       34         42
```

```
----------+------------------
65-74     |
      No  |      88          18
     Yes  |      36          19
----------+------------------
>= 75     |
      No  |      31
     Yes  |       8           5
----------+------------------
```

. cc *heavy cancer* [freq=*patients*], by(age)   {3}

```
      Age (years) |      OR      [95% Conf. Interval] M-H Weight
------------------+------------------------------------------------
          25-34 |        .          0           .            0   (exact)
          35-44 |  5.046154    .9268664    24.86538     .6532663   (exact)
          45-54 |  5.665025    2.632894    12.16536     2.859155   (exact)
          55-64 |  6.359477    3.299319    12.28473     3.793388   (exact)
          65-74 |  2.580247    1.131489     5.857261    4.024845   (exact)
          >= 75 |        .     2.761795           .            0   (exact)
------------------+------------------------------------------------
          Crude |  5.640085    3.937435     8.061794              (exact)  {4}
   M-H combined |  5.157623    3.562131     7.467743                        {5}
------------------+------------------------------------------------
```

Test of homogeneity (B-D)   chi2(5) =   9.32 Pr>chi2= 0.0968   {6}
                     Test that combined OR = 1:
                         Mantel-Haenszel chi2(1) =   85.01   {7}
                                       Pr>chi2 =   0.0000

Comments

1 This *table* command gives a cross tabulation of values of *heavy* by values of *cancer*. The 5.5.EsophagealCa.dta data set contains one record for each unique combination of the covariate values. The *patients* variable indicates the number of subjects in the study with these values. The [*freq=patients*] command qualifier tells Stata the number of subjects represented by each record. The variable *heavy* takes the numeric values 0 and 1, which denote daily alcohol consumption of <80 gm and ≥80 gm, respectively. The table shows the value labels that have been assigned to this variable rather than its underlying numeric values. Similarly, *cancer* takes the numeric values 0 and 1, which have been assigned the value labels *No* and *Yes*, respectively.

2 The *by(age)* option of the *table* command produces a separate table of

cancer by *heavy* for each distinct value of *age*. The *age* variable takes a different value for each stratum in the study, producing six subtables.

3 The *by(age)* option of the *cc* command causes odds ratios to be calculated for each age stratum. No estimate is given for the youngest strata because there were no moderate drinking cases. This results in division by zero when calculating the odds ratio. Similarly, no estimate is given for the oldest strata because there were no heavy drinking controls.

4 The crude odds ratio is 5.640, which we derived in the last chapter. This odds ratio is obtained by ignoring the age strata.

The exact 95% confidence interval consists of all values of the odds ratio that cannot be rejected at the $\alpha = 0.05$ level of statistical significance (see Section 1.4.7). The derivation of this interval uses a rather complex iterative formula (Dupont and Plummer, 1999).

5 The Mantel–Haenszel estimate of the common odds ratio within all age strata is 5.158. This is slightly lower than the crude estimate, and is consistent with a mild confounding of age and drinking habits on the risk of esophageal cancer (see Section 5.1). Stata uses the method of Robins et al. (1986) to estimate the 95% confidence interval for this common odds ratio, which is (3.56, 7.47).

6 Breslow and Day's test of homogeneity equals 9.32. This χ^2 statistic has five degrees of freedom giving a *P* value of 0.097.

7 We test the null hypothesis that the age-adjusted odds ratio equals 1. The Mantel–Haenszel test of this hypothesis equals 85.01. Stata calculates this statistic without the continuity correction. The associated *P* value is less than 0.00005.

5.6. Multiple Logistic Regression Model

The Mantel–Haenszel method works well when we have a single confounding variable that can be used to create fairly large strata. For a more general approach to modeling dichotomous response data we will need to use logistic regression.

Suppose that we observe an unbiased sample of *n* patients from some target population. Let

$$d_i = \begin{cases} 1: \text{if the } i^{\text{th}} \text{ patient suffers event of interest} \\ 0: \text{otherwise,} \end{cases}$$

and $x_{i1}, x_{i2}, \ldots, x_{iq}$ be *q* covariates that are measured on the ith patient. Let $\mathbf{x}_i = (x_{i1}, x_{i2}, \ldots, x_{iq})$ denote the values of all of the covariates for the ith patient. Then the multiple logistic regression model assumes that d_i has a Bernoulli distribution, and

$$\text{logit}\,[\text{E}\,[d_i \mid \mathbf{x}_i]] = \alpha + \beta_1 x_{i1} + \beta_2 x_{i2} + \cdots + \beta_q x_{iq}, \tag{5.11}$$

where

$\alpha, \beta_1, \beta_2, \ldots,$ and β_q are unknown parameters.

The probability that $d_i = 1$ given the covariates $\mathbf{x}_i$ is denoted $\pi\,[x_{i1}, x_{i2}, \ldots, x_{iq}] = \pi\,[\mathbf{x}_i]$ and equals $\text{E}\,[d_i \mid \mathbf{x}_i]$. The only difference between simple and multiple logistic regression is that the linear predictor is now $\alpha + \beta_1 x_{i1} + \beta_2 x_{i2} + \cdots + \beta_k x_{iq}$. As in simple logistic regression, the model has a logit link function and a Bernoulli random component.

The data may also be organized as one record per unique combination of covariate values. Suppose that there are n_j patients with identical covariate values $x_{j1}, x_{j2}, \ldots, x_{jq}$ and that d_j of these patients suffer the event of interest. Then the logistic regression model (5.11) can be rewritten

$$\text{logit}[\text{E}[d_j \mid \mathbf{x}_j]/n_j] = \alpha + \beta_1 x_{j1} + \beta_2 x_{j2} + \cdots + \beta_q x_{jq}. \tag{5.12}$$

(In equation (5.12) there is a different value of j for each distinct observed pattern of covariates while in equation (5.11) there is a separate value of i for each patient.) The statistic d_j is assumed to have a binomial distribution obtained from n_j independent dichotomous experiments with probability of success $\pi\,[x_{j1}, x_{j2}, \ldots, x_{jq}]$ on each experiment. Equation (5.12) implies that

$$\pi\,[x_{j1}, x_{j2}, \ldots, x_{jq}] = \frac{\exp[\alpha + \beta_1 x_{j1} + \beta_2 x_{j2} + \cdots + \beta_q x_{jq}]}{1 + \exp[\alpha + \beta_1 x_{j1} + \beta_2 x_{j2} + \cdots + \beta_q x_{jq}]}. \tag{5.13}$$

Choose any integer k between 1 and q. Suppose that we hold all of the covariates constant except x_{jk}, which we allow to vary. Then $\alpha' = \alpha + \beta_1 x_{j1} + \cdots + \beta_{k-1} x_{j,k-1} + \beta_{k+1} x_{j,k+1} + \cdots + \beta_q x_{jq}$ is a constant and equation (5.13) can be rewritten

$$\pi\,[x_{jk}] = \frac{\exp[\alpha' + \beta_k x_{jk}]}{1 + \exp[\alpha' + \beta_k x_{jk}]}, \tag{5.14}$$

which is the equation for a simple logistic regression model. This implies that β_k is the log odds ratio associated with a unit rise in x_{jk} while holding the values of all the other covariates constant (see Section 4.12). Thus, the β parameters in a multiple logistic regression model have an interpretation that is analogous to that for multiple linear regression. Each parameter equals the log odds ratio associated with a unit rise of its associated covariate adjusted for all of the other covariates in the model.

5.7. 95% Confidence Interval for an Adjusted Odds Ratio

Logistic regression provides maximum likelihood estimates of the model parameters in equation (5.11) or (5.12) together with estimates of their standard errors. Let $\hat{\beta}_k$ and se$[\hat{\beta}_k]$ denote the maximum likelihood estimate of β_k and its standard error, respectively. Then a 95% confidence interval for the odds ratio associated with a unit rise in x_{ik} adjusted for the other covariates in the model is

$$(\exp[\hat{\beta}_k - 1.96\mathrm{se}[\hat{\beta}_k]], \exp[\hat{\beta}_k + 1.96\mathrm{se}[\hat{\beta}_k]]). \tag{5.15}$$

5.8. Logistic Regression for Multiple 2 × 2 Contingency Tables

We will first consider a model that gives results that are similar to those of the Mantel–Haenszel method. Let us return to the Ille-et-Vilaine data from Section 5.1. Let d_{ij} and n_{ij} be defined as in Section 5.1 and let

J = the number of strata,

$$i = \begin{cases} 1: \text{for subjects who are heavy drinkers} \\ 0: \text{for those who are not,} \end{cases}$$

π_{ij} = the probability that a study subject from the jth age stratum has cancer given that he is $(i = 1)$, or is not $(i = 0)$, a heavy drinker, and α, β and α_j be model parameters.

Consider the logistic model

$$\mathrm{logit}[\mathrm{E}[d_{ij} \mid ij]/n_{ij}] = \begin{cases} \alpha + \beta \times i & : j = 1 \\ \alpha + \alpha_j + \beta \times i : j = 2, 3, \ldots, J, \end{cases} \tag{5.16}$$

where d_{ij} has a binomial distribution obtained from n_{ij} independent trials with success probability π_{ij} on each trial. For any age stratum j and drinking habit i $\mathrm{E}[d_{ij} \mid ij]/n_{ij} = \pi_{ij}$. For any $j > 1$,

$$\mathrm{logit}[\mathrm{E}[d_{0j} \mid i = 0, j]/n_{ij}] = \mathrm{logit}[\pi_{0j}] = \log[\pi_{0j}/(1 - \pi_{0j})] = \alpha + \alpha_j \tag{5.17}$$

is the log odds that a study subject from the jth stratum who is a moderate drinker will have cancer. Similarly,

$$\text{logit}[\,E[d_{1j} \mid i = 1, j]/n_{ij}] = \text{logit}[\pi_{1j}] = \log[\pi_{1j}/(1 - \pi_{1j})]$$

$$= \alpha + \alpha_j + \beta \tag{5.18}$$

is the log odds that a study subject from the jth stratum who is a heavy drinker will have cancer. Subtracting equation (5.17) from equation (5.18) gives us

$$\log[\pi_{j1}/(1 - \pi_{j1})] - \log[\pi_{j0}/(1 - \pi_{j0})] = \beta,$$

or

$$\log\left[\frac{\pi_{j1}/(1 - \pi_{j1})}{\pi_{j0}/(1 - \pi_{j0})}\right] = \log\psi = \beta. \tag{5.19}$$

A similar argument shows that equation (5.19) also holds when $j = 1$. Hence, this model implies that the odds ratio for esophageal cancer among heavy drinkers compared to moderate drinkers is the same in all strata and equals $\psi = \exp[\beta]$. Moreover, as explained in Section 4.23, ψ also equals this odds ratio for members of the target population.

In practice we fit model (5.16) by defining indicator covariates

$$age_j = \begin{cases} 1: \text{if subjects are from the } j^{th} \text{ age strata} \\ 0: \text{otherwise.} \end{cases}$$

Then (5.16) becomes

$$\text{logit}[\text{E}[d_{ij} \mid ij]/n_{ij}] = \alpha + \alpha_2 \times age_2 + \alpha_3 \times age_3 + \alpha_4 \times age_4$$

$$+ \alpha_5 \times age_5 + \alpha_6 \times age_6 + \beta \times i. \tag{5.20}$$

Note that this model places no restraints of the effect of age on the odds of cancer and only requires that the within-strata odds ratio be constant. For example, consider two study subjects from the first and j^{th} age strata who have similar drinking habits (i is the same for both men). Then the man from the jth stratum has log odds

$$\text{logit}[\,E(d_{ij} \mid ij)/n_{ij}] = \alpha + \alpha_j + \beta \times i, \tag{5.21}$$

while the man from the first age stratum has log odds

$$\text{logit}[\text{E}[d_{i1} \mid i, j = 1]/n_{i1}] = \alpha + \beta \times i. \tag{5.22}$$

Subtracting equation (5.22) from equation (5.21) gives that the log odds ratio for men with similar drinking habits from stratum j versus stratum 1 is α_j. Hence, each of strata 2 through 6 has a separate parameter that determines the odds ratio for men in that stratum relative to men with the same drinking habits from stratum 1.

An alternative model that we could have used is

$$\text{logit}[\text{E}[d_{ij} \mid ij]/n_{ij}] = \alpha \times j + \beta \times i. \tag{5.23}$$

However, this model imposes a linear relationship between age and the log odds for cancer. That is, the log odds ratio

for age stratum 2 vs. stratum 1 is $2\alpha - \alpha = \alpha$,
for age stratum 3 vs. stratum 1 is $3\alpha - \alpha = 2\alpha$, and
for age stratum 6 vs. stratum 1 is $6\alpha - \alpha = 5\alpha$.

As this linear relationship may not be valid, we are often better off using the more general model given by equation (5.20).

Performing the logistic regression defined by equation (5.20) gives $\hat{\beta} = 1.670$ with a standard error of $\text{se}[\hat{\beta}] = 0.1896$. Therefore, the age-adjusted estimate of the odds ratio for esophageal cancer in heavy drinkers compared to moderate drinkers is $\hat{\psi} = \exp[\hat{\beta}] = e^{1.670} = 5.31$. From equation (5.15) we have that the 95% confidence interval for ψ is $(\exp[1.670 - 1.96 \times 0.1896], \exp[1.670 + 1.96 \times 0.1896]) = (3.66, 7.70)$. The results of this logistic regression are similar to those obtained from the Mantel–Haenszel analysis. The age-adjusted odds ratio from this latter test was $\hat{\psi} = 5.16$ as compared to 5.31 from this logistic regression model.

5.9. Analyzing Multiple 2 × 2 Tables with Stata

The following log file and comments illustrate how to fit the logistic regression model (5.20) to the Ille-et-Vilaine data set.

```
. * 5.9.EsophagealCa.log
. *
. * Calculate age-adjusted odds ratio from the Ille-et-Vilaine study
. * of esophageal cancer and alcohol using logistic regression.
. *
. use C:\WDDtext\5.5.EsophagealCa.dta, clear
. *
. * First, define indicator variables for age strata 2 through 6
. *
. generate age2 = 0
. replace age2 = 1 if age == 2                                   {1}
(32 real changes made)
```

```
. generate age3 = 0

. replace age3 =1 if age == 3
(32 real changes made)

. generate age4 = 0

. replace age4 = 1 if age == 4
(32 real changes made)

. generate age5 = 0

. replace age5 = 1 if age == 5
(32 real changes made)

. generate age6 = 0

. replace age6 = 1 if age == 6
(32 real changes made)
```

. **logistic** *cancer age2 age3 age4 age5 age6 heavy* **[freq=***patients***]**   {2}

```
Logit estimates                             Number of obs   =       975
                                            LR chi2(6)      =    200.57
                                            Prob > chi2     =    0.0000
Log likelihood = -394.46094                 Pseudo R2       =    0.2027
```

cancer	Odds Ratio	Std. Err.	z	P>|z|	[95% Conf. Interval]	
age2	4.675303	4.983382	1.447	0.148	.5787862	37.76602 {3}
age3	24.50217	25.06914	3.126	0.002	3.298423	182.0131
age4	40.99664	41.75634	3.646	0.000	5.56895	301.8028
age5	52.81958	54.03823	3.877	0.000	7.111389	392.3155
age6	52.57232	55.99081	3.720	0.000	6.519386	423.9432
heavy	5.311584	1.007086	8.807	0.000	3.662981	7.702174 {4}

Comments

1 The numeric values of *age* are 1 through 6 and denote the age strata 25–34, 35–44, 45–54, 55–64, 65–74 and ≥ 75, respectively. We define *age2* = 1 for subjects from the second stratum and 0 otherwise; *age3* through *age6* are similarly defined for the other strata.

2 Regress *cancer* against *age2*, *age3*, *age4*, *age5*, *age6* and *heavy* using logistic regression. This command analyzes the model specified by equation (5.20). (See also Comment 1 from Section 5.5.)

3 The estimated cancer odds ratio for men from the second age stratum relative to men from the first with the same drinking habits is 4.68. This odds ratio equals $\exp[\hat{\alpha}_2]$. Note that the odds ratio rises steeply with increasing age until the fourth age stratum and then levels off. Hence, the model specified by equation (5.23) would do a poor job of modeling age for these data.

4 The age-adjusted estimated odds ratio for cancer in heavy drinkers relative to moderate drinkers is $\hat{\psi} = \exp[\hat{\beta}] = 5.312$. Hence, $\hat{\beta} = \log[5.312] = 1.670$. The logistic command does not give the value of $se[\hat{\beta}]$. However, the 95% confidence interval for $\hat{\psi}$ is (3.66, 7.70), which agrees with our hand calculations.

5.10. Handling Categorical Variables in Stata

In the Section 5.9 *age* is a categorical variable taking six values that are recoded as five separate indicator variables. It is very common to recode categorical variables in this way to avoid forcing a linear relationship on the effect of a variable on the response outcome. In the preceding example we did the recoding by hand. It can also be done much faster using the *xi:* command prefix. We illustrate this by repeating the preceding analysis of the model specified by equation (5.20).

```
. * 5.10.EsophagealCa.log
. *
. * Repeat the analysis in 5.9.EsophagealCa.log using
. * automatic recoding of the age classification variable
. *
. use C:\WDDtext\5.5.EsophagealCa.dta, clear
```

```
. xi: logistic cancer i.age heavy [freq=patients]                    {1}
i.age                    _Iage_1-6        (naturally coded; _Iage_1 omitted)
Logit estimates                           Number of obs   =      975
                                          LR chi2(6)      =   200.57
                                          Prob > chi2     =   0.0000
Log likelihood   = -394.46094             Pseudo R2       =   0.2027
```

cancer	Odds Ratio	Std. Err.	z	P>|z|	[95% Conf. Interval]	
_Iage_2	4.675303	4.983382	1.447	0.148	.5787862 37.76602	{2}
_Iage_3	24.50217	25.06914	3.126	0.002	3.298423 182.0131	

```
_Iage_4 |   40.99664    41.75634    3.646    0.000        5.56895    301.8028
_Iage_5 |   52.81958    54.03823    3.877    0.000       7.111389    392.3155
_Iage_6 |   52.57232    55.99081    3.720    0.000       6.519386    423.9432
  heavy |   5.311584    1.007086    8.807    0.000       3.662981    7.702174
```

Comments

1 The *xi:* prefix before an estimation command (like *logistic*) tells Stata that indicator variables will be created and used in the model; *i.age* indicates that a separate indicator variable is to be created for each distinct value of *age*. These variables are named *_Iage_1*, *_Iage_2*, *_Iage_3*, *_Iage_4*, *_Iage_5* and *_Iage_6*. Note that these variable names start with "*_I*". When specifying these variables they must be capitalized in exactly the same way they were defined. The variables *_Iage_2* through *_Iage_6* are identical to the variables *age2* through *age6* in Section 5.9. By default, the new variable associated with the smallest value of *age* (that is, *_Iage_1*) is deleted from the model. As a consequence, the model analyzed is that specified by equation (5.20).

2 Note that the output of this logistic regression analysis is identical to that in Section 5.9. The only difference is the names of the indicator variables that define the age strata.

5.11. Effect of Dose of Alcohol on Esophageal Cancer Risk

The Ille-et-Vilaine data set provides four different levels of daily alcohol consumption: 0–39 gm, 40–79 gm, 80–119 gm and $\geq$120 gm. To investigate the joint effects of dose of alcohol on esophageal cancer risk we analyze the model

$$\text{logit}[E[d_{ij} \mid ij]/n_{ij}] = \alpha + \sum_{h=2}^{6} \alpha_h \times age_h + \sum_{h=2}^{4} \beta_h \times alcohol_{ih}, \qquad (5.24)$$

where the terms are analogous to those in equation (5.20), only now

i denotes the drinking levels 1 through 4,
j denotes age strata 1 through 6, and

$$alcohol_{ih} = \begin{cases} 1\text{: if } i = h \\ 0\text{: otherwise.} \end{cases}$$

Deriving the age-adjusted cancer odds ratio for dose level *k* relative to dose level 1 is done using an argument similar to that given in Section 5.8. From equation (5.24) we have that the cancer log odds for a man at the first dose level is

$$\text{logit}[\,E(d_{1j} \mid i=1,\ j)/n_{1j}] = \log\left[\frac{\pi_{1j}}{1-\pi_{1j}}\right] = \alpha + \sum_{h=2}^{6} \alpha_h \times age_h$$

$$= \alpha + \alpha_j. \tag{5.25}$$

For a man from the same age stratum at the ith dose level, the log odds are

$$\log\left[\frac{\pi_{ij}}{1-\pi_{ij}}\right] = \alpha + \sum_{h=2}^{6} \alpha_h \times age_h + \sum_{h=2}^{4} \beta_h \times alcohol_{ih} = \alpha + \alpha_j + \beta_i. \tag{5.26}$$

Subtracting equation (5.25) from equation (5.26) gives that the age-adjusted log odds ratio for a man at the ith dose level relative to the first is

$$\log\left[\frac{\pi_{ij}/(1-\pi_{ij})}{\pi_{1j}/(1-\pi_{1j})}\right] = \log\left[\frac{\pi_{ij}}{1-\pi_{ij}}\right] - \log\left[\frac{\pi_{1j}}{1-\pi_{1j}}\right] = \beta_i. \tag{5.27}$$

Hence, the age-adjusted odds ratio for dose level i versus dose level 1 is $\exp[\beta_i]$. This model was used to estimate the odds ratios given in the top half of Table 5.3. For example, the odds ratio for the second dose level compared

Table 5.3. Effect of dose of alcohol and tobacco on the odds ratio for esophageal cancer in the Ille-et-Vilaine study. These odds ratios associated with alcohol are adjusted for age using the logistic regression model (5.24). A similar model is used for tobacco. The risk of esophageal cancer increases dramatically with increasing dose of both alcohol and tobacco.

Risk factor	Dose level i	Daily dose	Log odds ratio $\hat{\beta}_i$	Odds ratio $\hat{\psi}_i$	95% confidence interval for ψ_i	P value[†]
Alcohol						
	1	0–39 gm		1*		
	2	40–79 gm	1.4343	4.20	2.6–6.8	<0.0005
	3	80–119 gm	2.0071	7.44	4.3–13	<0.0005
	4	≥120 gm	3.6800	39.65	19–83	<0.0005
Tobacco						
	1	0–9 gm		1*		
	2	10–19 gm	0.6073	1.84	1.2–2.7	0.003
	3	20–29 gm	0.6653	1.95	1.2–3.2	0.008
	4	≥30 gm	1.7415	5.71	3.2–10	<0.0005

*Denominator (reference group) of following odds ratios
[†]Associated with the two-sided test of the null hypothesis that $\psi_i = 1$

to the first is $\exp[\hat{\beta}_2] = 4.20$. Clearly, the risk of esophageal cancer increases precipitously with increasing dose of alcohol.

5.11.1. Analyzing Model (5.24) with Stata

The following log file and comments explain how to analyze model (5.24) with Stata.

```
. * 5.11.1.EsophagealCa.log
. *
. * Estimate age-adjusted risk of esophageal cancer due to dose of alcohol.
. *
. use C:\WDDtext\5.5.EsophagealCa.dta, clear
. *
. * Show frequency tables of effect of dose of alcohol on esophageal cancer.
. *
. tabulate cancer alcohol [freq=patients], column                            {1}
```

```
Esophageal  |                Alcohol (gm/day)
   Cancer   |     0-39      40-79    80-119     >= 120   |     Total
------------+--------------------------------------------+----------
       No   |      386        280        87         22   |       775
            |    93.01      78.87     63.04      32.84   |     79.49
------------+--------------------------------------------+----------
      Yes   |       29         75        51         45   |       200
            |     6.99      23.13     36.96      67.16   |     20.51
------------+--------------------------------------------+----------
    Total   |      415        355       138         67   |       975
            |   100.00     100.00    100.00     100.00   |    100.00
```

```
. *
. * Analyze the Ille-et-Vilaine data using logistic regression model (5.24)
. *
. xi: logistic cancer i. age i. alcohol [freq=patients]
i.age       _Iage_1_6               (naturally coded; _Iage_1 omitted)
i.alcohol   _Ialcohol_1-4           (naturally coded; _Ialcohol_1 omitted)
Logit estimates                               Number of obs  =   975
                                              LR chi2(8)     = 274.07
                                              Prob > chi2    = 0.0000
Log likelihood = -363.70808                   Pseudo R2      = 0.2649
```

cancer	Odds Ratio	Std. Err.	z	P>|z|	[95% Conf.	Interval]	
_Iage_2	5.109602	5.518316	1.51	0.131	.6153163	42.43026	
_Iage_3	30.74859	31.9451	3.30	0.001	4.013298	235.5858	
_Iage_4	51.59663	53.38175	3.81	0.000	6.791573	391.9876	
_Iage_5	78.00528	81.22778	4.18	0.000	10.13347	600.4678	
_Iage_6	83.44844	91.07367	4.05	0.000	9.827359	708.5975	
_Ialcohol_2	4.196747	1.027304	5.86	0.000	2.597472	6.780704	{2}
_Ialcohol_3	7.441782	2.065952	7.23	0.000	4.318873	12.82282	
_Ialcohol_4	39.64689	14.92059	9.78	0.000	18.9614	82.8987	

Comments

1 The *tabulate* command produces one- and two-way frequency tables. The variable *alcohol* gives the dose level. The numeric values of this variable are 1, 2, 3, and 4. The *column* option expresses the number of observations in each cell as a percentage of the total number of observations in the associated column.

  It is always a good idea to produce such tables as a cross-check of the results of our regression analyses. Note that the proportion of cancer cases increase dramatically with increasing dose.

2 The indicator variables *_Ialcohol_2*, *_Ialcohol_3* and *_Ialcohol_4* are the covariates $alcohol_{i2}$, $alcohol_{i3}$ and $alcohol_{i4}$ in model (5.24). The shaded odds ratios and confidence intervals that are associated with these covariates are also given in Table 5.3.

5.12. Effect of Dose of Tobacco on Esophageal Cancer Risk

The Ille-et-Vilaine data set also provides four different levels of daily tobacco consumption: 0–9 gm, 10–19 gm, 20–29 gm and ≥30 gm. This risk factor is modeled in exactly the same way as alcohol. The log file named *5.12.EsophagealCa.log* on my web site illustrates how to perform this analysis in Stata. The bottom panel of Table 5.3 shows the effect of increasing tobacco dose on esophageal cancer risk. This risk increases significantly with increasing dose. Note, however, that the odds ratios associated with 10–19 gm and 20–29 gm are very similar. For this reason, it makes sense to combine subjects with these two levels of tobacco consumption into a single group. In subsequent models, we will recode tobacco dosage to permit tobacco to be modeled with two parameters rather than three. In general, it is a good idea to avoid having unnecessary parameters in our models as this reduces their statistical power.

5.13. Deriving Odds Ratios from Multiple Parameters

Model (5.24) also permits us to calculate the age-adjusted odds ratio for, say, alcohol dose level 4 relative to dose level 3. From equation (5.26) we have that the log odds of cancer for two men from the jth age stratum who are at dose levels 3 and 4 are

$$\log\left[\frac{\pi_{3j}}{1 - \pi_{3j}}\right] = \alpha + \alpha_j + \beta_3$$

and

$$\log\left[\frac{\pi_{4j}}{1 - \pi_{4j}}\right] = \alpha + \alpha_j + \beta_4.$$

Subtracting the first of these log odds from the second gives that the cancer log odds ratio for men at dose level 4 relative to dose level 3 is

$$\log\left[\frac{\pi_{4j}/(1 - \pi_{4j})}{\pi_{3j}/(1 - \pi_{3j})}\right] = \log\left[\frac{\pi_{4j}}{1 - \pi_{4j}}\right] - \log\left[\frac{\pi_{3j}}{1 - \pi_{3j}}\right] = \beta_4 - \beta_3,$$

and the corresponding odds ratio is $\exp[\beta_4 - \beta_3]$.

In more complex multiple logistic regression models we often need to make inferences about odds ratios that are estimated from multiple parameters. The preceding is a simple example of such an odds ratio. To derive confidence intervals and perform hypothesis tests on these odds ratios we need to be able to compute the standard errors of weighted sums of parameter estimates.

5.14. The Standard Error of a Weighted Sum of Regression Coefficients

Suppose that we have a model with q parameters $\beta_1, \beta_2, \ldots, \beta_q$. Let

$\hat{\beta}_1, \hat{\beta}2, \ldots, \hat{\beta}_q$ be estimates of these parameters,

$c_1, c_2, \ldots, c_q$ be a set of known weights,

$f = \sum c_j \beta_j$ be the weighted sum of the coefficients that equals some log odds ratio of interest, and

$\hat{f} = \sum c_j \hat{\beta}_j$ be an estimate of f.   (5.28)

For example, in model (5.24) there is the constant parameter α, the five age parameters $\alpha_2, \alpha_3, \ldots, \alpha_6$, and the three alcohol parameters β_2, β_3, and β_4, giving a total of $q = 9$ parameters. Let us reassign $\alpha, \alpha_2, \alpha_3, \alpha_4, \alpha_5$ and α_6 with the names $\beta_1, \beta_5, \beta_6, \beta_7, \beta_8$ and β_9. Let $c_4 = 1$, $c_3 = -1$, and $c_1 = c_2 = c_5 = c_6 = c_7 = c_8 = c_9 = 0$. Then $\hat{f} = \hat{\beta}_4 - \hat{\beta}_3$. From Table 5.3 we have that $\hat{\beta}_4 = 3.6800$ and $\hat{\beta}_3 = 2.0071$. Therefore, $\hat{f} = 3.6800 - 2.0071 = 1.6729$ and $\exp[\hat{f}] = \exp[1.6729] = 5.33$ is the estimated odds ratio of level 4 drinkers relative to level 3 drinkers. Let

s_{jj} be the estimated variance of $\hat{\beta}_j$ for $j = 1, \ldots, q$, and
s_{ij} be the estimated covariance of $\hat{\beta}_i$ and $\hat{\beta}_j$ for any $i \neq j$.

Then it can be shown that the variance of $\hat{f}$ may be estimated by

$$s_f^2 = \sum_{i=1}^{q} \sum_{j=1}^{q} c_i c_j s_{ij}. \tag{5.29}$$

5.15. Confidence Intervals for Weighted Sums of Coefficients

The estimated standard error of $\hat{f}$ is s_f. For large studies the 95% confidence interval for f is approximated by

$$\hat{f} \pm 1.96 s_f. \tag{5.30}$$

A 95% confidence interval for the odds ratio $\exp[f]$ is given by

$$(\exp[\hat{f} - 1.96 s_f], \exp[\hat{f} + 1.96 s_f]). \tag{5.31}$$

Equation (5.31) is an example of a Wald confidence interval (see Section 4.9.4).

In our example comparing level 4 drinkers to level 3 drinkers, our logistic regression program estimates $s_{33} = 0.07707$, $s_{34} = s_{43} = 0.04224$, and $s_{44} = 0.14163$. Hence, $s_f^2 = (-1)^2 s_{33} + (-1) \times 1 \times s_{34} + 1 \times (-1) s_{43} + 1^2 s_{44} = 0.07707 - 2 \times 0.04224 + 0.14163 = 0.13422$, which gives $s_f = 0.3664$. This is the standard error of the log odds ratio for level 4 drinking compared to level 3. Equation (5.31) gives the 95% confidence interval for this odds ratio to be $(\exp[1.6729 - 1.96 \times 0.3664], \exp[1.6729 + 1.96 \times 0.3664]) = (2.60, 10.9)$. Fortunately, Stata has a powerful post estimation command called *lincom*, which rarely makes it necessary for us to calculate equations (5.29) or (5.31) explicitly.

5.16. Hypothesis Tests for Weighted Sums of Coefficients

For large studies

$$z = \hat{f}/s_f \tag{5.32}$$

has an approximately standard normal distribution. Equation (5.32) is an example of a Wald test (see Section 4.9.4). We use this statistic to test the null hypothesis that $f = \sum c_j \beta_j = 0$, or equivalently, that $\exp[f] = 1$. For example, to test the null hypothesis that $\beta_4 - \beta_3 = 0$ we calculate $z = (1.6729/0.3664) = 4.57$. The P value associated with a two-sided test of this null hypothesis is $P = 0.000\ 005$. Note that this null hypothesis is equivalent to the hypothesis that $\exp[\beta_4 - \beta_3] = 1$ (i.e., that the odds ratio for level 4 drinkers relative to level 3 equals 1). Hence, we can reject the hypothesis that these two consumption levels are associated with equivalent cancer risks with overwhelming statistical significance.

5.17. The Estimated Variance–Covariance Matrix

The estimates of s_{ij} can be written in a square array

$$\begin{bmatrix} s_{11} & s_{12} & \cdots & s_{1q} \\ s_{21} & s_{22} & \cdots & s_{2q} \\ \vdots & \vdots & \ddots & \vdots \\ s_{q1} & s_{q2} & \cdots & s_{qq} \end{bmatrix},$$

which is called the estimated variance–covariance matrix. For any two variables x and y the covariance of x with y equals the covariance of y with x. Hence, $s_{ij} = s_{ji}$ for any i and j between 1 and q, and the variance–covariance matrix is symmetric about the main diagonal that runs from s_{11} to s_{qq}. For this reason it is common to display this matrix in the lower triangular form

$$\begin{bmatrix} s_{11} & & & \\ s_{21} & s_{22} & & \\ \vdots & \vdots & \ddots & \\ s_{q1} & s_{q2} & \cdots & s_{qq} \end{bmatrix}.$$

The Stata *vce* post estimation command introduced in Section 4.18 uses this format to display the variance–covariance matrix. We use this command whenever we wish to print the variance and covariance estimates for the parameters from our regression models.

5.18. Multiplicative Models of Two Risk Factors

Suppose that subjects either were or were not exposed to alcohol and tobacco and we do not adjust for age. Consider the model

$$\text{logit}[\text{E}[d_{ij} \mid ij]/n_{ij}] = \text{logit}[\pi_{ij}] = \alpha + \beta_1 \times i + \beta_2 \times j, \tag{5.33}$$

where $i = \begin{cases} 1: \text{if subject drank} \\ 0: \text{otherwise}, \end{cases}$

$j = \begin{cases} 1: \text{if subject smoked} \\ 0: \text{otherwise}, \end{cases}$

n_{ij} = the number of subjects with drinking status i and smoking status j,
d_{ij} = the number of cancer cases with drinking status i and smoking status j,
π_{ij} = the probability that someone with drinking status i and smoking status j develops cancer,

and α, β_1 and β_2 are model parameters.

Then the cancer log odds of a drinker with smoking status j is

$$\text{logit}[\text{E}[d_{1j} \mid i = 1, j]/n_{1j}] = \text{logit}[\pi_{1j}] = \alpha + \beta_1 + \beta_2 \times j. \tag{5.34}$$

The log-odds of a non-drinker with smoking status j is

$$\text{logit}[\text{E}[d_{0j} \mid i = 0, j]/n_{0j}] = \text{logit}[\pi_{0j}] = \alpha + \beta_2 \times j, \tag{5.35}$$

Subtracting equation (5.35) from (5.34) gives

$$\log\left[\frac{\pi_{1j}/(1-\pi_{1j})}{\pi_{0j}/(1-\pi_{0j})}\right] = \beta_1.$$

In other words, $\exp[\beta_1]$ is the cancer odds ratio in drinkers compared to non-drinkers adjusted for smoking. Note that this implies that the relative risk of drinking is the same in smokers and non-smokers. By an identical argument, $\exp[\beta_2]$ is the odds ratio for cancer in smokers compared to non-smokers adjusted for drinking.

For people who both drink and smoke the model is

$$\text{logit}[\text{E}[d_{11} \mid i = 1, j = 1]/n_{11}] = \text{logit}[\pi_{11}] = \alpha + \beta_1 + \beta_2, \tag{5.36}$$

while for people who neither drink nor smoke it is

$$\text{logit}[\text{E}[d_{00} \mid i = 0, j = 0]/n_{00}] = \text{logit}[\pi_{00}] = \alpha. \tag{5.37}$$

Subtracting equation (5.37) from (5.36) gives that the log odds ratio for people who both smoke and drink relative to those who do neither is $\beta_1 + \beta_2$. The corresponding odds ratio is $\exp[\beta_1 + \beta_2] = \exp[\beta_1] \times \exp[\beta_2]$. Thus, our model implies that the odds ratio of having both risk factors equals the product of the individual odds ratios for drinking and smoking. It is for this reason that this is called a **multiplicative model**.

5.19. Multiplicative Model of Smoking, Alcohol, and Esophageal Cancer

The multiplicative assumption is a very strong one that is often not justified. Let us see how it works with the Ille-et-Vilaine data set. The model that we will use is

$$\text{logit}[\text{E}[d_{ijk} \mid ijk]/n_{ijk}] = \alpha + \sum_{h=2}^{6} \alpha_h \times age_h + \sum_{h=2}^{4} \beta_h \times alcohol_{ih}$$

$$+ \sum_{h=2}^{3} \gamma_h \times smoke_{kh}, \tag{5.38}$$

where

i	is one of four dose levels of alcohol,
k	is one of three dose levels of tobacco,
n_{ijk}	is the number of subjects from the jth age stratum who are at the ith dose level of alcohol and the kth dose level of tobacco,
d_{ijk}	is the number of cancer cases from the jth age stratum who are at the ith dose level of alcohol and the kth dose level of tobacco,

α, α_h, age_h, β_h, and $alcohol_{ih}$ are as defined in equation (5.24),

γ_h is a parameter associated with the hth dose level of tobacco, and

$$smoke_{kh} = \begin{cases} 1: \text{if } k = h \\ 0: \text{otherwise.} \end{cases}$$

In Table 5.3 we found that the middle two levels of tobacco consumption were associated with similar risks of esophageal cancer. In this model we combine these levels into one; dose levels $k = 1$, 2, and 3 correspond to daily consumption levels 0–9 gm, 10–29 gm, and $\geq$30 gm, respectively.

Let ψ_{ik} be the odds ratio for men at alcohol dose level i and tobacco dose level k relative to men at level 1 for both drugs. Then for $i > 1$ and $j > 1$ we have by the same argument used in Section 5.18 that

$$\psi_{i1} = \exp[\beta_i],$$

Table 5.4. Effect of alcohol and tobacco on the risk of esophageal cancer in the Ille-et-Vilaine study. These estimates are based on the multiplicative model (5.38). This model requires that the odds ratio associated with the joint effects of alcohol and tobacco equal the product of the odds ratios for the individual effects of these risk factors.

| | Daily tobacco consumption | | | | | |
| | 0–9 gm | | 10–29 gm | | ≥ 30 gm | |
Daily alcohol consumption	Odds ratio	95% confidence interval	Odds ratio	95% confidence interval	Odds ratio	95% confidence interval
0–39 gm	1.0*		1.59	(1.1–2.4)	5.16	(2.6–10)
40–79 gm	4.21	(2.6–6.9)	6.71	(3.6–12)	21.7	(9.2–51)
80–119 gm	7.22	(4.1–13)	11.5	(5.9–22)	37.3	(15–91)
≥120 gm	36.8	(17–78)	58.6	(25–140)	190	(67–540)

*Denominator of odds ratios

$\psi_{1k} = \exp[\gamma_k]$, and

$\psi_{ik} = \exp[\beta_i] \times \exp[\gamma_k]$.

Solving model (5.38) yields maximum likelihood parameter estimates $\hat{\beta}_i$ and $\hat{\gamma}_k$, which can be used to generate Table 5.4 using the preceding formulas. For example, $\hat{\beta}_4 = 3.6053$ and $\hat{\gamma}_3 = 1.6408$. Therefore, $\hat{\psi}_{41} = \exp[3.6053] = 36.79$, $\hat{\psi}_{13} = \exp[1.6408] = 5.16$, and $\hat{\psi}_{43} = 36.79 \times 5.16 = 189.8$. The confidence intervals in this table are derived using equation (5.31).

If model (5.38) is to be believed, then the risk of esophageal cancer associated with the highest levels of alcohol and tobacco consumption are extraordinary. There is no biologic reason, however, why the odds ratio associated with the combined effects of two risk factors should equal the product of the odds ratios for the individual risk factors. Indeed, the joint risk is usually less than the product of the individual risks. To investigate whether this is the case here we will need to analyze a more general model. We will do this in Section 5.22.

5.20. Fitting a Multiplicative Model with Stata

In the following Stata log file we first combine subjects at smoking levels 2 and 3 into a single group. We then fit the age-adjusted multiplicative model (5.38) to estimate the effect of dose of alcohol and tobacco on the risk of esophageal cancer.

```
. * 5.20.EsophagealCa.log
. *
. * Regress esophageal cancers against age and dose of alcohol
. * and tobacco using a multiplicative model.
. *
. use C:\WDDtext\5.5.EsophagealCa.dta,clear

. *
. * Combine tobacco levels 2 and 3 in a new variable called smoke
. *
. generate smoke = tobacco
. recode smoke 3=2 4=3                                             {1}
(96 changes made)
. label variable smoke "Smoking (gm/day)"
. label define smoke 1 "0-9" 2 "10-29" 3 ">= 30"
. label values smoke smoke
. table smoke tobacco [freq=patients], row col                    {2}


----------+----------------------------------
 Smoking  |          Tobacco (gm/day)
 (gm/day) |   0-9   10-19   20-29   >= 30  Total
----------+----------------------------------
     0-9  |   525                           525
   10-29  |         236     132             368
   >= 30  |                          82      82
          |
   Total  |   525   236     132      82     975
----------+----------------------------------

. *
. * Regress cancer against age, alcohol and smoke
. * using a multiplicative model
. *
. xi: logistic cancer i.age i.alcohol i.smoke [freq=patients]     {3}
i.age          _Iage_ 1-6          (naturally coded; _Iage_1 omitted)
i.alcohol      _Ialcohol_1-4       (naturally coded; _Ialcohol_1 omitted)
i.smoke        _Ismoke_1-3         (naturally coded; _Ismoke_1 omitted)

Logit estimates                    Number of obs =        975
                                   LR chi2(10)   =     285.55
                                   Prob > chi2   =     0.0000
```

```
Log likelihood =  − 351.96823                    Pseudo R2 = 0.2886          {4}
```

cancer	Odds Ratio	Std. Err.	z	P>|z|	[95% Conf.	Interval]	
_Iage_2	7.262526	8.017364	1.796	0.072	.8344795	63.2062	
_Iage_3	43.65627	46.6239	3.536	0.000	5.382485	354.0873	
_Iage_4	76.3655	81.32909	4.071	0.000	9.470422	615.7792	
_Iage_5	133.7632	143.9718	4.549	0.000	16.22455	1102.81	
_Iage_6	124.4262	139.5027	4.302	0.000	13.82203	1120.088	
_Ialcohol_2	4.213304	1.05191	5.761	0.000	2.582905	6.872853	{5}
_Ialcohol_3	7.222005	2.053956	6.952	0.000	4.135937	12.61077	
_Ialcohol_4	36.7912	14.1701	9.361	0.000	17.29435	78.26787	
_Ismoke_2	1.592701	.3200883	2.316	0.021	1.074154	2.361576	
_Ismoke_3	5.159309	1.775205	4.769	0.000	2.628523	10.12678	

. **lincom** _Ialcohol_2 + _Ismoke_2, **or**   {See comment 6 below}

(1)   _Ialcohol_2 + _Ismoke_2 = 0.0

cancer	Odds Ratio	Std. Err.	z	P>|z|	[95% Conf.	Interval]
(1)	6.710535	2.110331	6.053	0.000	3.623022	12.4292

. **lincom** _Ialcohol_ 3 + _Ismoke_ 2, **or**

(1) _Ialcohol_3 + _Ismoke_2 = 0.0

cancer	Odds Ratio	Std. Err.	z	P>|z|	[95% Conf.	Interval]
(1)	11.5025	3.877641	7.246	0.000	5.940747	22.27118

. **lincom** _Ialcohol_4 + _Ismoke_2, **or**

(1) _Ialcohol_4 + _Ismoke_2 = 0.0

cancer	Odds Ratio	Std. Err.	z	P>|z|	[95% Conf.	Interval]
(1)	58.59739	25.19568	9.467	0.000	25.22777	136.1061

```
. lincom _Ialcohol_2 + _Ismoke_3, or

(1) _Ialcohol_2 + _Ismoke_3 = 0.0

------------------------------------------------------------------------
   cancer |  Odds Ratio   Std. Err.     z     P>|z|     [95% Conf. Interval]
----------+-------------------------------------------------------------
      (1) |    21.73774    9.508636   7.039   0.000    9.223106     51.23319
------------------------------------------------------------------------

. lincom _Ialcohol_3 + _Ismoke_3, or

(1) _Ialcohol_3 + _Ismoke_3 = 0.0

------------------------------------------------------------------------
   cancer |  Odds Ratio   Std. Err.     z     P>|z|     [95% Conf. Interval]
----------+-------------------------------------------------------------
      (1) |    37.26056   17.06685   7.899   0.000    15.18324     91.43957
------------------------------------------------------------------------

. lincom _Ialcohol_4 + _Ismoke_3, or                                    {6}

(1) _Ialcohol_4 + _Ismoke_3 = 0.0

------------------------------------------------------------------------
   cancer |  Odds Ratio   Std. Err.     z     P>|z|     [95% Conf. Interval]
----------+-------------------------------------------------------------
      (1) |   189.8171   100.9788   9.861   0.000    66.91353    538.4643
------------------------------------------------------------------------
```

Comments

1 We want to combine the 2nd and 3rd levels of tobacco exposure. We do this by defining a new variable called *smoke* that is identical to *tobacco* and then using the *recode* statement, which, in this example, changes values of *smoke* = 3 to *smoke* = 2, and values of *smoke* = 4 to *smoke* = 3.

2 This table statement gives a cross tabulation of values of *smoke* by values of *tobacco*. The *row* and *col* options specify that row and column totals are to be given. The resulting table shows that the previous *recode* statement had the desired effect.

3 This statement performs the logistic regression specified by model (5.38).

4 The maximum value of the log likelihood function is $-351.968\,23$. We will discuss this statistic in Section 5.24.

5 The highlighted odds ratios and confidence intervals are also given in Table 5.4. For example, _Ialcohol_4 and _Ismoke_3 are the covariates $alcohol_{i4}$ and $smoke_{k3}$, respectively, in model (5.38). The associated parameter estimates are $\hat{\beta}_4$ and $\hat{\gamma}_3$, which give odds ratio estimates

$\hat{\psi}_{41} = \exp[\hat{\beta}_4] = 36.7912$ and $\hat{\psi}_{13} = \exp[\hat{\gamma}_3] = 5.159\,309$. Hence $\hat{\beta}_4 = \log[36.7912] = 3.6053$, and $\hat{\gamma}_3 = \log[5.159\,309] = 1.6408$. The 95% confidence intervals for these odds ratios are calculated using equation (5.15).

6 The *lincom* post estimation command calculates any linear combination of parameter estimates, tests the null hypothesis that the true value of this combination equals zero, and gives a 95% confidence interval for this estimate. In this example, the parameters associated with _Ialcohol_4 and _Ismoke_3 are $\hat{\beta}_4$ and $\hat{\gamma}_3$, respectively, and the linear combination is $\hat{\beta}_4 + \hat{\gamma}_3$. When the *or* option is given, *lincom* exponentiates this sum in its output, giving the odds ratio $\hat{\psi}_{43} = \exp[\hat{\beta}_4 + \hat{\gamma}_3] = \exp[3.6053 + 1.6408] = 189.8$. The 95% confidence interval for $\hat{\psi}_{43}$ is (66.9–538). This interval is calculated using equation (5.31). The weights in equation (5.28) are 1 for $\hat{\beta}_4$ and $\hat{\gamma}_3$ and 0 for the other parameters in the model. Thus, the cancer odds ratio for men who consume more than 119 gm of alcohol and 29 gm of tobacco a day is 189.8 relative to men whose daily consumption is less than 40 gm of alcohol and 10 gm of tobacco. The test of the null hypothesis that this odds ratio equals 1 is done using the z statistic given in equation (5.32). This hypothesis is rejected with overwhelming statistical significance.

The results of this *lincom* command together with the other *lincom* commands given above are used to complete Table 5.4.

5.21. Model of Two Risk Factors with Interaction

Let us first return to the simple model of Section 5.18 where people either do, or do not, drink or smoke and where we do not adjust for age. Our multiplicative model was

$$\text{logit}[E[d_{ij} \mid ij]/n_{ij}] = \log\left[\frac{\pi_{ij}}{1 - \pi_{ij}}\right] = \alpha + \beta_1 \times i + \beta_2 \times j,$$

where

$i \quad = 1$ or 0 for people who do, or do not, drink,
$j \quad = 1$ or 0 for people who do, or do not, smoke, and
$\pi_{ij} =$ the probability that someone with drinking status i and smoking status j develops cancer.

We next allow alcohol and tobacco to have a synergistic effect on cancer odds by including a fourth parameter as follows:

$$\text{logit}[E[d_{ij} \mid ij]/n_{ij}] = \alpha + \beta_1 \times i + \beta_2 \times j + \beta_3 \times i \times j. \tag{5.39}$$

Note that β_3 only enters the model for people who both smoke and drink since for everyone else $i \times j = 0$. Under this model, subjects can be divided into four categories determined by whether they do, or do not, drink and whether they do, or do not, smoke. We can derive the cancer odds ratio associated with any one of these categories relative to any other by the type of argument that we have used in the preceding sections. Specifically, we write down the log odds for people in the numerator of the odds ratio, write down the log odds for people in the denominator of the odds ratio, and then subtract the denominator log odds from the numerator log odds. This gives us the desired log odds ratio. You should be able to show that

β_1 is the log odds ratio for cancer associated with alcohol among non-smokers,

β_2 is the log odds ratio for cancer associated with smoking among non-drinkers,

$\beta_1 + \beta_3$ is the log odds ratio for cancer associated with alcohol among smokers,

$\beta_2 + \beta_3$ is the log odds ratio for cancer associated with smoking among drinkers, and

$\beta_1 + \beta_2 + \beta_3$ is the log odds ratio for cancer associated with people who both smoke and drink compared to those who do neither.

Let ψ_{ij} be the odds ratio associated with someone with drinking status i and smoking status j relative to people who neither smoke nor drink. Then $\psi_{10} = \exp[\beta_1]$, $\psi_{01} = \exp[\beta_2]$ and $\psi_{11} = \exp[\beta_1 + \beta_2 + \beta_3] = \psi_{10}\psi_{01}\exp[\beta_3]$. Hence, if $\beta_3 = 0$, then the multiplicative model holds. We can test the validity of the multiplicative model by testing the null hypothesis that $\beta_3 = 0$. If $\beta_3 > 0$, then the risk of both smoking and drinking will be greater than the product of the risk of smoking but not drinking times that of drinking but not smoking. If $\beta_3 < 0$, then the risk of both habits will be less than that of this product.

5.22. Model of Alcohol, Tobacco, and Esophageal Cancer with Interaction Terms

In order to weaken the multiplicative assumption implied by model (5.38) we add interaction terms to the model. Specifically, we use the model

$$\text{logit}[E[d_{ijk} \mid ijk]/n_{ijk}] = \alpha + \sum_{h=2}^{6} \alpha_h \times age_h + \sum_{h=2}^{4} \beta_h \times alcohol_{ih}$$

$$+ \sum_{h=2}^{3} \gamma_h \times smoke_{kh} + \sum_{g=2}^{4} \sum_{h=2}^{3} \delta_{gh} \times alcohol_{ig} \times smoke_{kh}, \qquad (5.40)$$

where i, j, k, d_{ijk}, n_{ijk}, α, α_h, age_h, β_h, $alcohol_{ih}$, γ_h, and $smoke_{kh}$ are as defined in model (5.38), and δ_{gh} is one of six new parameters that we have added to the model. This parameter is an interaction term that only appears in the model when both $i = g$ and $k = h$. The log odds of cancer for a man from the jth age stratum who consumes alcohol level $i > 1$ and tobacco level $k > 1$ is

$$\log\left[\frac{\pi_{ijk}}{1 - \pi_{ijk}}\right] = \alpha + \alpha_j + \beta_i + \gamma_k + \delta_{ik}, \qquad (5.41)$$

where π_{ijk} is his probability of having cancer. The log odds of cancer for a man from this age stratum who consumes both alcohol and tobacco at the first level is

$$\log\left[\frac{\pi_{1j1}}{1 - \pi_{1j1}}\right] = \alpha + \alpha_j. \qquad (5.42)$$

Subtracting equation (5.42) from equation (5.41) gives that the age-adjusted log odds ratio for men at the ith and k^{th} levels of alcohol and tobacco exposure relative to men at the lowest levels of these drugs is

$$\log\left[\frac{\pi_{ijk}/(1 - \pi_{ijk})}{\pi_{1j1}/(1 - \pi_{1j1})}\right] = \beta_i + \gamma_k + \delta_{ik}. \qquad (5.43)$$

It is the presence of the δ_{ik} term in equation (5.43) that permits this log odds ratio to be unaffected by the size of the other log odds ratios that can be estimated by the model. By the usual argument, β_i is the log odds ratio for alcohol level i versus level 1 among men at tobacco level 1, and γ_k is the log odds ratio for tobacco level k versus level 1 among men at alcohol level 1.

Table 5.5 contains the age-adjusted odds ratios obtained by fitting model (5.40) to the Ille-et-Vilaine data set and then applying equation (5.43). The odds ratios in this table should be compared to those in Table 5.4. Note that among men who smoke less than 10 gm a day the odds ratios increase more rapidly with increasing dose of alcohol in Table 5.5 than in Table 5.4. For example, $\hat{\psi}_{41}$ equals 65.1 in Table 5.5 but only 36.8 in Table 5.4.

Table 5.5. Effect of alcohol and tobacco on the risk of esophageal cancer in the Ille-et-Vilaine study. These estimates are based on model (5.40). This model contains interaction terms that permit the joint effects of alcohol and tobacco to vary from those dictated by the multiplicative model. Compare these results with those of Table 5.4.

| | Daily tobacco consumption | | | | | |
| | 0–9 gm | | 10–29 gm | | $\geq$ 30 gm | |
Daily alcohol consumption	Odds ratio	95% confidence interval	Odds ratio	95% confidence interval	Odds ratio	95% confidence interval
0–39 gm	1.0*		3.8	(1.6–9.2)	8.65	(2.4–31)
40–79 gm	7.55	(3.4–17)	9.34	(4.2–21)	32.9	(10–110)
80–119 gm	12.7	(5.2–31)	16.1	(6.8–38)	72.3	(15–350)
$\geq$120 gm	65.1	(20–210)	92.3	(29–290)	196	(30–1300)

*Denominator of odds ratios

A similar comparison can be made among men at the lowest level of alcohol consumption with regard to rising exposure to tobacco. In Table 5.5 the odds ratios associated with the combined effects of different levels of alcohol and tobacco consumption are uniformly less than the product of the corresponding odds ratios for alcohol and tobacco alone. Note, however, that both models indicate a dramatic increase in cancer risk with increasing dose of alcohol and tobacco. The confidence intervals are wider in Table 5.5 than in Table 5.4 because they are derived from a model with more parameters and because some of the interaction parameter estimates have large standard errors due to the small number of subjects with the corresponding combined levels of alcohol and tobacco consumption.

5.23. Fitting a Model with Interaction using Stata

We next fit model (5.40) to the Ille-et-Vilaine data set. The *5.20.Esophageal Ca.log* log file that was started in Section 5.20 continues as follows.

```
. *
. * Regress cancer against age, alcohol and smoke.
. * Include alcohol-smoke interaction terms.
. *
```

```
. xi: logistic cancer i.age i.alcohol*i.smoke [freq=patients]                {1}
i.age              _Iage_1—6        (naturally coded; _Iage_1 omitted)
i.alcohol          _Ialcohol_1—4    (naturally coded; _Ialcohol_1 omitted)
i.smoke            _Ismoke_1—3      (naturally coded; _Ismoke_1 omitted)
i.alc~l*i.smoke    _IalcXsmo_#-#    (coded as above)
```

```
Logit estimates                          Number of obs    =        975
                                         LR chi2(16)      =     290.90
                                         Prob > chi2      =     0.0000
Log likelihood = -349.29335              Pseudo R2        =     0.2940
---------------------------------------------------------------------
      cancer | Odds Ratio  Std. Err.    z     P>|z|  [95% Conf. Interval]
---------------------------------------------------------------------
     _Iage_2 |   6.697614   7.410168  1.719   0.086  .7658787   58.57068
     _Iage_3 |    40.1626   42.67237  3.476   0.001   5.00528   322.2665
     _Iage_4 |   69.55115   73.73317  4.001   0.000  8.708053   555.5044
     _Iage_5 |  123.0645   131.6687   4.498   0.000  15.11535   1001.953
     _Iage_6 |  118.8368   133.2476   4.261   0.000  13.19858   1069.977
 _Ialcohol_2 |   7.554406   3.043768  5.019   0.000  3.429574   16.64027    {2}
 _Ialcohol_3 |   12.71358   5.825001  5.550   0.000  5.179307   31.20787
 _Ialcohol_4 |   65.07188   39.54144  6.871   0.000  19.77671   214.1079
    _Ismoke_2 |   3.800862   1.703912  2.978   0.003  1.578671   9.151083    {3}
    _Ismoke_3 |   8.651205   5.569299  3.352   0.001  2.449668   30.55245
 _IalcXsm~2_2 |   .3251915   .1746668 -2.091   0.036  .1134859   .9318291    {4}
 _IalcXsm~2_3 |   .5033299   .4154535 -0.832   0.406  .0998303   2.537716
 _IalcXsm~3_2 |   .3341452   .2008274 -1.824   0.068  .1028839   1.085233
 _IalcXsm~3_3 |    .657279   .6598906 -0.418   0.676  .0918684    4.70255
 _IalcXsm~4_2 |   .3731549   .3018038 -1.219   0.223  .0764621   1.821093
 _IalcXsm~4_3 |   .3489097   .4210271 -0.873   0.383  .0327773   3.714089
---------------------------------------------------------------------
```

```
lincom _Ialcohol_2 + _Ismoke_2 + _IalcXsmo_2_2, or                           {5}
( 1) _Ialcohol_2 + _Ismoke_2 + _IalcXsmo_2_2 = 0.0
---------------------------------------------------------------------
  cancer | Odds Ratio  Std. Err.    z    P>|z|    [95% Conf. Interval]
---------+-----------------------------------------------------------
     (1) |   9.337306   3.826162  5.452  0.000   4.182379    20.84586
---------------------------------------------------------------------

. lincom _Ialcohol_2 + _Ismoke_3 + _IalcXsmo_2_3, or
( 1) _Ialcohol_2 + _Ismoke_3 + _IalcXsmo_2_3 = 0.0
```

```
--------------------------------------------------------------------
cancer | Odds Ratio  Std. Err.     z    P>|z|    [95% Conf. Interval]
-------+------------------------------------------------------------
   (1) |   32.89498   19.73769   5.822  0.000    10.14824    106.6274
--------------------------------------------------------------------
```

. lincom _Ialcohol_3 + _Ismoke_2 + _IalcXsmo_3_2, or

(1) _Ialcohol_3 + _Ismoke_2 + _IalcXsmo_3_2 = 0.0

```
--------------------------------------------------------------------
cancer | Odds Ratio  Std. Err.     z    P>|z|    [95% Conf. Interval]
-------+------------------------------------------------------------
   (1) |   16.14675   7.152595   6.280  0.000    6.776802    38.47207
--------------------------------------------------------------------
```

. lincom _Ialcohol_3 + _Ismoke_3 + _IalcXsmo_3_3, or

(1) _Ialcohol_3 + _Ismoke_3 + _IalcXsmo_3_3 = 0.0

```
--------------------------------------------------------------------
cancer | Odds Ratio  Std. Err.     z    P>|z|    [95% Conf. Interval]
-------+------------------------------------------------------------
   (1) |   72.29267   57.80896   5.353  0.000    15.08098    346.5446
--------------------------------------------------------------------
```

. lincom _Ialcohol_4 + _Ismoke_2 + _IalcXsmo_4_2, or

(1) _Ialcohol_4 + _Ismoke_2 + _IalcXsmo_4_2 = 0.0

```
--------------------------------------------------------------------
cancer | Odds Ratio  Std. Err.     z    P>|z|    [95% Conf. Interval]
-------+------------------------------------------------------------
   (1) |   92.29212   53.97508   7.737  0.000    29.33307    290.3833
--------------------------------------------------------------------
```

. lincom _Ialcohol_4 + _Ismoke_3 + _IalcXsmo_4_3, or

(1) _Ialcohol_4 + _Ismoke_3 + _IalcXsmo_4_3 = 0.0

```
--------------------------------------------------------------------
cancer | Odds Ratio  Std. Err.     z    P>|z|    [95% Conf. Interval]
-------+------------------------------------------------------------
   (1) |   196.4188   189.1684   5.483  0.000    29.74417    1297.072
--------------------------------------------------------------------
```

Comments

1 This command performs the logistic regression specified by model (5.40). The Stata variable *age* equals j in this model, *alcohol* $= i$, and *smoke* $= k$. The syntax *i.alcohol*i.smoke* defines the following categorical variables that are included in the model:

$$\_Ialcohol\_2 = alcohol_{i2} = \begin{cases} 1: \text{if } alcohol = 2 \\ 0: \text{otherwise,} \end{cases}$$

$$\_Ialcohol\_3 = alcohol_{i3} = \begin{cases} 1: \text{if } alcohol = 3 \\ 0: \text{otherwise,} \end{cases}$$

$$\_Ialcohol\_4 = alcohol_{i4} = \begin{cases} 1: \text{if } alcohol = 4 \\ 0: \text{otherwise,} \end{cases}$$

$$\_Ismoke\_2 = smoke_{k2} = \begin{cases} 1: \text{if } smoke = 2 \\ 0: \text{otherwise,} \end{cases}$$

$$\_Ismoke\_3 = smoke_{k3} = \begin{cases} 1: \text{if } smoke = 3 \\ 0: \text{otherwise,} \end{cases}$$

$$\_IalcXsmo\_2\_2 = alcohol_{i2} \times smoke_{k2} = \_Ialcohol\_2 \times \_Ismoke\_2,$$

$$\_IalcXsmo\_2\_3 = alcohol_{i2} \times smoke_{k3} = \_Ialcohol\_2 \times \_Ismoke\_3,$$

$$\_IalcXsmo\_3\_2 = alcohol_{i3} \times smoke_{k2} = \_Ialcohol\_3 \times \_Ismoke\_2,$$

$$\_IalcXsmo\_3\_3 = alcohol_{i3} \times smoke_{k3} = \_Ialcohol\_3 \times \_Ismoke\_3,$$

$$\_IalcXsmo\_4\_2 = alcohol_{i4} \times smoke_{k2} = \_Ialcohol\_4 \times \_Ismoke\_2, \quad \text{and}$$

$$\_IalcXsmo\_4\_3 = alcohol_{i4} \times smoke_{k3} = \_Ialcohol\_4 \times \_Ismoke\_3.$$

A separate parameter is fitted for each of these variables. In addition, the model specifies five parameters for the five age indicator variables and a constant parameter.

2 The parameter associated with the covariate $\_Ialcohol\_2 = alcohol_{i2}$ is β_2; $\hat{\psi}_{21} = \exp[\hat{\beta}_2] = 7.5544$ is the estimated age-adjusted odds ratio for men at alcohol level 2 and tobacco level 1 relative to men at alcohol level 1 and tobacco level 1. The odds ratios and confidence intervals highlighted in this output were used to produce Table 5.5.

3 The parameter associated with the covariate $\_Ismoke\_2 = smoke_{k2}$ is γ_2; $\hat{\psi}_{12} = \exp[\hat{\gamma}_2] = 3.8009$ is the estimated age-adjusted odds ratio for men at alcohol level 1 and tobacco level 2 relative to men at alcohol level 1 and tobacco level 1.

4 The parameter associated with the covariate $\_IalcXsmo\_2\_2 = alcohol_{i2} \times smoke_{k2}$ is δ_{22}. Note that due to lack of room, Stata abbreviates this covariate in the left hand column as $\_IalcXsmo{\sim}2\_2$. This interaction parameter does not equal any specific odds ratio. Nevertheless, Stata outputs $\exp[\hat{\delta}_{22}] = 0.3252$ in the odds ratio column.

5 This statement uses equation (5.43) to calculate $\hat{\psi}_{22} = \exp[\hat{\beta}_2 + \hat{\gamma}_2 + \hat{\delta}_{22}] = 9.3373$. This is the age-adjusted odds ratio for men at the second level of alcohol and tobacco consumption relative to men at the first level of both of these variables.

5.24. Model Fitting: Nested Models and Model Deviance

A model is said to be **nested** within a second model if the first model is a special case of the second. For example, the multiplicative model (5.34) was

$$\text{logit}[E[d_{ij} \mid ij]/n_{ij}] = \alpha + \beta_1 \times i + \beta_2 \times j,$$

while model (5.39), which contained an interaction term, was

$$\text{logit}[E[d_{ij} \mid ij]/n_{ij}] = \alpha + \beta_1 \times i + \beta_2 \times j + \beta_3 \times i \times j.$$

Model (5.34) is nested within model (5.39) since model (5.34) is a special case of model (5.39) with $\beta_3 = 0$.

The model **deviance** D is a statistic derived from the likelihood function that measures goodness of fit of the data to the model. Suppose that a model has parameters $\beta_1, \beta_2, \ldots, \beta_q$. Let $L[\beta_1, \beta_2, \ldots, \beta_q]$ denote the likelihood function for this model and let $\hat{L} = L[\hat{\beta}_1, \hat{\beta}_2, \ldots, \hat{\beta}_q]$ denote the maximum value of the likelihood function over all possible values of the parameters. Then the model deviance is

$$D = K - 2\log[\hat{L}], \tag{5.44}$$

where K is a constant. The value of K is always the same for any two models that are nested. D is always non-negative. Large values of D indicate poor model fit; a perfect fit has $D = 0$.

Suppose that D_1 and D_2 are the deviances from two models and that model 1 is nested within model 2. Let $\hat{L}_1$ and $\hat{L}_2$ denote the maximum values of the likelihood functions for these models. Then it can be shown that if model 1 is true,

$$\Delta D = D_1 - D_2 = 2(\log[\hat{L}_2] - \log[\hat{L}_1]) \tag{5.45}$$

has an approximately χ^2 distribution with the number of degrees of freedom equal to the difference in the number of parameters between the two models. We use this reduction in deviance as a guide to building reasonable models for our data. Equation (5.45) is an example of a likelihood ratio test (see Section 4.9.1).

To illustrate the use of this test consider the Ile-et-Villain data. The multiplicative model (5.38) of alcohol and tobacco levels is nested within model

(5.40). The log file given in Sections 5.20 and 5.23 show that the maximum log likelihoods for models (5.38) and (5.40) are

$$\log[\hat{L}_1] = -351.968 \text{ and } \log[\hat{L}_2] = -349.293, \text{ respectively.}$$

Therefore, the reduction in deviance is

$$\Delta D = 2(\log[\hat{L}_2] - \log[\hat{L}_1]) = 2(-349.293 + 351.968) = 5.35.$$

Since there are six more parameters in the interactive model than the multiplicative model, ΔD has a χ^2 distribution with six degrees of freedom if the multiplicative model is true. The probability that this χ^2 statistic exceeds 5.35 is $P = 0.50$. Thus, there is no statistical evidence to suggest that the multiplicative model is false, or that any meaningful improvement in the model fit can be obtained by adding interaction terms to the model.

There are no hard and fast guidelines to model building other than that it is best not to include uninteresting variables in the model that have a trivial effect on the model deviance. In general, I am guided by deviance reduction statistics when deciding whether to include variables that may, or may not, be true confounders, but that are not intrinsically of interest. It is important to bear in mind, however, that failure to reject the null hypothesis that the nested model is true does not prove the validity of this model. We will discuss this further in the next section.

5.25. Effect Modifiers and Confounding Variables

An **effect modifier** is a variable that influences the effect of a risk factor on the outcome variable. In the preceding example, smoking is a powerful effect modifier of alcohol and vice versa. The key difference between confounding variables and effect modifiers is that confounding variables are not of primary interest in our study while effect modifiers are. A variable is an important effect modifier if there is a meaningful interaction between it and the exposure of interest on the risk of the event under study. Clearly, any variable that requires an interaction term in a regression model is an effect modifier. It is common practice to be fairly tolerant of the multiplicative model assumption for confounding variables but less tolerant of this assumption when we are considering variables of primary interest. For example, model (5.40) assumes that age and either of the other two variables have a multiplicative effect on the cancer odds ratio. Although this assumption may not be precisely true, including age in the model in this way does adjust to a considerable extent for the confounding effects of age on the relationship between alcohol, smoking, and esophageal cancer. Similarly, if you only wanted to present the effects of alcohol on esophageal cancer adjusted for age and smoking, or the effects of smoking on esophageal cancer adjusted for age and alcohol, then the multiplicative model (5.38) would do just fine. The lack of significance of the deviance reduction statistic between models (5.38) and (5.40) provides ample justification for using model (5.38) to adjust for the confounding effects of age and smoking on the cancer risk associated with alcohol consumption. On the other hand, when we present a table such as Table 5.5, we need to be careful to neither overestimate nor underestimate the joint effects of two risk factors on the outcome of interest. For this reason, I recommend that you include an interaction term when presenting the joint effects of two variables unless there is strong evidence that the multiplicative assumption is true. Hence, my personal preference is for Table 5.5 over Table 5.4 even though we are unable to reject model (5.38) in favor of model (5.40) with statistical significance.

5.26. Goodness-of-Fit Tests

We need to be able to determine whether our model gives a good fit to our data, and to detect outliers that have an undue effect on our inferences. Many of the concepts that we introduced for linear regression have counterparts in logistic regression.

5.26.1. The Pearson χ^2 Goodness-of-Fit Statistic

Let us return to the general multiple logistic regression model (5.12). Suppose that there are J distinct covariate patterns and that d_j events occur among n_j patients with the covariate pattern $x_{j1}, x_{j2}, \ldots, x_{jq}$. Let $\pi_j = \pi[x_{j1}, x_{j2}, \ldots, x_{jq}]$ denote the probability that a patient with the jth pattern of covariate values suffers an event, which is given by equation (5.13). Then d_j has a binomial distribution with expected value $n_j \pi_j$ and standard error $\sqrt{n_j \pi_j (1 - \pi_j)}$. Hence

$$(d_j - n_j \pi_j)/\sqrt{n_j \pi_j (1 - \pi_j)} \tag{5.46}$$

will have a mean of 0 and a standard error of 1. Let

$$\hat{\pi}_j = \frac{\exp[\alpha + \hat{\beta}_1 x_{j1} + \hat{\beta}_2 x_{j2} + \cdots + \hat{\beta}_q x_{jq}]}{1 + \exp[\hat{\alpha} + \hat{\beta}_1 x_{j1} + \hat{\beta}_2 x_{j2} + \cdots + \hat{\beta}_q x_{jq}]} \tag{5.47}$$

be the estimate of π_j obtained by substituting the maximum likelihood parameter estimates into equation (5.13). Then the **residual** for the jth

covariate pattern is $d_j - n_j\hat{\pi}_j$. Substituting $\hat{\pi}_j$ for π_j in the equation (5.46) gives the **Pearson residual,** which is

$$r_j = (d_j - n_j\hat{\pi}_j)/\sqrt{n_j\hat{\pi}_j(1 - \hat{\pi}_j)}. \qquad (5.48)$$

If model (5.12) is correct and n_j is sufficiently large, then

$$\chi^2 = \sum_j r_j^2 \qquad (5.49)$$

will have a chi-squared distribution with $J - (q + 1)$ degrees of freedom. Equation (5.49) is the **Pearson chi-squared goodness-of-fit statistic**. It can be used as a goodness-of-fit test of model (5.12) as long as J, the number of distinct covariate patterns, is small in comparison to the number of study subjects. A conservative rule of thumb is that the estimated expected number of events $n_j\hat{\pi}_j$ should be at least 5 and not greater than $n_j - 5$ for each distinct pattern of covariates. In this case, we can reject model (5.12) if the P value associated with this chi-squared statistic is less than 0.05.

It should be noted that the meaning of $\hat{\pi}_j$ depends on whether we are analyzing data from a prospective or case-control study. In an unbiased prospective study, $\hat{\pi}_j$ estimates the probability that someone from the underlying population with the jth covariate pattern will suffer the event of interest. In a case-control study we are unable to estimate this probability (see Sections 4.19.2 and 4.23). Nevertheless, we can still perform valid goodness-of-fit tests and residual analyses even though the value of $\hat{\pi}_j$ is greatly affected by our study design and is not directly related to the probability of disease in the underlying population.

5.27. Hosmer–Lemeshow Goodness-of-Fit Test

When some of the covariates are continuous we may have a unique covariate pattern for each patient, and it is likely that the number of covariate patterns will increase with increasing sample size. In this situation, equation (5.49) will not provide a valid goodness-of-fit test. Hosmer and Lemeshow (1980, 1989) proposed the following test for this situation. First, sort the covariate patterns by increasing values of $\hat{\pi}_j$. Then, divide the patients into g groups containing approximately equal numbers of subjects in such a way that subjects with the lowest values of $\hat{\pi}_j$ are in group 1, subjects with the next lowest values of $\hat{\pi}_j$ are in group 2, and so on – the last group consisting of subjects with the largest values of $\hat{\pi}_j$. Summing within each group, let $m_k = \sum n_j$ and $o_k = \sum d_j$ be the total number of subjects and events in the kth group, respectively. Let $\bar{\pi}_k = \sum n_j\hat{\pi}_j/m_k$ be a weighted average of the values of $\bar{\pi}_j$ in the kth group. Then the **Hosmer–Lemeshow goodness-of-fit statistic** is

$$\hat{C} = \sum_{k=1}^{g} \frac{(o_k - m_k \bar{\pi}_k)^2}{m_k \bar{\pi}_k (1 - \bar{\pi}_k)}. \tag{5.50}$$

If model (5.12) is true, then $\hat{C}$ has an approximately chi-squared distribution with $g - 2$ degrees of freedom. We reject this model if $\hat{C}$ exceeds the critical value associated with the 0.05 significance level of a chi-squared statistic with $g - 2$ degrees of freedom. A value of $g = 10$ is often used in this test.

5.27.1. An Example: The Ille-et-Vilaine Cancer Data Set

In Section 5.22 we fitted model (5.40) to the Ille-et-Vilaine esophageal cancer data set. Under this model there are 68 distinct covariate patterns in the data. The number of patients associated with these patterns varies considerably from pattern to pattern. For example, there is only one subject age 25–34 who drank 80–119 grams of alcohol and smoked 10–29 grams of tobacco each day, while there were 34 subjects age 65–74 who drank 40–79 grams of alcohol and smoked 0–9 grams of tobacco a day. Let's designate this latter group as having the jth covariate pattern. Then in this group there were $d_j = 17$ esophageal cancer cases among $n_j = 34$ subjects. Under model (5.40), the estimated probability that a subject in this group was a case is $\hat{\pi}_j = 0.393\,38$. Hence, the expected number of esophageal cancers is $n_j \hat{\pi}_j = 34 \times 0.393\,38 = 13.375$ and the residual for this pattern is

$$d_j - n_j \hat{\pi}_j = 17 - 13.375 = 3.625.$$

The Pearson residual is

$$r_j = (d_j - n_j \hat{\pi}_j)/\sqrt{n_j \hat{\pi}_j (1 - \hat{\pi}_j)}$$

$$= \frac{3.625}{\sqrt{34 \times 0.393\,38 \times (1 - 0.393\,38)}} = 1.2727.$$

Performing similar calculations for all of the other covariate patterns and summing the square of these residuals gives

$$\chi^2 = \sum_{j=1}^{68} r_j^2 = 55.85.$$

As there are $q = 16$ covariates in model (5.40) this Pearson goodness-of-fit statistic will have $68 - 16 - 1 = 51$ degrees of freedom. The probability that such a statistic exceeds 55.85 equals 0.30.

In this example there are 27 covariate patterns in which the expected number of cancers is less than one and there are 51 patterns in which the expected number of cancers is less than five. This raises serious doubts as to whether we can assume that the Pearson goodness-of-fit statistic has a chi-squared distribution under the null hypothesis that model (5.40) is true. For this reason, the Hosmer–Lemeshow goodness-of-fit test is a better statistic for this model. Sorting the covariate patterns by the values of $\hat{\pi}_j$ gives probabilities that range from $\hat{\pi}_1 = 0.000\,697$ to $\hat{\pi}_{68} = 0.944\,011$. To calculate this test with $g = 10$ we first divide the covariate patterns into ten groups with approximately equal numbers of patients in each group. There are 975 patients in the study so we would prefer to have 97 or 98 patients in each group. We may be forced to deviate from this target in order to keep all patients with the same pattern in the same group. For example, the three lowest cancer probabilities associated with distinct covariate patterns are $\hat{\pi}_1 = 0.000\,697$, $\hat{\pi}_2 = 0.002\,6442$, and $\hat{\pi}_3 = 0.004\,65$. The number of patients with these patterns are $n_1 = 40$, $n_2 = 16$, and $n_3 = 60$. Now $n_1 + n_2 + n_3 = 116$ is closer to 97.5 than $n_1 + n_2 = 56$. Hence, we choose the first of the ten groups to consist of the 116 patients with the three lowest estimated cancer probabilities. The remaining nine groups are chosen similarly. Among patients with the three covariate patterns associated with the smallest cancer probabilities, there were no cancer cases giving $d_1 = d_2 = d_3 = 0$. Hence, for the first group

$$m_1 = n_1 + n_2 + n_3 = 116, \quad o_1 = d_1 + d_2 + d_3 = 0,$$

$$\bar{\pi}_1 = (n_1\hat{\pi}_1 + n_2\hat{\pi}_2 + n_3\hat{\pi}_3)/m_1 = (40 \times 0.000\,697$$

$$+ \, 16 \times 0.002\,644 + 60 \times 0.004\,65)/116 = 0.003\,01,$$

and

$$\frac{(o_1 - m_1\bar{\pi}_1)^2}{m_1\bar{\pi}_1(1 - \bar{\pi}_1)} = (0 - 116 \times 0.003\,01)^2/(116 \times 0.003\,01$$

$$\times \, (1 - 0.003\,01)) = 0.350.$$

Performing the analogous computations for the other nine groups and summing the standardized squared residuals gives

$$\hat{C} = \sum_{k=1}^{10} \frac{(o_k - m_k\bar{\pi}_k)^2}{m_k\bar{\pi}_k(1 - \bar{\pi}_k)} = 4.728.$$

This Hosmer–Lemeshow test statistic has eight degrees of freedom. The probability that a chi-squared statistic with eight degrees of freedom exceeds 4.728 is $P = 0.7862$. Hence, this test provides no evidence to reject model (5.40).

5.28. Residual and Influence Analysis

Of course, the failure to reject a model by a goodness-of-fit test does not prove that the model is true or fits the data well. For this reason, residual analyses are always advisable for any results that are to be published. A residual analysis for a logistic regression model is analogous to one for linear regression. Although the standard error of d_j is $se[d_j] = \sqrt{n_j \pi_j (1 - \pi_j)}$, the standard error of the residual $d_j - n_j \hat{\pi}_j$ is less than $se[d_j]$ due to the fact that the maximum likelihood values of the parameter estimates tend to shift $n_j \hat{\pi}_j$ in the direction of d_j. The ability of an individual covariate pattern to reduce the standard deviation of its associated residual is measured by the **leverage** h_j (Pregibon, 1981). The formula for h_j is complex and not terribly edifying. For our purposes, we can define h_j by the formula

$$\text{var}[d_j - n_j \hat{\pi}_j] = n_j \hat{\pi}_j (1 - \hat{\pi}_j)(1 - h_j) \cong \text{var}[d_j - n_j \pi_j](1 - h_j).$$

(5.51)

In other words, $100(1 - h_j)$ is the percent reduction in the variance of the jth residual due to the fact that the estimate of $n_j \hat{\pi}_j$ is pulled towards d_j. The value of h_j lies between 0 and 1. When h_j is very small, d_j has almost no effect on its estimated expected value $n_j \hat{\pi}_j$. When h_j is close to one, then $d_j \cong n_j \hat{\pi}_j$. This implies that both the residual $d_j - n_j \hat{\pi}_j$ and its variance will be close to zero. This definition of leverage is highly analogous to that given for linear regression. See, in particular, equation (2.24).

5.28.1. Standardized Pearson Residual

The **standardized Pearson residual** for the jth covariate pattern is the residual divided by its standard error. That is,

$$r_{sj} = \frac{d_j - n_j \pi_j}{\sqrt{n_j \hat{\pi}_j (1 - \hat{\pi}_j)(1 - h_j)}} = \frac{r_j}{\sqrt{1 - h_j}}.$$

(5.52)

This residual is analogous to the standardized residual for linear regression (see equation 2.25). The key difference between equation (2.25) and equation (5.52) is that the standardized residual has a known t distribution under the linear model. Although r_{sj} has mean zero and standard error one it does not have a normally shaped distribution when n_j is small. The square of the standardized Pearson residual is denoted by

$$\Delta X_j^2 = r_{sj}^2 = r_j^2 / (1 - h_j).$$

(5.53)

We will use the critical value $(z_{0.025})^2 = 1.96^2 = 3.84$ as a very rough guide to identifying large values of ΔX_j^2. Approximately 95% of these squared residuals should be less than 3.84 if the logistic regression model is correct.

5.28.2. $\Delta \hat{\beta}_j$ Influence Statistic

Covariate patterns that are associated with both high leverage and large residuals can have a substantial influence on the parameter estimates of the model. The $\Delta \hat{\beta}_j$ **influence statistic** is a measure of the influence of the jth covariate pattern on all of the parameter estimates taken together (Pregibon, 1981), and equals

$$\Delta \hat{\beta}_j = r_{sj}^2 h_j / (1 - h_j). \tag{5.54}$$

Note that $\Delta \hat{\beta}_j$ increases with both the magnitude of the standardized residual and the size of the leverage. It is analogous to Cook's distance for linear regression (see Section 3.20.2). Covariate patterns associated with large values of ΔX_j^2 and $\Delta \hat{\beta}_j$ merit special attention.

5.28.3. Residual Plots of the Ille-et-Vilaine Data on Esophageal Cancer

Figure 5.1 shows a plot of the squared residuals ΔX_j^2 against the estimated cancer probability for model (5.40). Each circle represents the squared residual associated with a unique covariate pattern. The area of each circle is proportional to $\Delta \hat{\beta}_j$. Black circles are used to indicate positive residuals while gray circles indicate negative residuals. Hosmer and Lemeshow (1989) first suggested this form of residual plot. They recommend that the area of the plotted circles be 1.5 times the magnitude of $\Delta \hat{\beta}_j$. Figure 5.1 does not reveal any obvious relationship between the magnitude of the residuals and the values of $\hat{\pi}_j$. There are 68 unique covariate patterns in this data set. Five percent of 68 equals 3.4. Hence, if model (5.40) is correct we would expect three or four squared residuals to be greater than 3.84. There are six such residuals with two of them being close to 3.84. Thus, the magnitude of the residuals is reasonably consistent with model (5.40).

There are two large squared residuals in Figure 5.1 that have high influence. These squared residuals are labeled A and B in this figure. Residual A is associated with patients who are age 55–64 and consume, on a daily basis, at least 120 gm of alcohol and 0–9 gm of tobacco. Residual B is associated with patients who are age 55–64 and consume, on a daily basis, 0–39 gm of alcohol and at least 30 gm of tobacco. The $\Delta \beta_j$ influence statistics associated

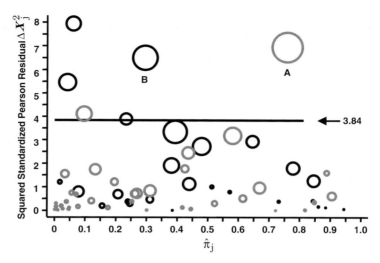

Figure 5.1 Squared residual plot of $\triangle X_j^2$ against $\hat{\pi}_j$ for the esophageal cancer data analyzed with model (5.40). A separate circle is plotted for each distinct covariate
pattern. The area of each circle is proportional to the influence statistic $\triangle \hat{\beta}_j$.
$\triangle X_j^2$ is the squared standardized Pearson residual for the jth covariate pattern;
$\hat{\pi}_j$ is the estimated probability that a study subject with this pattern is one of
the case patients. Black and gray circles indicate positive and negative residuals, respectively. Two circles associated with covariate patterns having large
influence and big squared residuals are labeled A and B (see text).

with residuals A and B are 6.16 and 4.15, respectively. Table 5.6 shows the
effects of deleting patients with these covariate patterns from the analysis.
Column 3 of this table repeats the odds ratio given in Table 5.5. Columns 5
and 7 show the odds ratios that result when patients with covariate patterns
A and B are deleted from model (5.40). Deleting patients with pattern A
increases the odds ratio for men who smoke 0–9 gm and drink ≥120 gm
from 65.1 to 274. This is a 321% increase that places this odds ratio outside
of its 95% confidence interval based on the complete data. The other odds
ratios in Table 5.5 are not greatly changed by deleting these patients. Deleting the patients associated with covariate pattern B causes a 78% reduction
in the odds ratio for men who smoke at least 30 gm and drink 0–39 gm a
day. Their deletion does not greatly affect the other odds ratios in this table.

   How should these analyses guide the way in which we present these results? Here, reasonable investigators may disagree on the best way to proceed. My own inclination would be to publish Table 5.5. This table provides
compelling evidence that tobacco and alcohol are strong independent risk

Table 5.6. Effects on odds ratios from model (5.40) due to deleting patients with covariates A and B identified in Figure 5.1 (see text).

		Complete data		Deleted covariate pattern			
				A[†]		B[‡]	
Daily drug consumption			95%		Percent change		Percent change
Tobacco	Alcohol	Odds ratio	confidence interval	Odds ratio	from complete data	Odds ratio	from complete data
0–9 gm	0–39 gm	1.0*		1.0*		1.0*	
0–9 gm	40–79 gm	7.55	(3.4–17)	7.53	−0.26%	7.70	2.0%
0–9 gm	80–119 gm	12.7	(5.2–31)	12.6	−0.79%	13.0	2.4%
0–9 gm	≥120 gm	65.1	(20–210)	274	321%	66.8	2.6%
10–29 gm	0–39 gm	3.80	(1.6–9.2)	3.77	−0.79%	3.86	1.6%
10–29 gm	40–79 gm	9.34	(4.2–21)	9.30	−0.43%	9.53	2.0%
10–29 gm	80–119 gm	16.1	(6.8–38)	16.0	−0.62%	16.6	3.1%
10–29 gm	≥120 gm	92.3	(29–290)	95.4	3.4%	94.0	1.8%
≥30 gm	0–39 gm	8.65	(2.4–31)	8.66	0.12%	1.88	−78%
≥30 gm	40–79 gm	32.9	(10–110)	33.7	2.4%	33.5	1.8%
≥30 gm	80–119 gm	72.3	(15–350)	73.0	0.97%	74.2	2.6%
≥30 gm	≥120 gm	196	(30–1300)	198	1.02%	203	3.6%

* Denominator of odds ratios
[†] Patients age 55–64 who drink at least 120 gm a day and smoke 0–9 gm a day deleted
[‡] Patients age 55–64 who drink 0–39 gm a day and smoke at least 30 gm a day deleted

factors for esophageal cancer and indicates an impressive synergy between these two risk factors. Deleting patients with covariate patterns A and B does not greatly alter this conclusion, although it does profoundly alter the size of two of these odds ratios. On the other hand, the size of some of the $\Delta \hat{\beta}_j$ influence statistics in Figure 5.1 and the width of the confidence intervals in Table 5.5 provide a clear warning that model (5.40) is approaching the upper limit of complexity that is reasonable for this data set. A more conservative approach would be to not report the combined effects of alcohol and smoking, or to use just two levels of consumption for each drug rather than three or four. Model (5.38) could be used to report the odds ratios associated with different levels of alcohol consumption adjusted for tobacco usage. This model could also be used to estimate odds ratios associated with different tobacco levels adjusted for alcohol.

Residual analyses in logistic regression are in many ways similar to those for linear regression. There is, however, one important difference. In linear regression, an influential observation is made on a single patient and there is always the possibility that this result is invalid and should be discarded from the analysis. In logistic regression, an influential observation usually is due to the response from multiple patients with the same covariate pattern. Hence, deleting these observations is not an option. Nevertheless, residual analyses are worthwhile in that they help us evaluate how well the model fits the data and can indicate instabilities that can arise from excessively complicated models.

5.29. Using Stata for Goodness-of-Fit Tests and Residual Analyses

We next perform the analyses discussed in the preceding sections. The *5.20.EsophagealCa.log* that was discussed in Sections 5.20 and 5.23 continues as follows:

```
. *
. * Perform Pearson chi-squared and Hosmer-Lemeshow tests of
. * goodness of fit.
. *
. lfit                                                              {1}

Logistic model for cancer, goodness-of-fit test

        number of observations =      975
 number of covariate patterns =       68
           Pearson chi2(51) =        55.85
                Prob > chi2 =        0.2977

. lfit, group(10) table                                            {2}

Logistic model for cancer, goodness-of-fit test
(Table collapsed on quantiles of estimated probabilities)
```

_Group	_Prob	_Obs_1	_Exp_1	_Obs_0	_Exp_0	_Total
1	0.0046	0	0.3	116	115.7	116
2	0.0273	2	2.0	118	118.0	120
3	0.0418	4	3.1	76	76.9	80
4	0.0765	4	5.1	87	85.9	91
5	0.1332	5	7.8	81	78.2	86
6	0.2073	21	20.2	91	91.8	112
7	0.2682	22	22.5	65	64.5	87
8	0.3833	32	28.5	56	59.5	88
9	0.5131	46	41.6	52	56.4	98
10	0.9440	64	68.9	33	28.1	97

```
      number of observations =       975
             number of groups =       10
      Hosmer-Lemeshow chi2(8) =       4.73
                 Prob > chi2 =      0.7862
```

```
. *
. * Perform residual analysis
. *
. predict p, p                                                    {3}

. predict dx2, dx2                                                {4}
(57 missing values generated)

. predict rstandard, rstandard                                   {5}
(57 missing values generated)

. generate dx2_pos = dx2 if rstandard >= 0                        {6}
(137 missing values generated)

. generate dx2_neg = dx2 if rstandard < 0
(112 missing values generated)

.  predict dbeta, dbeta                                           {7}
(57 missing values generated)

. generate bubble= 1.5*dbeta
(57 missing values generated)

. graph dx2_pos dx2_neg p [weight=bubble], symbol(OO) xlabel(0.1 to 1.0)   {8}
> xtick (0.05 0.1 to 0.95) ylabel(0 1 to 8) ytick (.5 1 to 7.5) yline(3.84)

. save temporary, replace                                        {9}
file temporary.dta saved

. drop if patients == 0                                          {10}
(57 observations deleted)

. generate ca_no = cancer*patients

. collapse (sum) n = patients ca = ca_no, by(age alcohol smoke dbeta dx2 p)
                                                                 {11}
. *
. * Identify covariate patterns associated with large squared residuals
. *
. list n ca age alcohol smoke dbeta dx2 p if dx2 > 3.84, nodisplay   {12}
        n     ca    age    alcohol   smoke    dbeta        dx2         p
11.     2      1    25-34   >= 120   10-29   1.335425    7.942312   .060482
17.    37      4    35-44    40-79   10-29   1.890465    5.466789   .041798
22.     3      2    35-44   >= 120    0-9    .9170162    3.896309   .2331274
```

```
25.   28     0    45-54      0-39    10-29    1.564479    4.114906    .0962316
38.    6     4    55-64      0-39    >= 30    4.159096    6.503713    .2956251
45.   10     5    55-64    >= 120     0-9     6.159449    6.949361    .7594333
```

. *

. * *Rerun analysis without the covariate pattern A*

. *

. use *temporary, clear*   {13}

. drop if *age == 4 alcohol == 4 smoke == 1*   {14}
(2 observations deleted)

. xi: logistic *cancer i.age i.alcohol*i.smoke [freq=patients]*   {15}
                                                              {Output omitted}
----
      cancer | Odds Ratio   Std. Err.   z   P>|z| [95% Conf. Interval]
-------------+---
                                                              {Output omitted}
  _Ialcohol_2 | 7.525681   3.032792   5.008   0.000   3.416001   16.57958
  _Ialcohol_3 | 12.62548   5.790079   5.529   0.000   5.139068   31.01781
  _Ialcohol_4 | 273.8578   248.0885   6.196   0.000   46.38949   1616.705
    _Ismoke_2 | 3.76567   1.6883   2.957   0.003   1.563921   9.067132
    _Ismoke_3 | 8.65512   5.583627   3.345   0.001   2.444232   30.64811
                                                              {Output omitted}
```

. lincom *_Ialcohol_2 + _Ismoke_2 + _IalcXsmo_2_2, or*

                                                              {Output omitted}
```
----
cancer | Odds Ratio   Std. Err.   z   P>|z| [95% Conf. Interval]
----
   (1) | 9.298176   3.811849   5.439   0.000   4.163342   20.76603

```

. lincom *_Ialcohol_2 +_Ismoke_3 + _IalcXsmo_2_3, or*

                                                              {Output omitted}
```
   (1) | 33.6871   20.40138   5.808   0.000   10.27932   110.3985

```

. lincom *_Ialcohol_3 + _Ismoke_2 + _IalcXsmo_3_2, or*

                                                              {Output omitted}
```
   (1) | 16.01118   7.097924   6.256   0.000   6.715472   38.1742

```
```

```
. lincom _Ialcohol_3 + _Ismoke_3 + _IalcXsmo_3_3, or

                                                    {Output omitted}
   (1) |   73.00683    58.92606    5.316    0.000    15.00833    355.1358
--------------------------------------------------------------------------

. lincom _Ialcohol_4 + _Ismoke_2 + _IalcXsmo_4_2, or

                                                    {Output omitted}
   (1) |   95.43948    56.55247    7.693    0.000    29.87792    304.8638
--------------------------------------------------------------------------

. lincom _Ialcohol_4 + _Ismoke_3 + _IalcXsmo_4_3, or

                                                    {Output omitted}
   (1) |   197.7124   192.6564    5.426    0.000    29.28192    1334.96
--------------------------------------------------------------------------

. *
. * Rerun analysis without the covariate pattern B
. *
. use temporary, clear                                          {16}

. drop if age == 4 & alcohol == 1 & smoke == 3                  {17}
(2 observations deleted)

. xi: logistic cancer i.age i.alcohol*i.smoke [freq=patients]   {18}
                                                    {Output omitted}
--------------------------------------------------------------------------
     cancer |  Odds Ratio  Std. Err.    z    P>|z|    [95% Conf. Interval]
------------+-------------------------------------------------------------
                                                    {Output omitted}
_Ialcohol_2 |   7.695185   3.109016  5.051  0.000    3.485907   16.98722
_Ialcohol_3 |   13.04068   5.992019  5.589  0.000    5.298882   32.09342
_Ialcohol_4 |   66.83578  40.63582   6.912  0.000   20.29938   220.057
  _Ismoke_2 |   3.864114   1.735157  3.010  0.003    1.602592    9.317017
  _Ismoke_3 |   1.875407   2.107209  0.560  0.576   .2073406    16.96315
                                                    {Output omitted}

. lincom _Ialcohol_2 + _Ismoke_2 + _IalcXsmo_2_2, or

                                                    {Output omitted}
--------------------------------------------------------------------------
     cancer |  Odds Ratio  Std. Err.    z    P>|z|    [95% Conf. Interval]
------------+-------------------------------------------------------------
   (1) |   9.526812   3.914527  5.486  0.000    4.25787   21.31586
--------------------------------------------------------------------------
```

```
. lincom _Ialcohol_2 + _Ismoke_3 + _IalcXsmo_2_3, or
```
{Output omitted}

```
  (1) |    33.48594   20.08865   5.853   0.000        10.33274       108.5199
------------------------------------------------------------------------------
```

```
. lincom _Ialcohol_3 + _Ismoke_2 + _IalcXsmo_3_2, or
```
{Output omitted}

```
  (1) |    16.58352   7.369457   6.320   0.000        6.940903       39.62209
------------------------------------------------------------------------------
```

```
. lincom _Ialcohol_3 + _Ismoke_3 + _IalcXsmo_3_3, or
```
{Output omitted}

```
  (1) |    74.22997   59.24187   5.397   0.000        15.53272       354.7406
------------------------------------------------------------------------------
```

```
. lincom _Ialcohol_4 + _Ismoke_2 + _IalcXsmo_4_2, or
```
{Output omitted}

```
  (1) |    94.0049    54.92414   7.776   0.000        29.91024       295.448
------------------------------------------------------------------------------
```

```
. lincom _Ialcohol_4 + _Ismoke_3 + _IalcXsmo_4_3, or
```
{Output omitted}

```
  (1)  |   202.6374   194.6184   5.530   0.000        30.84628       1331.179
------------------------------------------------------------------------------
```

Comments

1 The *lfit* command is a post-estimation command that can be used with logistic regression. Without options it calculates the Pearson chi-squared goodness-of-fit test for the preceding logistic regression analysis. In this example, the preceding logistic command analyzed model (5.40) (see Section 5.23). As indicated in Section 5.27.1, this statistic equals 55.85 and has 51 degrees of freedom. The associated P value is 0.30.

2 The *group(10)* option causes *lfit* to calculate the Hosmer–Lemeshow goodness-of-fit test with the study subjects subdivided into $g = 10$ groups. The *table* option displays information about these groups. The columns in the subsequent table are defined as follows: $\_Group = k$ is the group number, $\_Prob$ is the maximum value of $\hat{\pi}_j$ in the kth group, $\_Obs\_1 = o_k$ is the observed number of events in the kth group, $\_Exp\_1 = \sum n_j \hat{\pi}_j$ is the expected number of events in the kth group, $\_Obs\_0 = m_k - o_k =$ the number of subjects who did not have events in the kth group, $\_Exp\_0 = m_k - \sum n_j \hat{\pi}_j$ is the expected number of subjects who did not have events in the kth group, and $\_Total = m_k$ is the total number of subjects in the kth group. The Hosmer–Lemeshow goodness-of-fit statistic

equals 4.73 with eight degrees of freedom. The P value associated with this test is 0.79.

3 The p option in this *predict* command defines the variable p to equal $\hat{\pi}_j$. In this and the next two *predict* commands the name of the newly defined variable is the same as the command option.

4 Define the variable *dx2* to equal ΔX_j^2. All records with the same covariate pattern are given the same value of *dx2*.

5 Define *rstandard* to equal the standardized Pearson residual r_{sj}.

6 We are going to draw a scatterplot of ΔX_j^2 against $\hat{\pi}_j$. We would like to color code the plotting symbols to indicate whether the residual is positive or negative. This command defines *dx2_pos* to equal ΔX_j^2 if and only if r_{sj} is non-negative. The next command defines *dx2_neg* to equal ΔX_j^2 if r_{sj} is negative. See comment 8 below.

7 Define the variable *dbeta* to equal $\Delta \hat{\beta}_j$. The values of *dx2*, *dbeta* and *rstandard* are affected by the number of subjects with a given covariate pattern, and the number of events that occur to these subjects. They are not affected by the number of records used to record this information. Hence, it makes no difference whether there is one record per patient or just two records specifying the number of subjects with the specified covariate pattern who did, or did not, suffer the event of interest.

8 This graph produces a scatterplot of ΔX_j^2 against $\hat{\pi}_j$ that is similar to Figure 5.1. The *[weight =bubble]* command modifier causes the plotting symbols to be circles whose area is proportional to the variable bubble. (We set *bubble* equal to $1.5 \times \Delta \hat{\beta}_j$ following the recommendation of Hosmer and Lemeshow (1989) for these residual plots.) We plot both *dx2_pos* and *dx2_neg* against p in order to be able to assign different pen colors to values of ΔX_j^2 that are associated with positive or negative residuals.

9 We need to identify and delete patients with covariate patterns A and B in Figure 5.1. Before doing this we save the current data file so that we can restore it to its current form when needed. This save command saves the data in a file called *temporary*, which is located in the Stata default file folder.

10 Delete covariate patterns that do not pertain to any patients in the study.

11 The *collapse (sum)* command reduces the data to one record for each unique combination of values for the variables listed in the *by* option. This command defines n and *ca* to be the sum of *patients* and *ca_no*, respectively over all records with identical values of *age*, *alcohol*, *smoke* *dbeta*, *dx2* and *p*. In other words, for each specific pattern of these covariates, n is the number of patients and *ca* is the number of cancer

cases with this pattern. All other covariates that are not included in the *by* option are deleted from memory. The covariates *age*, *alcohol* and *smoke* uniquely define the covariate pattern. The variables *dbeta*, *dx2* and *p* are the same for all patients with the same covariate pattern. However, we include them in this *by* statement in order to be able to list them in the following command.

12 List the covariate values and other variables for all covariate patterns for which $\Delta X_j^2 > 3.84$. The two largest values of $\Delta \beta_j$ are highlighted. The record with $\Delta \beta_j = 6.16$ corresponds to squared residual A in Figure 5.1. Patients with the covariate pattern associated with this residual are age 55–64, drink at least 120 gm of alcohol and smoke less than 10 gm of tobacco a day. Squared residual B has $\Delta \beta_j = 4.16$. The associated residual pattern is for patients aged 55–64 who drink 0–39 gm alcohol and smoke $\geq$30 gm tobacco a day.

    The *nodisplay* option forces the output to be given in tabular format rather than display format. Display format looks better when there are lots of variables but requires more lines per patient.

13 Restore the complete data file that we saved earlier.

14 Delete records with covariate pattern A. That is, the record is deleted if *age* = 4 and *alcohol* = 4 and *smoke* = 1. These coded values correspond to age 55–64, $\geq$120 gm alcohol, and 0–9 gm tobacco, respectively.

15 Analyze the data with covariate pattern A deleted using model (5.40). The highlighted odds ratios in the subsequent output are also given in column 5 of Table 5.6.

16 Restore complete database.

17 Delete records with covariate pattern B.

18 Analyze the data with covariate pattern B deleted using model (5.40). The highlighted odds ratios in the subsequent output are also given in column 7 of Table 5.6.

5.30. Frequency Matched Case-Control Studies

We often have access to many more potential control patients than case patients for case-control studies. If the distribution of some important confounding variable, such as age, differs markedly between cases and controls, we may wish to adjust for this variable when designing the study. One way to do this is through **frequency matching**. The cases and potential controls are stratified into a number of groups based on, say, age. We then randomly select from each stratum the same number of controls as there are cases in the stratum. The data can then be analyzed by logistic regression with a classification variable to indicate these strata.

It is important, however, to keep the strata fairly large if logistic regression is to be used for the analysis. Otherwise the estimates of the parameters of real interest may be seriously biased. Breslow and Day (1980) recommend that the strata be large enough so that each stratum contains at least ten cases and ten controls when the true odds ratio is between one and two. They show that even larger strata are needed to avoid appreciable bias when the true odds ratio is greater than two.

5.31. Conditional Logistic Regression

Sometimes there is more than one important confounder that we would like to adjust for in the design of our study. In this case we typically match each case patient to one or more controls with the same values of the confounding variables. This approach is often quite reasonable. However, it usually leads to strata (matched pairs or sets of patients) that are too small to be analyzed accurately with logistic regression. In this case, an alternative technique called **conditional logistic regression** should be used. This technique is discussed in Breslow and Day (1980). In Stata, the *clogit* command may be used to implement these analyses. The syntax of the *clogit* command is similar to that for *logistic*. A mandatory "option" for this command is

```
group(varname)
```

where *varname* is a variable that links cases to their matched controls. That is, each case and her matched control share a unique value of *varname*.

5.32. Analyzing Data with Missing Values

Frequently, data sets will contain missing values of some covariates. Most regression programs, including those of Stata, deal with missing values by excluding all records with missing values in any of the covariates. This can result in the discarding of substantial amounts of information and a considerable loss of power. Some statisticians recommend using methods of **data imputation** to estimate the values of missing covariates. The basic idea of these methods is as follows. Suppose that x_{ij} represents the jth covariate value on the ith patient, and that x_{kj} is missing for the kth patient. We first identify all patients who have non-missing values of both the jth covariate and all other covariates that are available on the kth patient. Using this patient subset, we regress x_{ij} against these other covariates. We use the results of this regression to predict the value of x_{kj} from the other known covariate values of the kth patient. This predicted value is called the **imputed value** of x_{kj}. This process is then repeated for all of the other missing covariates in the data set. The imputed covariate values are then used in the final regression in place of the missing values.

These methods work well if the values of x_{ij} that are available are a representative sample from the entire target population. Unfortunately, this is often not the case in medical studies. Consider the following example.

5.32.1. Cardiac Output in the Ibuprofen in Sepsis Study

An important variable for assessing and managing severe pulmonary morbidity is oxygen delivery, which is the rate at which oxygen is delivered to the body by the lungs. Oxygen delivery is a function of cardiac output and several other variables (Marini and Wheeler, 1997). Unfortunately, cardiac output can only be reliably measured by inserting a catheter into the pulmonary artery. This is an invasive procedure that is only performed in the sickest patients. In the Ibuprofen in Sepsis study, baseline oxygen delivery was measured in 37% of patients. However, we cannot assume that the oxygen delivery was similar in patients who were, or were not, catheterized. Hence, any analysis that assesses the influence of baseline oxygen delivery on 30 day mortality must take into account the fact that this covariate is only known on a biased sample of study subjects.

Let us restrict our analyses to patients who are either black or white. Consider the model

$$\text{logit}[E[d_i \mid x_i, y_i]] = \alpha + \beta_1 x_i + \beta_2 y_i, \tag{5.55}$$

where

$$d_i = \begin{cases} 1: \text{if the } i^{th} \text{ patient dies within 30 days} \\ 0: \text{otherwise,} \end{cases}$$

$$x_i = \begin{cases} 1: \text{if the } i^{th} \text{ patient is black} \\ 0: \text{otherwise,} \end{cases}$$

and y_i is the rate of oxygen delivery for the ith patient. The analysis of model (5.55) excludes patients with missing oxygen delivery. This, together with the exclusion of patients of other race, restricts this analysis to 161 of the 455 subjects in the study. The results of this analysis are given in the

Table 5.7. Effect of race and baseline oxygen delivery on mortality in the Ibuprofen in Sepsis study. Oxygen delivery can only be reliably measured in patients with pulmonary artery catheters. In the analysis of model (5.55) 262 patients were excluded because of missing oxygen delivery. These patients were retained in the analysis of model (5.56). In this latter model, black patients had a significantly higher mortality than white patients, and uncatheterized patients had a significantly lower mortality than those who were catheterized. In contrast, race did not significantly affect mortality in the analysis of model (5.55) (see text).

	Model (5.55)			Model (5.56)		
Risk factor	Odds ratio	95% confidence interval	P value	Odds ratio	95% confidence interval	P value
Race						
White	1.0*			1.0*		
Black	1.38	0.60–3.2	0.45	1.85	1.2–2.9	0.006
Unit increase in oxygen delivery[†]	0.9988	0.9979–0.9997	0.01	0.9988	0.9979–0.9997	0.01
Pulmonary artery catheter						
Yes				1.0*		
No				0.236	0.087–0.64	0.005

*Denominator of odds ratio
[†]Oxygen delivery is missing in patients who did not have a pulmonary artery catheter

left-hand side of Table 5.7. The mortality odds ratio for blacks of 1.38 is not significantly different from one, and the confidence interval for this odds ratio is wide. As one would expect, survival improves with increasing oxygen delivery ($P = 0.01$).

In this study, oxygen delivery was measured in every patient who received a pulmonary artery catheter. Hence, a missing value for oxygen delivery indicates that the patient was not catheterized. A problem with model (5.55) is that it excludes 262 patients of known race because they did not have their oxygen delivery measured. A better model is

$$\text{logit}[\text{E}[d_i \mid x_i, y_i', z_i]] = \alpha + \beta_1 x_i + \beta_2 y_i' + \beta_3 z_i, \tag{5.56}$$

where

d_i and x_i and are as in model(5.55),

$$y_i' = \begin{cases} \text{oxygen delivery for the } i^{\text{th}} \text{ patient if measured} \\ 0: \text{if oxygen delivery was not measured, and} \end{cases}$$

$$z_i = \begin{cases} 1: \text{if oxygen delivery was not measured for } i^{\text{th}} \text{ patient} \\ 0: \text{otherwise.} \end{cases}$$

An analysis of model (5.56) gives the odds ratio estimates in the right half of Table 5.7. Note that the mortal odds ratio for blacks is higher than in model (5.55) and is significantly different from one. The confidence interval for this odds ratio is substantially smaller than in model (5.56) due to the fact that it is based on all 423 subjects rather than just the 161 patients who where catheterized. The odds ratio associated with oxygen delivery is the same in both models. This is because β_2 only enters the likelihood function through the linear predictor, and y_i' is always 0 when oxygen delivery is missing. Hence, in model (5.56), patients with missing oxygen delivery have no influence on the maximum likelihood estimate of β_2.

It is particularly noteworthy that the odds ratio associated with z_i is both highly significant and substantially less than one. This means that patients who were not catheterized were far less likely to die than patients who were catheterized. Thus, we need to be very cautious in interpreting the meaning of the significant odds ratio for oxygen consumption. We can only say that increased oxygen delivery was beneficial among those patients in whom it was measured. The effect of oxygen delivery on mortality among other uncatheterized patients may be quite different since this group had a much better prognosis. For example, it is possible that oxygen delivery in the uncatheterized is sufficiently good that variation in the rate of oxygen delivery has little effect on mortality. Using a data imputation method for these data would be highly inappropriate.

This analysis provides evidence that blacks have a higher mortality rate from sepsis than whites and catheterized patients have higher mortality than uncatheterized patients. It says nothing, however, about why these rates differ. As a group, blacks may differ from whites with respect to the etiology of their sepsis and the time between onset of illness and admission to hospital. Certainly, critical care physicians do not catheterize patients unless they consider it necessary for their care, and it is plausible that patients who are at the greatest risk of death are most likely to be monitored in this way.

5.32.2. Modeling Missing Values with Stata

The following Stata log file regresses death within 30 days against race and baseline oxygen delivery in the Ibuprofen in Sepsis study using models (5.55) and (5.56).

```
. * 5.32.2.Sepsis.log
. *
. * Regress fate against race and oxygen delivery in black and
. * white patients from the Ibuprofen in Sepsis study (Bernard et al., 1997).
. *
. use C:\WDDtext\1.4.11.Sepsis.dta, clear
```

```
. keep if race <2                                                    {1}
(32 observations deleted)
```

```
. logistic fate race o2del                                          {2}
 Logit estimates                        Number of obs    =      161
                                        LR chi2(2)       =     7.56
                                        Prob > chi2      =   0.0228
 Log likelihood = -105.19119            Pseudo R2        =   0.0347

--------------------------------------------------------------------------------
 fate  |  Odds Ratio   Std. Err.      z     P>|z|      [95% Conf. Interval]
-------+------------------------------------------------------------------------
 race  |   1.384358    .5933089    0.759   0.448      .5976407     3.206689
 o2del |   .9988218    .0004675   -2.519   0.012      .9979059     .9997385
--------------------------------------------------------------------------------
```

```
. *
. * Let o2mis indicate whether o2del is missing. Set o2del1 = o2del when
. * oxygen delivery is available and = 0 when it is not.
. *
. generate o2mis = 0
```

```
. replace o2mis = 1 if o2del == .                                    {3}
(262 real changes made)
```

```
. generate o2del1 = o2del
(262 missing values generated)
```

```
. replace o2del1 = 0 if o2del == .
(262 real changes made)
```

```
. logistic fate race o2del1 o2mis                                    {4}
Logit estimates                         Number of obs    =      423
                                        LR chi2(3)       =    14.87
                                        Prob > chi2      =   0.0019
Log likelihood = -276.33062             Pseudo R2        =   0.0262
```

```
----------------------------------------------------------------------------
  fate  |  Odds Ratio   Std. Err.     z     P>|z|       [95% Conf. Interval]
--------+-------------------------------------------------------------------
  race  |   1.847489    .4110734    2.759   0.006       1.194501    2.857443
 o2del1 |    .9987949   .0004711   -2.557   0.011        .9978721    .9997186
  o2mis |    .2364569   .1205078   -2.829   0.005        .0870855    .6420338
----------------------------------------------------------------------------
```

Comments

1 The values of *race* are 0 and 1 for whites and blacks, respectively. This statement excludes patients of other races from our analyses.

2 The variable *o2del* denotes baseline oxygen delivery. We regress *fate* against *race* and *o2del* using model (5.55).

3 Missing values are represented in Stata by a period; "*o2del* ==." is true when *o2del* is missing.

4 We regress *fate* against *race*, *o2del1* and *o2mis* using model (5.56).

5.33. Additional Reading

Breslow and Day (1980) provide additional breadth and depth on logistic regression in general and the analysis of the Ille-et-Vilaine data set in particular. They also provide an excellent presentation of classical methods for case-control studies.

Hosmer and Lemeshow (1989) is another standard reference work on logistic regression. It provides an extensive discussion of model fitting, goodness-of-fit tests, residual analysis, and influence analysis for logistic regression.

Marini and Wheeler (1997) provide a good overview of the biology and treatment of acute pulmonary disease.

Dupont and Plummer (1999) explain how to derive an exact confidence interval for the odds ratio from a 2×2 case-control study.

Hosmer and Lemeshow (1980) is the original reference for the Hosmer–Lemeshow goodness-of-fit test.

Mantel and Haenszel (1959) is another classic original reference that is discussed by many authors, including Pagano and Gauvreau (2000).

Pregibon (1981) is the original reference for the $\Delta\hat{\beta}_j$ influence statistic.

Tuyns et al. (1977) is the original reference on the Ille-et-Vilaine study.

Robins et al. (1986) derived the confidence interval for the Mantel–Haenszel odds ratio given in equation (5.7).

5.34. Exercises

1 In Section 5.21 we said that β_1 is the log odds ratio for cancer associated with alcohol among non-smokers, β_2 is the log odds ratio for cancer associated with smoking among non-drinkers, $\beta_1 + \beta_3$ is the log odds ratio for cancer associated with alcohol among smokers, $\beta_2 + \beta_3$ is the log odds ratio for cancer associated with smoking among drinkers, and $\beta_1 + \beta_2 + \beta_3$ is the log odds ratio for cancer associated with people who both smoke and drink compared to those who do neither. Write down the log odds for the appropriate numerator and denominator groups for each of these odds ratios. Subtract the denominator log odds from the numerator log odds to show that these statements are all true.

The following exercises are based on a study by Scholer et al. (1997). This was a nested case-control study obtained from a cohort of children age 0 through 4 years in Tennessee between January 1, 1991 and December 31, 1995. Case patients consist of all cohort members who suffered injury deaths. Control patients were frequency matched to case patients by birth year. The data set that you will need for these exercises is posted on my web site and is called *5.ex.InjuryDeath.dta*. The variables in this file are

$byear$ = year of birth,

$$injflag = \begin{cases} 1: \text{if subject died of injuries} \\ 0: \text{otherwise,} \end{cases}$$

$$pnclate = \begin{cases} 1: \text{if no prenatal care was received in the first four months} \\ \quad\quad \text{of pregnancy} \\ 0: \text{if such care was given, or if information is missing,} \end{cases}$$

$$illegit = \begin{cases} 1: \text{if born out of wedlock} \\ 0: \text{otherwise.} \end{cases}$$

2 Calculate the Mantel–Haenszel estimate of the birth-year adjusted odds ratio for injury death among children with unmarried mothers compared to those with married mothers. Test the homogeneity of this odds ratio across birth-year strata. Is it reasonable to estimate a common odds ratio across these strata?

3 Using logistic regression, calculate the odds ratio for injury death of children with unmarried mothers compared to married mothers, adjusted for birth year. What is the 95% confidence interval for this odds ratio?

4 Fit a multiplicative model of the effect of illegitimacy and prenatal care on injury death adjusted for birth year. Complete the following table.

(Recall that for rare events the odds ratio is an excellent estimate of the corresponding relative risk.)

Numerator of relative risk	Denominator of relative risk	Relative risk	95% confidence interval
Unmarried mother	Married mother		
Inadequate prenatal care	Adequate prenatal care		
Married mother	Unmarried mother		

5 Add an interaction term to your model in question 4 for the effect of being illegitimate and not having adequate prenatal care. Complete the following table.

Numerator of relative risk	Denominator of relative risk	Relative risk	95% confidence interval
Married mother without prenatal care	Married mother with prenatal care		
Unmarried mother with prenatal care	Married mother with prenatal care		
Unmarried mother without prenatal care	Married mother with prenatal care		
Unmarried mother without prenatal care	Unmarried mother with prenatal care		
Unmarried mother without prenatal care	Married mother without prenatal care		

6 Are your models in questions 4 and 5 nested? Derive the difference in deviance between them. Is this difference significant? If you were writing a paper on the effects of illegitimacy and adequate prenatal care on the risk of injury death, which model would you use?

7 Generate a squared residual plot similar to Figure 5.1 only using model (5.38). What does this plot tell you about the adequacy of this model?

6

Introduction to Survival Analysis

Survival analysis is concerned with prospective studies of patients. We start with a cohort of patients and then follow them forwards in time to determine some clinical outcome. The covariates in a survival analysis are treatments or attributes of the patient when they are first recruited. Follow-up continues for each patient until either some event of interest occurs, the study ends, or further observation becomes impossible. The response variables in a survival analysis consist of the patient's fate and length of follow-up at the end of the study. A critical aspect of survival analysis is that the outcome of interest may not occur to all patients during follow-up. For such patients, we know only that this event did not occur while the patient was being followed. We do not know whether or not it will occur at some later time.

6.1. Survival and Cumulative Mortality Functions

Suppose we have a cohort of n patients who we wish to follow. Let

t_i be the time that the ith person dies,

$m[t]$ be the number of patients for whom $t < t_i$, and

$d[t]$ be the number of patients for whom $t_i \leq t$.

Then $m[t]$ is the number of patients who we know survived beyond time t while $d[t]$ is the number who are known to have died by this time. The **survival function** is

$S[t] = \Pr[t_i > t] =$ the probability of surviving until at least time t.

The **cumulative mortality function** is

$D[t] = \Pr[t_i \leq t] =$ the probability of dying by time t.

If t_i is known for all members of the cohort we can estimate $S(t)$ and $D(t)$ by

$\hat{S}[t] = m[t]/n$, the proportion of subjects who are alive at time t, and

$\hat{D}[t] = d[t]/n$, the proportion of subjects who have died by time t.

Table 6.1. Survival and mortality in the Ibuprofen in Sepsis study. In this study, calculating the proportion of patients who have survived a given number of days is facilitated by the fact that all patients were followed until death or 30 days, and no patients were lost to follow-up before death.

Days since entry t	Number of patients alive $m[t]$	Number of deaths since entry $d[t]$	Proportion alive $\hat{S}[t] = m[t]/n$	Proportion dead $\hat{D}[t] = d[t]/n$
0	455	0	1.00	0.00
1	431	24	0.95	0.05
2	416	39	0.91	0.09
.	.	.	.	.
.	.	.	.	.
.	.	.	.	.
28	284	171	0.62	0.38
29	282	173	0.62	0.38
30	279	176	0.61	0.39

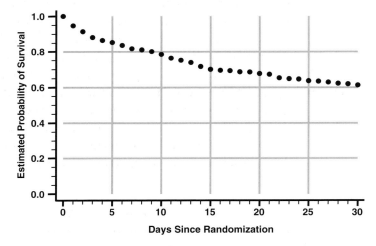

Figure 6.1   Estimated survival function $\hat{S}[t]$ for patients in the Ibuprofen in Sepsis trial. In this study all patients were followed until death or thirty days. Hence, $S[t]$ is estimated by the number of patients alive at time t divided by the total number of study subjects.

For example, Table 6.1 shows the values of $\hat{S}[t]$ and $\hat{D}[t]$ for patients from the Ibuprofen in Sepsis study. Figure 6.1 shows a plot of the survival function for this study.

Often the outcome of interest is some morbid event rather than death, and t_i is the time that the ith patient suffers this event. In this case, $S[t]$ is called the **disease free survival curve** and is the probability of surviving until time t without suffering this event. $D[t]$ is called the **cumulative morbidity curve** and is the probability of suffering the event of interest by time t. The equations used to estimate morbidity and mortality curves are the same.

6.2. Right Censored Data

In clinical studies, patients are typically recruited over a recruitment interval and then followed for an additional period of time (see Figure 6.2). Patients are followed forward in time until some event of interest, say death, occurs. For each patient, the follow-up interval runs from her recruitment until her death or the end of the study. Patients who are alive at the end of follow-up are said to be **right censored**. This means that we know that they survived their follow-up interval but do not know how much longer they lived thereafter (further to the right on the survival graph). In survival studies we are usually concerned with elapsed time since recruitment rather than calendar time. Figure 6.3 shows the same patients as in Figure 6.2 only with the x-axis showing time since recruitment. Note that the follow-up time is highly variable, and that some patients are censored before others die. With censored data, the proportion of patients who are known to have died by time t underestimates the true cumulative mortality by this time. This is because some patients may die after their censoring times but before time t. In the next section, we will introduce a method of calculating the survival function that provides unbiased estimates from censored survival data. Patients who are censored are also said to be **lost to follow-up**.

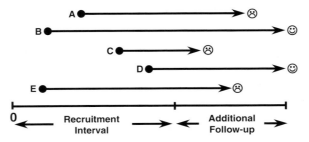

Figure 6.2   Schematic diagram showing the time of recruitment and length of follow-up for five patients in a hypothetical clinical trial. The ☹ and ☺ symbols denote death or survival at the end of follow-up, respectively. The length of follow-up can vary widely in these studies. Note that patient E, who dies, has a longer follow-up time than patient D, who survives.

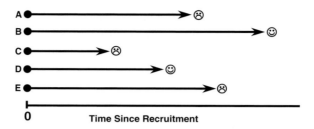

Figure 6.3

Figure 6.2 is redrawn with the x-axis denoting time since recruitment. Note that patient D is censored before patients A and E die. Such censoring must be taken into account when estimating the survival function since some censored patients may die after their follow-up ends.

6.3. Kaplan–Meier Survival Curves

Suppose that we have censored survival data on a cohort of patients. We divide the follow-up into short time intervals, say days, that are small enough that few patients die in any one interval. Let

n_i be the number of patients known to be at risk at the beginning of the ith day, and

d_i be the number of patients who die on day i.

Then for the patients alive at the beginning of the ith day, the estimated probability of surviving the day given that d_i of them will die is

$$p_i = \frac{n_i - d_i}{n_i}. \tag{6.1}$$

The probability that a patient survives the first t days is the joint probability of surviving days $1, 2, \ldots, t-1$, and t. This probability is estimated by

$$\hat{S}[t] = p_1 p_2 p_3 \cdots p_t.$$

Note that $p_i = 1$ on all days when no deaths are observed. Hence, if t_k denotes the kth death day then

$$\hat{S}(t) = \prod_{\{k : t_k < t\}} p_k. \tag{6.2}$$

This estimate is the **Kaplan–Meier survival function** (Kaplan and Meier, 1958). It is also sometimes referred to as the **product limit survival function**. The **Kaplan–Meier cumulative mortality function** is

$$\hat{D}[t] = 1 - \hat{S}[t]. \tag{6.3}$$

The Kaplan–Meier survival and mortality functions avoid bias that might be induced by censored patients because patients censored before the kth day are not included in the denominator of equation (6.1).

Equations (6.2) and (6.3) are also used to estimate disease free survival and cumulative morbidity curves. The only difference is that n_i is now the number of patients who are known to have not suffered the event by the beginning of the ith day, and d_i is the number of these patients who suffer the event on day i.

Tabulated values of t_j, n_j, d_j, and $\hat{S}[t_j]$ are often called **life tables**. These tables are typically given for times t_i at which patients die or are censored. This term is slightly old fashioned but is still used.

6.4. An Example: Genetic Risk of Recurrent Intracerebral Hemorrhage

O'Donnell et al. (2000) have studied the effect of the apolipoprotein E gene on the risk of recurrent lobar intracerebral hemorrhage in patients who have survived such a hemorrhage. Follow-up was obtained for 70 patients who had survived a lobar intracerebral hemorrhage and whose genotype was known. There are three common alleles for the apolipoprotein E gene: $\varepsilon 2$, $\varepsilon 3$, and $\varepsilon 4$. The genotype of all 70 patients was composed of these three alleles. Patients were classified as either being homozygous for $\varepsilon 3$ (Group 1), or as having at least one of the other two alleles (Group 2). Table 6.2 shows the follow-up for these patients. There were four recurrent hemorrhages among the 32 patients in Group 1 and 14 hemorrhages among the 38 patients in Group 2. Figure 6.4 shows the Kaplan–Meier disease free survival function for these two groups of patients. These curves were derived

Table 6.2. Length of follow-up and fate for patients in the study by O'Donnell et al. (2000). Patients are divided into two groups defined by their genotype for the apolipoprotein E gene. Follow-up times marked with an asterisk indicate patients who had a recurrent lobar intracerebral hemorrhage at the end of follow-up. All other patients did not suffer this event during follow-up

Length of follow-up (months)									
Homozygous $\varepsilon 3/\varepsilon 3$ (Group 1)									
0.23*	1.051	1.511	3.055*	8.082	12.32*	14.69	16.72	18.46	18.66
19.55	19.75	24.77*	25.56	25.63	26.32	26.81	32.95	33.05	34.99
35.06	36.24	37.03	37.75	38.97	39.16	42.22	42.41	45.24	46.29
47.57	53.88								
At least one $\varepsilon 2$ or $\varepsilon 4$ allele (Group 2)									
1.38	1.413*	1.577	1.577*	3.318*	3.515*	3.548*	4.041	4.632	4.764*
8.444	9.528*	10.61	10.68	11.86	13.27	13.60	15.57*	17.84	18.04
18.46	18.46	19.15*	20.11	20.27	20.47	24.87*	28.09*	30.52	33.61*
37.52*	38.54	40.61	42.78	42.87*	43.27	44.65	46.88		

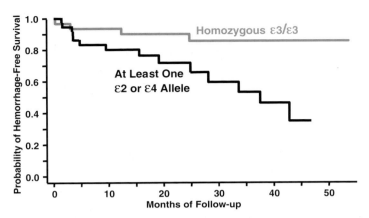

Figure 6.4

Kaplan–Meier estimates of hemorrhage-free survival functions for patients who had previously survived a lobular intracerebral hemorrhage. Patients are subdivided according to their apolipoprotein E genotype. Patients who were homozygous for the $\varepsilon3$ allele of this gene had a much better prognosis than other patients (O'Donnell et al., 2000).

using equation (6.2). For example, suppose that we wish to calculate the disease free survival function at 15 months for the 32 patients in Group 1. Three hemorrhages occurred in this group before 15 months at 0.23, 3.055 and 12.32 months. Therefore,

$$\hat{S}[15] = p_1 p_2 p_3 = \prod_{k=1}^{3} p_k,$$

where p_k is the probability of avoiding a hemorrhage on the kth day on which hemorrhages occurred. At 12.3 months there are 27 patients at risk; two of the original 32 have already had hemorrhages and three have been censored. Hence, $p_3 = (27-1)/27 = 0.9629$. Similarly, $p_1 = (32-1)/32 = 0.9688$ and $p_2 = (29-1)/29 = 0.9655$. Therefore, $\hat{S}[15] = 0.9688 \times 0.9655 \times 0.9629 = 0.9007$. $\hat{S}[t]$ is constant and equals 0.9007 from $t = 12.32$ until just before the next hemorrhage in Group 1, which occurs at time 24.77.

In Figure 6.4, the estimated disease free survival functions are constant over days when no hemorrhages are observed and drop abruptly on days when hemorrhages occur. If the time interval is short enough that there is rarely more than one death per interval, then the height of the drop at each death day indicates the size of the cohort remaining on that day. The accuracy of the survival curve gets less as we move towards the right, as it is based on fewer and fewer patients. Large drops in these curves are warnings of decreasing accuracy of our survival estimates due to diminishing numbers of study subjects.

If there is no censoring and there are q death days before time t then

$$\hat{S}(t) = \left(\frac{n_1 - d_1}{n_1}\right)\left(\frac{n_2 - d_2}{n_1 - d_1}\right)\cdots\left(\frac{n_q - d_q}{n_{q1} - d_{q1}}\right)$$
$$= \frac{n_q - d_q}{n_1} = \frac{m(t)}{n}.$$

Hence the Kaplan–Meier survival curve reduces to the proportion of patients alive at time t if there is no censoring.

6.5. 95% Confidence Intervals for Survival Functions

The variance of $\hat{S}(t)$ is estimated by Greenwood's formula (Kalbfleisch and Prentice, 1980), which is

$$s^2_{\hat{S}(t)} = \hat{S}(t)^2 \sum_{\{k:\, t_k < t\}} \frac{d_k}{n_k(n_k - d_k)}. \tag{6.4}$$

A 95% confidence interval for $S(t)$ could be estimated by $\hat{S}(t) \pm 1.96 s_{\hat{S}(t)}$. However, this interval is unsatisfactory when $\hat{S}(t)$ is near 0 or 1. This is because $\hat{S}(t)$ has a skewed distribution near these extreme values. The true survival curve is never less than zero or greater than one, and we want our confidence intervals to never exceed these bounds. For this reason we calculate the statistic $\log[-\log[\hat{S}(t)]]$, which has variance

$$\hat{\sigma}^2(t) = \frac{\displaystyle\sum_{\{k:\, t_k < t\}} \frac{d_k}{n_k(n_k - d_k)}}{\left[\displaystyle\sum_{\{k:\, t_k < t\}} \log\left[\frac{(n_k - d_k)}{d_k}\right]\right]^2} \tag{6.5}$$

(Kalbfleisch and Prentice, 1980). A 95% confidence interval for this statistic is

$$\log[-\log[\hat{S}(t)]] \pm 1.96\hat{\sigma}(t). \tag{6.6}$$

Exponentiating equation (6.6) twice gives a 95% confidence interval for $\hat{S}(t)$ of

$$\hat{S}(t)^{\exp(\mp 1.96\hat{\sigma}(t))}. \tag{6.7}$$

Equation (6.7) provides reasonable confidence intervals for the entire range of values of $\hat{S}(t)$. Figure 6.5 shows these confidence intervals plotted for the hemorrhage-free survival curve of patients with an $\varepsilon 2$ or $\varepsilon 4$ allele in

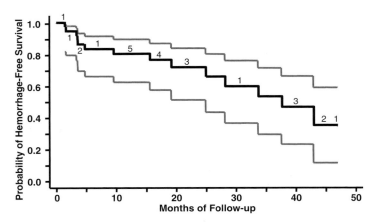

Figure 6.5
The thick black curve is the Kaplan–Meier survival function for patients with an $\varepsilon 2$ or $\varepsilon 4$ allele in the study by O'Donnell et al. (2000). The gray lines give 95% confidence intervals for this curve. The digits near the survival curve indicate numbers of patients who are lost to follow-up. Note that the confidence intervals widen with increasing time. This indicates the reduced precision of the estimated survival function due to the reduced numbers of patients with lengthy follow-up.

O'Donnell et al. (2000). If we return to the homozygous $\varepsilon 3$ patients in Section 6.4 and let $t = 15$ then

$$\sum_{\{k\,:\,t_k<15\}} \frac{d_k}{n_k(n_k - d_k)} = \frac{1}{32 \times 31} + \frac{1}{29 \times 28} + \frac{1}{27 \times 26} = 0.003\,66 \text{ and}$$

$$\sum_{\{k\,:\,t_k<15\}} \log\left[\frac{(n_k - d_k)}{d_k}\right] = \log\left[\frac{32-1}{32}\right] + \log\left[\frac{29-1}{29}\right] + \log\left[\frac{27-1}{27}\right]$$

$$= -0.104\,58.$$

Therefore, $\hat{\sigma}^2(15) = 0.003\,66/(-0.104\,58)^2 = 0.335$, and a 95% confidence interval for $\hat{S}[15]$ is $0.9007^{\exp(\mp 1.96 \times \sqrt{0.335})} = (0.722, 0.967)$. This interval remains constant from the previous Group 1 hemorrhage recurrence at time 12.32 until just before the next at time 24.77.

6.6. Cumulative Mortality Function

The 95% confidence interval for the cumulative mortality function $D[t] = 1 - S(t)$ is estimated by

$$1 - \hat{S}(t)^{\exp(\pm 1.96 \hat{\sigma}(t))}. \tag{6.8}$$

Figure 6.6 shows the cumulative morbidity function for the homozygous $\varepsilon 3/\varepsilon 3$ patients of O'Donnell et al. (2000). Plotting cumulative morbidity

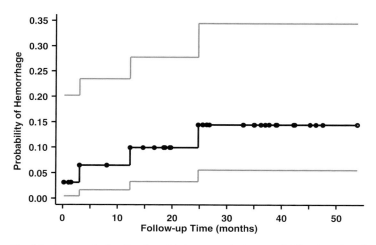

Figure 6.6

The black curve is the Kaplan–Meier cumulative morbidity function for homozygous $\varepsilon3/\varepsilon3$ patients from the study of O'Donnell et al. (2000). The First black dot on each horizontal segment of this line indicates a time that a patient suffered a hemorrhage. Other dots indicate censoring times. The gray lines give 95% confidence intervals for this morbidity curve.

rather than disease-free survival is a good idea when the total morbidity is low. This is because the y-axis can be plotted on a larger scale and need only extend up to the maximum observed morbidity. An alternative to Figure 6.6 would have been to plot the hemorrhage free survival curve with the y-axis ranging from 0.65 to 1.00. Although this would achieve the same magnification of the y-axis as Figure 6.6, it tends to exaggerate the extent of the morbidity, particularly if the reader does not notice that the y-axis starts at 0.65.

6.7. Censoring and Bias

A Kaplan–Meier survival curve will provide an appropriate estimate of the true survival curve as long as
1 the patients are representative of the underlying population, and
2 patients who are censored have the same risk of subsequently suffering the event of interest as patients who are not.
If censored patients are more likely to die than uncensored patients with equal follow-up, then our survival estimates will be biased. Such bias can occur for many reasons, not the least of which is that dead patients do not return for follow-up visits.

Survival curves are often derived for some endpoint other than death. In this case, some deaths may be treated as censoring events. For example, if the event of interest is developing of breast cancer, then we may treat death due to heart disease as a censoring event. This is reasonable as long as there is no relationship between heart disease and breast cancer. That is, when we censor a woman who died of heart disease, we are assuming that she would have had the same subsequent risk of breast cancer as other women if she had lived. If we were studying lung cancer and smoking, however, then treating death from heart disease as a censoring event would bias our results since smoking increases the risk of both lung cancer morbidity and cardiovascular mortality.

6.8. Logrank Test

Suppose that two treatments have survival functions $S_1[t]$ and $S_2[t]$. We wish to know whether these functions are equal. One approach that we could take is to test whether $S_1[t_0] = S_2[t_0]$ at some specific time point t_0. The problem with doing this is that it is difficult to know how to chose t_0. It is tempting to choose the value of t_0 where the estimated survival functions are most different. However, this results in underestimating the true P value of the test, and hence, overestimating the statistical significance of the difference in survival curves. A better approach is to test the null hypothesis

$$H_0: \ S_1[t] = S_2[t] \text{ for all } t.$$

Suppose that on the kth death day there are n_{1k} and n_{2k} patients at risk on treatments 1 and 2 and that d_{1k} and d_{2k} deaths occur in these groups on this day. Let $N_k = n_{1k} + n_{2k}$ and $D_k = d_{1k} + d_{2k}$ denote the total number of patients at risk and observed deaths on the kth death day. Then the observed death rate on the kth death day is D_k/N_k. If the null hypothesis H_0 is true, then the expected number of deaths among patients on treatment 1 given that D_k deaths occurred in both groups is

$$E[d_{1k} \mid D_k] = n_{1k}(D_k/N_k). \tag{6.9}$$

The greater the difference between d_{1k} and $E[d_{1k} \mid D_k]$, the greater the evidence that the null hypothesis is false.

Mantel (1966) proposed the following test of this hypothesis. For each death day, create a 2 × 2 table of the number of patients who die or survive on each treatment (see Table 6.3). Then perform a Mantel–Haenszel test on these tables. In other words, apply equation (5.5) to strata defined by the

Table 6.3. To test the null hypothesis of equal survivorship we form the following 2×2 table for each day on which a death occurs. This table gives the numbers of patients at risk and the number of deaths for each treatment on that day. We then perform a Mantel–Haenszel chi-squared test on these tables (see text).

k^{th} death day	Treatment 1	Treatment 2	Total
Died	d_{1k}	d_{2k}	D_k
Survived	$n_{1k} - d_{1k}$	$n_{2k} - d_{2k}$	$N_k - D_k$
Total at risk at the start of the day	n_{1k}	n_{2k}	N_k

different death days. This gives

$$\chi_1^2 = \left(\left| \sum d_{1k} - \sum E[d_{1k} \mid D_k] \right| - 0.5 \right)^2 \Big/ \sum \text{var}[d_{1k} \mid D_k], \qquad (6.10)$$

which has a chi-squared distribution with one degree of freedom if H_0 is true. In equation (6.10) the estimated variance of d_{1k} given a total of D_k deaths and assuming that H_0 is true is

$$\text{var}[d_{1k} \mid D_k] = \frac{n_{1k} n_{2k} D_k (N_k - D_k)}{N_k^2 (N_k - 1)}. \qquad (6.11)$$

Equation (6.11) is equation (5.4) rewritten in the notation of this section.

In the intracerebral hemorrhage study the tenth hemorrhage among both groups occurs at time 12.32 months. Prior to this time, two patients have hemorrhages and three patients are lost to follow-up in Group 1 (the homozygous patients). In Group 2, seven patients have hemorrhages and eight patients are lost to follow-up before time 12.32. Therefore, just prior to the tenth hemorrhage there are $n_{1,10} = 32 - 2 - 3 = 27$ patients at risk in Group 1, and $n_{2,10} = 38 - 7 - 8 = 23$ patients are at risk in Group 2, giving a total of $N_{10} = 27 + 23 = 50$ patients at risk of hemorrhage. The tenth hemorrhage occurs in Group 1 and there are no hemorrhages in Group 2 at the same time. Therefore $d_{1,10} = 1$, $d_{2,10} = 0$ and $D_{10} = 1 + 0 = 1$. Under the null hypothesis H_0 of equal risk in both groups,

$$E[d_{1,10} \mid D_{10}] = n_{1,10}(D_{10}/N_{10}) = 27 \times 1/50 = 0.54$$

and $\text{var}[d_{1,10} \mid D_{10}] = \dfrac{n_{1,10} n_{2,10} D_{10}(N_{10} - D_{10})}{N_{10}^2(N_{10} - 1)} = \dfrac{27 \times 23 \times 1 \times 49}{50^2 \times (50 - 1)}$

$= 0.2484.$

Performing similar calculations for all of the other recurrence times and summing over recurrence days gives that $\sum E[d_{1k} \mid D_k] = 9.277$ and

$\sum \text{var}[d_{1k} \mid D_k] = 4.433$. There are a total of $\sum d_{1k} = 4$ recurrences in Group 1. Therefore, equation (6.10) gives us $\chi_1^2 = (|4 - 9.277| - 0.5)^2 / 4.433 = 5.15$. Without the continuity correction this statistic equals 6.28. The probability that a chi-squared statistic with one degree of freedom exceeds 6.28 equals 0.01. Hence, Group 1 patients have significantly fewer recurrent hemorrhages than Group 2 patients.

Equation (6.10) is sometimes called the **Mantel–Haenszel test for survival data**. It was renamed the **logrank test** by Peto and Peto (1972) who studied its mathematical properties. If the time interval is short enough so that $d_k \leq 1$ for each interval, then the test of H_0 depends only on the order in which the deaths occur and not on their time of occurrence. It is in this sense that this statistic is a rank order test. It can also be shown that the logrank test is a score test (see Section 4.9.4). Today, the most commonly used name for this statistic is the logrank test.

It should also be noted that we could also perform a simple 2×2 chi-squared test on the total number of recurrences in the two patient groups (see Section 4.19.4). However, differences in survivorship are affected by time to death as well as the number of deaths, and the simple test does not take time into consideration. Consider the hypothetical survival curves shown in Figure 6.7. These curves are quite different, with Group 1 patients dying sooner than Group 2 patients. However, the overall mortality at the end of follow-up is the same in both groups. The 2×2 chi-squared test would not be able to detect this difference in survivorship. For a sufficiently large study, the logrank test would be significant.

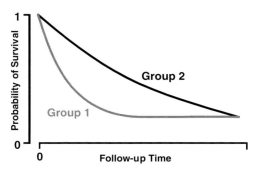

Figure 6.7   In these hypothetical survival curves the total mortality at the end of follow-up is the same in both groups. Mortality, however, tends to happen sooner in Group 1 than in Group 2. This difference in time to death may be detected by the logrank test but will not be detected by a 2×2 chi-squared test of overall mortality in the two groups.

6.9. Using Stata to Derive Survival Functions and the Logrank Test

The following log file and comments illustrate how to perform the preceding analyses with Stata.

```
. * 6.9. Hemorrhage.do
. *
. * Plot Kaplan—Meier Survival functions for recurrent lobar intracerebral
. * hemorrhage in patients who are, or are not, homozygous for the epsilon3
. * allele of the apolipoprotein E gene (O'Donnell et al. 2000).
. *
. use   C:\WDDtext\6.9.Hemorrhage.dta, clear
. summarize                                                                    {1}

Variable |    Obs         Mean     Std. Dev.        Min          Max
---------+-----------------------------------------------------------------
genotype |     70    .5428571     .5017567          0            1
    time |     71    22.50051     15.21965    .2299795     53.88091
   recur |     71    .2676056     .4458618          0            1

. table genotype recur, col row                                               {2}
------------+-------------------
Apolipopro |
tein E     |    Recurrence
Genotype   |   No    yes   Total
------------+-------------------
     e3/e3 |   28     4      32
e2+ or e4+ |   24    14      38
     Total |   52    18      70
------------+-------------------

. stset   time, failure(recur)                                                {3}
    failure event:  recur ~= 0 & recur ~= .
obs. time interval:  (0, time]
 exit on or before:  failure
--------------------------------------------------------------------
      71  total obs.
       0  exclusions
--------------------------------------------------------------------
      71  obs. remaining, representing
      19  failures in single record/single failure data
```

```
1597.536   total analysis time at risk, at risk from t =        0
                              earliest observed entry t =        0
                              last observed exit t = 53.88091
. set textsize 120
. *
. * Graph survival function by genotype
. *
. sts graph, by(genotype) ylabel(0 .2 to 1) ytick(.1 .3  to .9)            {4}
> xlabel(0 10 to 50) xtick(5 15 to 45)
> l1title("Probability of Hemorrhage-Free Survival")
> b2title("Months of Follow-up") gap(2) noborder
```
                                                    {Graph omitted, see Figure 6.4}
```
          failure_d: recur
  analysis time_t: time
. *
. * List survival statistics
. *
. sts list, by(genotype)                                                  {5}
          failure_d: recur
  analysis time_t: time
```

| | Beg. | | Net | Survivor | Std. | | |
Time	Total	Fail	Lost	Function	Error	[95% Conf. Int.]	
e3/e3							
.23	32	1	0	0.9688	0.0308	0.7982	0.9955
1.051	31	0	1	0.9688	0.0308	0.7982	0.9955
1.511	30	0	1	0.9688	0.0308	0.7982	0.9955
3.055	29	1	0	0.9353	0.0443	0.7651	0.9835
8.082	28	0	1	0.9353	0.0443	0.7651	0.9835
12.32	27	1	0	0.9007	0.0545	0.7224	0.9669
						{Output omitted}	
24.77	20	1	0	0.8557	0.0679	0.6553	0.9441
						{Output omitted}	
53.88	1	0	1	0.8557	0.0679	0.6553	0.9441
e2+ or e4+							
1.38	38	0	1	1.0000	.	.	.
1.413	37	1	0	0.9730	0.0267	0.8232	0.9961
1.577	36	1	1	0.9459	0.0372	0.8007	0.9862
3.318	34	1	0	0.9181	0.0453	0.7672	0.9728
3.515	33	1	0	0.8903	0.0518	0.7335	0.9574

3.548	32	1	0	0.8625	0.0571	0.7005	0.9404
4.041	31	0	1	0.8625	0.0571	0.7005	0.9404
4.632	30	0	1	0.8625	0.0571	0.7005	0.9404
4.764	29	1	0	0.8327	0.0624	0.6646	0.9213
8.444	28	0	1	0.8327	0.0624	0.6646	0.9213
9.528	27	1	0	0.8019	0.0673	0.6280	0.9005
10.61	26	0	1	0.8019	0.0673	0.6280	0.9005
10.68	25	0	1	0.8019	0.0673	0.6280	0.9005
11.86	24	0	1	0.8019	0.0673	0.6280	0.9005
13.27	23	0	1	0.8019	0.0673	0.6280	0.9005

{Output omitted}

| 46.88 | 1 | 0 | 1 | 0.3480 | 0.1327 | 0.1174 | 0.5946 |

```
. *
. * Graph survival functions by genotype with 95% confidence intervals.
. * Show loss to follow-up.
. *
. sts graph, by(genotype) lost gwood ylabel(0 .2 to 1) ytick(.1 .3 to .9)     {6}
> xlabel(0 10 to 50) xtick(5 15 to 45)
> l1title("Probability of Hemorrhage-Free Survival")
> b2title("Months of Follow-up") gap(2) noborder
```
{Graph omitted, See Figure 6.5}

```
        failure_d: recur
  analysis time_t: time

. *
. * Calculate cumulative morbidity for homozygous epsilon3 patients
. * together with 95% confidence intervals for this morbidity.
. *
. sts generate s0 = s if  genotype == 0                                       {7}

. sts generate lb_s0 = lb(s) if genotype == 0

. sts generate ub_s0 = ub(s) if genotype == 0

. generate  d0 = 1 - s0                                                        {8}
(39 missing values generated)

. generate lb_d0 = 1 - ub_s0                                                   {9}
(39 missing values generated)

. generate ub_d0 = 1 - lb_s0
(39 missing values generated)
```

```
. *
. * Plot cumulative morbidity for homozygous epsilon3 patients.
. * Show 95% confidence intervals and loss to follow-up
. *
. graph lb_d0 ub_d0 d0 time, symbol(ii0) connect(JJJ) ylabel(0 0.05 to 0.35)   {10}
> xlabel(0 10 to 50) xtick(5 15 to 45) l1title("Probability of Hemorrhage") gap(3)
```
                                  {Graph omitted, see Figure 6.6}

```
. *
. * Compare survival functions for the two genotypes using the logrank test.
. *
. sts test genotype                                                           {11}

       failure_d: recur
  analysis time_t: time

Log-rank test for equality of survivor functions
-------------------------------------------------
           | Events
genotype   | observed          expected
-----------+------------------------------
e3/e3      |      4                9.28
e2+ or e4+ |     14                8.72
-----------+------------------------------
Total      |     18               18.00
               chi2(1)  =        6.28
               Pr>chi2  =      0.0122
```

Comments

1 The hemorrhage data set contains three variables on 71 patients. The variable *time* denotes length of follow-up in months; *recur* records whether the patient had a hemorrhage (*recur* = 1) or was censored (*recur* = 0) at the end of follow-up; *genotype* divides the patients into two groups determined by their genotype. The value of *genotype* is missing on one patient who did not give a blood sample.

2 This command tabulates study subjects by hemorrhage recurrence and genotype. The value labels of these two variables are shown.

3 This *stset* command specifies that the data set contains survival data. Each patient's follow-up time is denoted by *time*; her fate at the end of follow-up is denoted by *recur*. Stata interprets *recur* = 0 to mean that the patient is censored and *recur* ≠ 0 to mean that she suffered the event of interest at exit. A *stset* command must be specified

before other survival commands such as *sts list, sts graph, sts test* or *sts generate.*

4 The *sts graph* command plots Kaplan–Meier survival curves; *by (genotype)* specifies that separate plots will be generated for each value of *genotype.* By default, the *sts graph* command does not title the *y*-axis and titles the *x*-axis "*analysis time*". The *l1title* and *b2title* options provides the titles "*Probability of Hemorrhage-Free Survival*" and "*Months of Follow-up*" for the *y*- and *x*-axes, respectively. The *noborder* option prevents a border from being drawn on the top and right side of the graph. The resulting graph is similar to Figure 6.4.

5 This command lists the values of the survival functions that are plotted by the preceding command. The *by(genotype)* option specifies that a separate survival function is to be calculated for each value of *genotype.* The number of patients at risk prior to each failure or loss to follow-up is also given, together with the 95% confidence interval for the survival function. The highlighted values agree with the hand calculations in Sections 6.4 and 6.5.

6 Stata also permits users to graph confidence bounds for $\hat{S}(t)$ and indicate the number of subjects lost to follow-up. This is done with the *gwood* and *lost* options, respectively. In this example, a separate plot is generated for each value of genotype. Figure 6.5 is similar to one of these two plots.

7 The *sts generate* command creates regular Stata variables from survival analyses. Here, $s0 = s$ defines $s0$, to equal the survival function for patients with genotype $= 0$ (i.e. homozygous $\varepsilon3/\varepsilon3$ patients). In the next two commands $lb\_s0 = lb(s)$ and $ub\_s0 = ub(s)$ define lb_s0 and ub_s0 to be the lower and upper bounds of the 95% confidence interval for $s0$.

8 The variable $d0$ is the cumulative morbidity function (see equation (6.3)).

9 The variables lb_d0 and ub_d0 are the lower and upper bounds of the 95% confidence interval for $d0$. Note the lower bound equals one minus the upper bound for $s0$ and vice versa.

10 This command produces a graph that is similar to Figure 6.6. The *J* symbol in the *connect* option produces the stepwise connections that are needed for a morbidity or survival function. The *O* symbol in the *symbol* option produces dots at times when patients have hemorrhages or are censored.

11 Perform a logrank test for the equality of survivor functions in patient groups defined by different values of *genotype.* In this example, patients who are homozygous for the $\varepsilon3$ allele are compared to other patients. The highlighted chi-squared statistic and *P* value agree with our hand calculations for the uncorrected test.

6.10. Logrank Test for Multiple Patient Groups

The logrank test generalizes to allow the comparison of survival in several groups. The test statistic has an asymptotic chi-squared distribution with one degree of freedom less than the number of patient groups being compared. In Stata, these groups are defined by the number of distinct levels taken by the variable specified in the *sts test* command. If, in the hemorrhage study, a variable named *geno6* indicated each of the six possible genotypes that can result from three alleles for one gene, then *sts test geno6* would compare the six survival curves for these groups of patients; the test statistic would have five degrees of freedom.

6.11. Hazard Functions

Our next topic is the estimation of relative risks in survival studies. Before doing this we need to introduce the concept of a hazard function. Suppose that a patient is alive at time t and that her probability of dying in the next short time interval $(t, t + \Delta t)$ is $\lambda[t]\Delta t$. Then $\lambda[t]$ is said to be the **hazard function** for the patient at time t. In other words

$$\lambda(t) = \frac{\Pr[\text{Patient dies by time } t + \Delta t \mid \text{Patient alive at time } t]}{\Delta t}. \tag{6.12}$$

Of course, both the numerator and denominator of equation (6.12) approach zero as Δt gets very small. However, the ratio of numerator to denominator approaches $\lambda[t]$ as Δt approaches zero. For a very large population,

$$\lambda[t]\Delta t \cong \frac{\text{The number of deaths in the interval } (t, t + \Delta t)}{\text{Number of people alive at time } t}.$$

The hazard function $\lambda[t]$ is the instantaneous rate per unit time at which people are dying at time t; $\lambda[t] = 0$ implies that there is no risk of death and $S[t]$ is flat at time t. Large values of $\lambda[t]$ imply a rapid rate of decline in $S[t]$. The hazard function is related to the survival function through the equation $S[t] = \exp[-\int_0^t \lambda[x]\,dx]$, where $\int_0^t \lambda[x]\,dx$ is the area under the curve $\lambda[t]$ between 0 and t. The simplest hazard function is a constant, which implies that a patients risk of death does not vary with time. If $\lambda[t] = k$, then the area under the curve between 0 and t is kt and the survival function is $S[t] = e^{-kt}$. Examples of constant hazard functions and the corresponding survival curves are given in Figure 6.8.

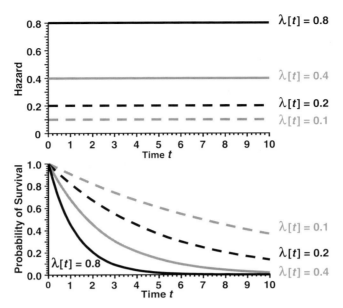

Figure 6.8   The hazard function equals the rate of instantaneous mortality for study subjects. This graph shows the relationship between different constant hazard functions and the associated survival curves. If $\lambda[t] = k$ then $S[t] = \exp[-kt]$. The higher the hazard function the more rapidly the probability of survival drops to zero with increasing time.

6.12. Proportional Hazards

Suppose that $\lambda_0[t]$ and $\lambda_1[t]$ are the hazard functions for patients on control and experimental treatments, respectively. Then these treatments have **proportional hazards** if

$$\lambda_1[t] = R\lambda_0[t]$$

for some constant R. The proportional hazards assumption places no restrictions on the shape of $\lambda_0(t)$ but requires that

$$\lambda_1[t]/\lambda_0[t] = R$$

at all times t. Figure 6.9 provides an artificial example that may help to increase your intuitive understanding of hazard functions, survival functions and the proportional hazards assumption. In this figure, $\lambda_0[t] = 0.1$ when $t = 0$. It decreases linearly until it reaches 0 at $t = 3$; is constant at 0 from $t = 3$ until $t = 6$ and then increases linearly until it reaches 0.1 at $t = 9$. The hazard functions $\lambda_0[t]$, $\lambda_1[t]$, $\lambda_2[t]$, and $\lambda_3[t]$ meet the proportional hazards assumption in that $\lambda_1[t] = 2.5\lambda_0[t]$, $\lambda_2[t] = 5\lambda_0[t]$, and $\lambda_3[t] = 10\lambda_0[t]$.

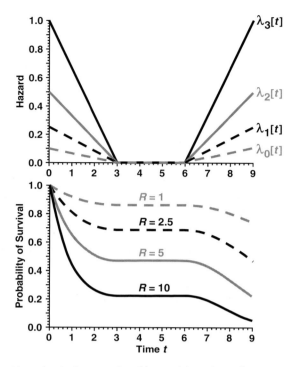

Figure 6.9

Hypothetical example of hazard functions that meet the proportional hazards assumption. Although the hazard functions themselves vary with time the ratio of any two hazard functions is constant. The associated survival functions are shown in the lower panel. The relative risks R of patients with hazards $\lambda_1[t]$, $\lambda_2[t]$, and $\lambda_3[t]$ compared to $\lambda_0[t]$ are given in the lower panel.

The associated survival functions are also shown in Figure 6.9. The fact that these hazard functions all equal zero between 3 and 6 imply that no one may die in this interval. For this reason, the associated survival functions are constant from 3 to 6. Regardless of the shape of the hazard function, the survival curve is always non-increasing, and is always between one and zero. The rate of decrease of the survival curve increases with increasing hazard and with increasing size of the survival function itself.

6.13. Relative Risks and Hazard Ratios

Suppose that the risks of death by time $t + \Delta t$ for patients on control and experimental treatments who are alive at time t are $\lambda_0[t]\Delta t$ and $\lambda_1[t]\Delta t$, respectively. Then the risk of experimental subjects at time t relative to controls is

$$\frac{\lambda_1[t]\Delta t}{\lambda_0[t]\Delta t} = \frac{\lambda_1[t]}{\lambda_0[t]}.$$

If $\lambda_1[t] = R\lambda_0[t]$ at all times, then this relative risk is

$$\frac{\lambda_1[t]}{\lambda_0[t]} = \frac{R\lambda_0[t]}{\lambda_0[t]} = R.$$

Thus, the ratio of two hazard functions can be thought of as an instantaneous relative risk. If the proportional hazards assumption is true, then this hazard ratio remains constant over time and equals the relative risk of experimental subjects compared to controls. In Figure 6.9, the hazard ratios $\lambda_1[t]/\lambda_0[t]$, $\lambda_2[t]/\lambda_0[t]$, and $\lambda_3[t]/\lambda_0[t]$ equal 2.5, 5, and 10, respectively. Therefore, the relative risks of patients with hazard functions $\lambda_1[t]$, $\lambda_2[t]$ and $\lambda_3[t]$ relative to patients with hazard function $\lambda_0[t]$ are 2.5, 5, and 10.

6.14. Proportional Hazards Regression Analysis

Suppose that patients are randomized to an experimental or control therapy. Let

$\lambda_0[t]$ be the hazard function for patients on the control therapy, and

$$x_i = \begin{cases} 1: & \text{if the } i^{\text{th}} \text{ patient receives the experimental therapy} \\ 0: & \text{if she receives the control therapy.} \end{cases}$$

Then the **simple proportional hazards model** assumes that the ith patient has hazard

$$\lambda_i[t] = \lambda_0[t] \exp[\beta x_i], \tag{6.13}$$

where β is an unknown parameter. Note that if the ith patient is on the control therapy then $\beta x_i = 0$ and $\lambda_i[t] = \lambda_0[t]e^0 = \lambda_0[t]$. If she is on the experimental therapy, then $\beta x_i = \beta$ and $\lambda_i[t] = \lambda_0[t]e^\beta$. This model is said to be **semi-nonparametric** in that it makes no assumptions about the shape of the control hazard function $\lambda_0[t]$. Under this model, the relative risk of experimental therapy relative to control therapy is $\lambda_0[t]e^\beta/\lambda_0[t] = e^\beta$. Hence, β is the log relative risk of the experimental therapy relative to the control therapy. Cox (1972) developed a regression method for survival data that uses the proportional hazards model. This method is in many ways similar to logistic regression. It provides an estimate, $\hat{\beta}$, of β together with an estimate, se $[\hat{\beta}]$, of the standard error of $\hat{\beta}$. For large studies $\hat{\beta}$ has an approximately normal distribution. We use these estimates in the same way that we used the analogous estimates from logistic regression. The estimated relative risk of experimental therapy relative to control therapy is

$$\hat{R} = \exp[\hat{\beta}]. \tag{6.14}$$

A 95% confidence interval for this relative risk is

$$\hat{R}\exp[\pm 1.96\text{se}[\hat{\beta}]]. \tag{6.15}$$

The two therapies will be equally efficacious if $R = 1$, or equivalently, if $\beta = 0$. Hence, testing the null hypothesis that $\beta = 0$ is equivalent to testing the null hypothesis of equal treatment efficacy. Under this null hypothesis

$$z = \hat{\beta}/\text{se}[\hat{\beta}] \tag{6.16}$$

has an approximately standard normal distribution. Equations (6.15) and (6.16) are a Wald confidence interval and Wald test, respectively (see Section 4.9.4).

6.15. Hazard Regression Analysis of the Intracerebral Hemorrhage Data

Let $\lambda_i[t]$ be the hemorrhage hazard function for the ith patient in the study of O'Donnell et al. (2000). Let $\lambda_0[t]$ be the hazard for patients who are homozygous for the $\varepsilon 3$ allele, and let

$$x_i = \begin{cases} 1: & \text{if the } i^{\text{th}} \text{ patient has an } \varepsilon 2 \text{ or } \varepsilon 4 \text{ allele} \\ 0: & \text{otherwise.} \end{cases}$$

We will assume the proportional hazards model $\lambda_i[t] = \lambda_0[t]\exp[\beta x_i]$. Performing a hazard regression analysis on these data gives an estimate of $\hat{\beta} = 1.3317$ with a standard error of $\text{se}[\hat{\beta}] = 0.5699$. Therefore, the relative risk of recurrence for patients with an $\varepsilon 2$ or $\varepsilon 4$ allele relative to homozygous $\varepsilon 3/\varepsilon 3$ patients is $\exp[1.3317] = 3.79$. A 95% confidence interval for this relative risk is $3.79\exp[\pm 1.96 \times 0.5699] = (1.2, 12)$. To test the null hypothesis that the two patient groups are at equal risk of recurrence, we calculate $z = 1.3317/0.5699 = 2.34$. The probability that a standard normal random variable is less than -2.34 or more than 2.34 is $P = 0.019$. Hence, the hemorrhage recurrence rate is significantly greater in patients with an $\varepsilon 2$ or $\varepsilon 4$ allele compared with homozygous $\varepsilon 3/\varepsilon 3$ patients. This P value is similar to that obtained from the logrank test, which is testing the same null hypothesis.

6.16. Proportional Hazards Regression Analysis with Stata

The following log file and comments illustrate a simple proportional hazards regression analysis that compares two groups of patients

```
. * 6.16. Hemorrhage.log

. *

. * Perform a proportional hazards regression analysis of recurrent lobar
. * intracerebral hemorrhage in patients who are, or are not, homozygous for
. * the epsilon3 allele of the apolipoprotein E gene (O'Donnell et al., 2000).
. *
. use C:\WDDtext\6.9. Hemorrhage.dta, clear

. stset time, failure(recur)
```
                                                    {Output omitted, see 6.8.Hemorrhage.log}
```
. stcox genotype                                                                    {1}
        failure_d: recur
  analysis time_t: time
```
                                                                          {Output omitted}
```
Cox regression -- no ties

No. of subjects =            70          Number of obs    =            70
No. of failures =            18
Time at risk     = 1596.320341
                                          LR chi2(1)       =          6.61
Log likelihood   =  -63.370953           Prob > chi2      =        0.0102
-----------------------------------------------------------------------------
       _t |
       _d |   Haz. Ratio  Std. Err.     z     P> |z|    [95% Conf. Interval]
----------+------------------------------------------------------------------
 genotype |    3.787366   2.158422   2.337   0.019     1.239473    11.57278    {2}
----------+------------------------------------------------------------------
```

Comments

1 This command fits the proportional hazards regression model

$$\lambda(t, \text{genotype}) = \lambda_0(t) \exp(\beta \times \text{genotype}).$$

That is, we fit model (6.13) using *genotype* as the covariate x_i. A *stset* command must precede the *stcox* command to define the fate and follow-up variables.

2 The *stcox* command outputs the hazard ratio $\exp[\hat{\beta}] = 3.787$ and the associated 95% confidence interval using equation (6.15). This hazard

ratio is the relative risk of patients with an $\varepsilon2$ or $\varepsilon4$ allele compared with homozygous $\varepsilon3/\varepsilon3$ patients. The z statistic is calculated using equation (6.16). Note that the highlighted output agrees with our hand calculations given in the preceding section.

6.17. Tied Failure Times

The most straightforward computational approach to the proportional hazards model can produce biased parameter estimates if a large proportion of the failure times are identical. For this reason, it is best to record failure times as precisely as possible to avoid ties in this variable. If there are extensive ties in the data, there are other approaches which are computationally intensive but which can reduce this bias (see StataCorp, 2001). An alternative approach is to use Poisson regression, which will be discussed in Chapters 8 and 9.

6.18. Additional Reading

Cox and Oakes (1984),

Kalbfleish and Prentice (1980), and

Lawless (1982) are three standard references on survival analysis. These texts all assume that the reader has a solid grounding in statistics.

Cox (1972) is the original reference on proportional hazards regression.

Greenwood (1926) is the original reference on Greenwood's formula for the variance of the survival function.

O'Donnell et al. (2000) studied the relationship between apolipoprotein E genotype and intracerebral hemorrhage. We used their data to illustrate survival analysis in this chapter.

Kaplan and Meier (1958) is the original reference on the Kaplan–Meier survival curve.

Mantel (1966) is the original reference on the Mantel–Haenszel test for survival data that is also known as the logrank test.

Peto and Peto (1972) studied the mathematical properties of the Mantel–Haenszel test for survival data, which they renamed the logrank test.

6.19. Exercises

The following exercises are based on a study by Dupont and Page (1985). A cohort of 3303 Nashville women underwent benign breast biopsies between 1950 and 1968. We obtained follow-up information from these women or their next of kin. You will find a data set on my web page called *6.ex.breast.dta* that contains some of the information from this cohort. The variables in this file are

id = patient identification number,

entage = age at entry biopsy,

follow = years of follow-up,

pd = diagnosis of entry biopsy

$$= \begin{cases} 0: \text{ no proliferative disease (No PD)} \\ 1: \text{ proliferative disease without atypia (PDWA)} \\ 2: \text{ atypical hyperplasia (AH),} \end{cases}$$

fate = fate at end of follow-up $= \begin{cases} 0: \text{ censored} \\ 1: \text{ invasive breast cancer,} \end{cases}$

fh = first degree family history of breast cancer $= \begin{cases} 0: \text{ no} \\ 1: \text{ yes.} \end{cases}$

1 Plot Kaplan–Meier breast cancer free survival curves for women with entry diagnoses of AH, PDWA, and No PD as a function of years since biopsy. Is this a useful graphic? If not, why not?

2 Plot the cumulative breast cancer morbidity in patient groups defined by entry histology. What is the estimated probability that a woman with PDWA will develop breast cancer within 15 years of her entry biopsy? Give a 95% confidence interval for this probability.

3 Derive the logrank test to compare the cumulative morbidity curves for women with these three diagnoses. Are these morbidity curves significantly different from each other? Is the cumulative incidence curve for women with AH significantly different from the curve for women with PDWA? Is the curve for women with PDWA significantly different from the curve for women without PD?

4 Calculate the breast cancer risk of women with AH relative to women without PD. Derive a 95% confidence interval for this relative risk. Calculate this relative risk for women with PDWA compared to women without PD.

5 What are the mean ages of entry biopsy for these three diagnoses? Do they differ significantly from each other? Does your answer complicate the interpretation of the preceding results?

7

Hazard Regression Analysis

In the last chapter we introduced the concept of proportional hazards regression analysis to estimate the relative risk associated with a single risk factor from survival data. In this chapter we generalize this technique. We will regress survival outcome against multiple covariates. The technique can be used to deal with multiple confounding variables or effect modifiers in precisely the same way as in logistic or linear regression. Indeed, many of the basic principles of multiple regression using the proportional hazards model have already been covered in previous chapters.

7.1. Proportional Hazards Model

We expand the simple proportional hazards model to handle multiple covariates as follows. Suppose we have a cohort of n patients who we follow forward in time as described in Chapter 6. Let

t_i be the time from entry to exit for the ith patient,

$$f_i = \begin{cases} 1: \text{if the } i^{\text{th}} \text{ patient dies at exit} \\ 0: \text{if the } i^{\text{th}} \text{ patient is censored at exit, and} \end{cases}$$

$x_{i1}, x_{i2}, \ldots, x_{iq}$ be the value of q covariates for the ith patient.

Let $\lambda_0[t]$ be the hazard function for patients with covariates $x_{i1} = x_{i2} = \cdots = x_{iq} = 0$. Then the proportional hazards model assumes that the hazard function for the ith patient is

$$\lambda_i[t] = \lambda_0[t] \exp[\beta_1 x_{i1} + \beta_2 x_{i2} + \cdots + \beta_q x_{iq}]. \tag{7.1}$$

7.2. Relative Risks and Hazard Ratios

Suppose that patients in risk groups 1 and 2 have covariates $x_{11}, x_{12}, \ldots, x_{1q}$ and $x_{21}, x_{22}, \ldots, x_{2q}$, respectively. Then the relative risk of patients in Group 2 with respect to those in Group 1 in the time interval $(t, t + \Delta t)$ is

$$\frac{\lambda_2\,[t]\,\Delta t}{\lambda_1\,[t]\,\Delta t} = \frac{\lambda_0[t]\,\exp[x_{21}\beta_1 + x_{22}\beta_2 + \cdots + x_{2q}\beta_q]}{\lambda_0[t]\,\exp[x_{11}\beta_1 + x_{12}\beta_2 + \cdots + x_{1q}\beta_q]}$$

$$= \exp[(x_{21} - x_{11})\beta_1 + (x_{22} - x_{12})\beta_2 + \cdots + (x_{2q} - x_{1q})\beta_q].$$

$$(7.2)$$

Note that $\lambda_0[t]$ drops out of this equation, and that this instantaneous relative risk remains constant over time. Thus, if the proportional hazards model is reasonable, we can interpret

$$(x_{21} - x_{11})\beta_1 + (x_{22} - x_{12})\beta_2 + \cdots + (x_{2q} - x_{1q})\beta_q \qquad (7.3)$$

as being the log relative risk associated with Group 2 patients as compared to Group 1 patients. Proportional hazards regression provides maximum likelihood estimates $\hat{\beta}_1, \hat{\beta}_2, \ldots, \hat{\beta}_q$ of the model parameters $\beta_1, \beta_2, \ldots \beta_q$. We use these estimates in equation (7.2) to estimate relative risks from the model.

It should be noted that there are strong similarities between logistic regression and proportional hazards regression. Indeed, if the patients in risk groups $i = 1$ or 2 followed the multiple logistic model

$$\text{logit}[\text{E}[d_i \mid \mathbf{x}_i]] = \log[\pi_i/(1 - \pi_i)] = \alpha + \beta_1 x_{i1} + \beta_2 x_{i2} + \cdots + \beta_q x_{iq},$$

then subtracting the log odds for Group 1 from Group 2 gives us

$$\log\left[\frac{\pi_2/(1 - \pi_2)}{\pi_1/(1 - \pi_1)}\right] = (x_{21} - x_{11})\,\beta_1 + (x_{22} - x_{12})\,\beta_2 + \cdots$$
$$+ (x_{2q} - x_{1q})\beta_q.$$

Hence, the only difference in the interpretation of logistic and proportional hazards regression models is that in logistic regression equation (7.3) is interpreted as a log odds ratio while in proportional hazards regression it is interpreted as a log relative risk.

Proportional hazards regression also provides an estimate of the variance–covariance matrix for $\hat{\beta}_1, \hat{\beta}_2, \ldots, \hat{\beta}_q$ (see Sections 5.14 and 5.15). The elements of this matrix are s_{ij}, the estimated covariance between $\hat{\beta}_i$ and $\hat{\beta}_j$ and s_{ii}, the estimated variance of $\hat{\beta}_i$. These variance and covariance terms are used in the same way as in Chapter 5 to calculate confidence intervals and to test hypotheses. Changes in model deviance between nested models are also used in the same way as in Chapter 5 as a guide to model building. I recommend that you read Chapter 5 prior to this chapter.

7.3. 95% Confidence Intervals and Hypothesis Tests

Suppose that $f = \Sigma c_j \beta_j$ is a weighted sum of the model coefficients and that $\hat{f} = \Sigma c_j \hat{\beta}_j$ is as in equation (5.28). Then the variance of $\hat{f}$ is estimated by $s_{\hat{f}}^2$ in equation (5.29). If $\exp[f]$ is a relative risk, then the 95% confidence interval for this risk is given by equation (5.31). We test the null hypotheses that $\exp[f] = 1$ using the z statistic defined in equation (5.32).

7.4. Nested Models and Model Deviance

We fit appropriate models to the data by comparing the change in model deviance between nested models. The model deviance is defined by equation (5.44). Suppose that we are considering two models and that model 1 is nested within model 2. Then the change in deviance ΔD between these models is given by equation (5.45). Under the null hypothesis that model 1 is true, ΔD will have an approximately chi-squared distribution whose degrees of freedom equal the difference in the number of parameters in the two models.

7.5. An Example: The Framingham Heart Study

Let us return to the Framingham didactic data set introduced in Sections 2.19.1 and 3.10. This data set contains long-term follow-up and cardiovascular outcome data on a large cohort of men and women. We will investigate the effects of gender and baseline diastolic blood pressure (DBP) on coronary heart disease (CHD) adjusted for other risk factors. Analyzing a complex real data set involves a considerable degree of judgment, and there is no single correct way to proceed. The following, however, includes the typical components of such an analysis.

7.5.1. Univariate Analyses

The first step is to perform a univariate analysis on the effects of DBP on CHD. Figure 7.1 shows a histogram of baseline DBP in this cohort. The range of blood pressures is very wide. Ninety-five per cent of the observations lie between 60 and 110 mm Hg. However, the data set is large enough that there are still 150 subjects with DBP ≤ 60 and 105 patients with pressures greater than 110. We subdivide the study subjects into seven groups based on their DBPs. Group 1 consists of patients with DBP ≤ 60, Group 2 has DBPs between 61 and 70, Group 3 has DBPs between 71 and 80, et cetera. The last

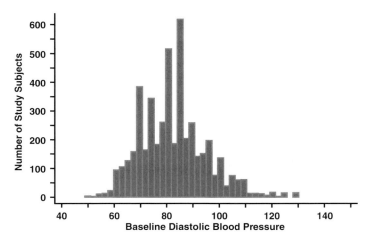

Figure 7.1

Histogram of baseline diastolic blood pressure among subjects from the Framingham Heart Study (Levy et al., 1999). These pressures were collected prior to the era of effective medical control of hypertension.

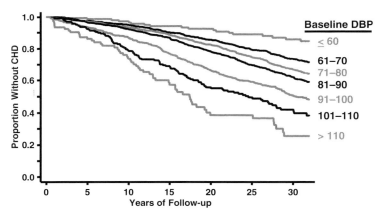

Figure 7.2

Effect of baseline diastolic blood pressure (DBP) on the risk of subsequent coronary heart disease (CHD). The proportion of subjects who subsequently develop CHD increases steadily with increasing DBP. This elevation in risk persists for over 30 years (Framingham Heart Study, 1997).

group (Group 7) has DBPs greater than 110. Figure 7.2 shows the Kaplan–Meier CHD free survival curves for these groups. The risk of CHD increases markedly with increasing DBP. The logrank χ^2 statistic equals 260 with six degrees of freedom ($P < 10^{-52}$). Hence, we can reject the hypothesis that the survival curves for these groups are all equal with overwhelming statistical significance. Moreover, the logrank tests of each adjacent pair of survival curves are also statistically significant. Hence, the data provides clear evidence that even modest increases in baseline DBP are predictive of increased risk of CHD.

Estimating the relative risks associated with different baseline blood pressures proceeds in exactly the same way as for estimating odds ratios in logistic regression. Let

$$dbp_{ij} = \begin{cases} 1: \text{if the } i^{\text{th}} \text{ patient is in DBP Group } j \\ 0: \text{otherwise.} \end{cases}$$

Then a simple proportional hazards model for estimating the relative risks associated with these blood pressures is

$$\lambda_i[t] = \lambda_0[t] \exp[\beta_2 \times dbp_{i2} + \beta_3 \times dbp_{i3} + \beta_4 \times dbp_{i4} + \beta_5 \times dbp_{i5}$$

$$+ \beta_6 \times dbp_{i6} + \beta_7 \times dbp_{i7}]. \tag{7.4}$$

For a patient in DBP Group 1, the hazard equals $\lambda_0[t] \exp[\beta_2 \times 0 + \beta_3 \times 0 + \cdots + \beta_7 \times 0] = \lambda_0[t]$. For a patient in Group j, the hazard is $\lambda_0[t] \exp[\beta_j \times 1]$ for $2 \leq j \leq 7$. Dividing $\lambda_0[t] \exp[\beta_j]\Delta t$ by $\lambda_0[t]\Delta t$ gives the relative risk for patients in DBP Group j relative to Group 1, which is $\exp[\beta_j]$. The log relative risk for Group j compared to Group 1 is β_j. Let $\hat{\beta}_j$ denote the maximum likelihood estimate of β_j and let $\text{se}[\hat{\beta}_j] = \sqrt{s_{jj}}$ denote the estimated standard error of $\hat{\beta}_j$. Then the estimated relative risk for subjects in Group j relative to those in Group 1 is $\exp[\hat{\beta}_j]$. The 95% confidence interval for this risk is

$$(\exp[\hat{\beta}_j - 1.96\text{se}[\hat{\beta}_j]], \ \exp[\hat{\beta}_j + 1.96\text{se}[\hat{\beta}_j]]). \tag{7.5}$$

Table 7.1 shows the estimates of β_j together with the corresponding relative risk estimates and 95% confidence intervals that result from model (7.4). These estimates are consistent with Figure 7.2 and confirm the importance of DBP as a predictor of subsequent risk of coronary heart disease.

Figure 7.3 shows the Kaplan–Meier CHD morbidity curves for men and women from the Framingham Heart Study. The logrank statistic for comparing these curves has one degree of freedom and equals 155. This statistic is also highly significant ($P < 10^{-34}$). Let

$$male_i = \begin{cases} 1: \text{if } i^{\text{th}} \text{ subject is a man} \\ 0: \text{if } i^{\text{th}} \text{ subject is a woman.} \end{cases}$$

Then a simple hazard regression model for estimating the effects of gender

7.5. An example: The Framingham Heart Study

Table 7.1. Effect of baseline diastolic blood pressure on coronary heart disease. The Framingham Heart Study data were analyzed using model (7.4).

Baseline diastolic blood pressure	Number of subjects	Cases of coronary heart disease	$\hat{\beta}_j$	Relative risk	95% confidence interval
≤60 mm Hg	150	18		1.0*	
61 – 70 mm Hg	774	182	0.677	1.97	(1.2 – 3.2)
71 – 80 mm Hg	1467	419	0.939	2.56	(1.6 – 4.1)
81 – 90 mm Hg	1267	404	1.117	3.06	(1.9 – 4.9)
91 –100 mm Hg	701	284	1.512	4.54	(2.8 – 7.3)
101 – 110 mm Hg	235	110	1.839	6.29	(3.8 – 10)
>110 mm Hg	105	56	2.247	9.46	(5.6 – 16)
Total	4699	1473			

*Denominator of relative risk

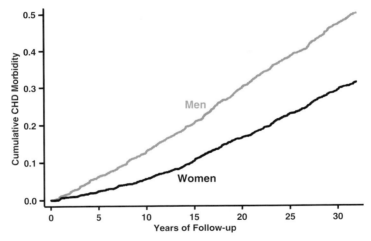

Figure 7.3 Cumulative incidence of coronary heart disease (CHD) in men and women from the Framingham Heart Study (Levy et al., 1999).

on CHD is

$$\lambda_i[t] = \lambda_0[t] \exp[\beta \times male_i]. \tag{7.6}$$

This model gives $\hat{\beta} = 0.642$ with standard error se$[\hat{\beta}] = 0.0525$. Therefore, the estimated relative risk of CHD in men relative to women is $\exp[0.642] = 1.90$. We calculate the 95% confidence interval for this risk to be $(1.71–2.11)$ using equation (7.5).

7.5.2. Multiplicative Model of DBP and Gender on Risk of CHD

The next step is to fit a multiplicative model of DBP and gender on CHD (see Section 5.18). Consider the model

$$\lambda_i[t] = \lambda_0[t] \exp\left[\sum_{h=2}^{7} \beta_h \times dbp_{ih} + \gamma \times male_i\right]. \tag{7.7}$$

The interpretation of this model is precisely analogous to that for model (5.38) in Section 5.19. To derive any relative risk under this model, write down the hazards for patients in the numerator and denominator of the desired relative risk. Then, divide the numerator hazard by the denominator hazard. You should be able to convince yourself that

- β_h is the log relative risk of women in DBP Group h relative to women in DBP Group 1,
- γ is the log relative risk of men in DBP Group 1 relative to women in DBP Group 1, and
- $\beta_h + \gamma$ is the log relative risk of men in DBP Group h relative to women in DBP Group 1.
- If R_h is the relative risk of being in Group h vs. Group 1 among women, and R_m is the relative risk of men vs. women among people in Group 1, then the relative risk of men in Group h relative to women in Group 1 equals $R_h \times R_m$. In other words, the effects of gender and blood pressure in model (7.7) are multiplicative.

Model (7.7) was used to produce the relative risk estimates in Table 7.2. Note that model (7.4) is nested within model (7.7). That is, if $\gamma = 0$ then model (7.7) reduces to model (7.4). This allows us to use the change in model deviance to test whether adding gender improves the fit of the model to the data. This change in deviance is $\Delta D = 133$, which has an approximately chi-squared distribution with one degree of freedom under the null hypothesis that $\gamma = 0$. Hence, we can reject this null hypothesis with overwhelming statistical significance ($P < 10^{-30}$).

7.5.3. Using Interaction Terms to Model the Effects of Gender and DBP on CHD

We next add interaction terms to weaken the multiplicative assumption in model (7.7) (see Sections 5.18 and 5.19). Let

$$\lambda_i[t] = \lambda_0[t] \exp\left[\sum_{h=2}^{7} \beta_h \times dbp_{ih} + \gamma \times male_i + \sum_{h=2}^{7} \delta_h \times dbp_{ih} \times male_i\right]. \tag{7.8}$$

This model is analogous to model (5.40) for esophageal cancer. For men in DBP Group h, the hazard is $\lambda_0[t] \exp[\beta_h + \gamma + \delta_h]$. For women in

Table 7.2. Effect of gender and baseline diastolic blood pressure on coronary heart disease. The Framingham Heart Study data are analyzed using the multiplicative model (7.7).

	Gender			
	Women		Men	
Baseline diastolic blood pressure	Relative risk	95% confidence interval	Relative risk	95% confidence interval
≤60 mm Hg	1.0*		1.83	(1.7–2.0)
61–70 mm Hg	1.91	(1.2–3.1)	3.51	(2.1–5.7)
71–80 mm Hg	2.43	(1.5–3.9)	4.46	(2.8–7.2)
81–90 mm Hg	2.78	(1.7–4.5)	5.09	(3.2–8.2)
91–100 mm Hg	4.06	(2.5–6.5)	7.45	(4.6–12)
101–110 mm Hg	5.96	(3.6–9.8)	10.9	(6.6–18)
>110 mm Hg	9.18	(5.4 – 15)	16.8	(9.8 – 29)

*Denominator of relative risk

Group 1, the hazard is $\lambda_0[t]$. Hence, the relative risk for men in DBP Group h relative to women in DBP Group 1 is $(\lambda_0[t] \exp[\beta_h + \gamma + \delta_h])/\lambda_0[t] = \exp[\beta_h + \gamma + \delta_h]$. This model was used to generate the relative risks in Table 7.3. Note the marked differences between the estimates in Table 7.2 and 7.3. Model (7.8) indicates that the effect of gender on the risk of CHD is greatest for people with low or moderate blood pressure and diminishes as blood pressure rises. Gender has no effect on CHD for people with a DBP above 110 mm Hg.

Model (7.7) is nested within model (7.8). Hence, we can use the change in the model deviance to test the null hypothesis that the multiplicative model is correct. This change in deviance is $\Delta D = 21.23$. Model (7.8) has six more parameters than model (7.7). Therefore, under the null hypothesis ΔD has an approximately chi-squared distribution with six degrees of freedom. The probability that this statistic exceeds 21.23 is $P = 0.002$. Thus, the evidence of interaction between DBP and gender on CHD risk is statistically significant.

7.5.4. Adjusting for Confounding Variables

So far we have not adjusted our results for other confounding variables. Of particular importance is age at baseline exam. Figure 7.4 shows that this age varied widely among study subjects. As both DBP and risk of CHD increases

Table 7.3. Effect of gender and baseline diastolic blood pressure on coronary heart disease. The Framingham Heart Study data are analyzed using model (7.8), which includes interaction terms for the joint effects of gender and blood pressure.

Baseline diastolic blood pressure	Women		Men	
	Relative risk	95% confidence interval	Relative risk	95% confidence interval
≤60 mm Hg	1.0*		2.37	(0.94–6.0)
61–70 mm Hg	1.83	(0.92–3.6)	4.59	(2.3–9.1)
71–80 mm Hg	2.43	(1.2–4.7)	5.55	(2.9–11)
81–90 mm Hg	3.52	(1.8–6.9)	5.28	(2.7–10)
91–100 mm Hg	4.69	(2.4–9.3)	8.28	(4.2–16)
101–110 mm Hg	7.64	(3.8–15)	10.9	(5.4–22)
>110 mm Hg	13.6	(6.6–28)	13.0	(5.9–29)

*Denominator of relative risk

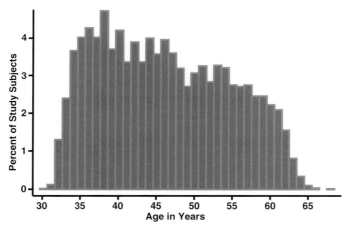

Figure 7.4   Histogram showing the age at baseline exam of subjects in the Framingham Heart Study (Levy et al., 1999).

markedly with age, we would expect age to strongly confound the effect of DBP on CHD. Other potential confounding variables that we may wish to consider include body mass index and serum cholesterol. Let age_i, bmi_i, and scl_i denote the age, body mass index, and serum cholesterol of the ith patient. We add these variables one at a time giving models

$$\lambda_i[t] = \lambda_0[t] \exp\left[\sum_{h=2}^{7} \beta_h \times dbp_{ih} + \gamma \times male_i + \sum_{h=2}^{7} \delta_h \times dbp_{ih} \right.$$

$$\left. \times male_i + \theta_1 \times age_i \right], \tag{7.9}$$

$$\lambda_i[t] = \lambda_0[t] \exp\left[\sum_{h=2}^{7} \beta_h \times dbp_{ih} + \gamma \times male_i + \sum_{h=2}^{7} \delta_h \times dbp_{ih} \right.$$

$$\left. \times male_i + \theta_1 \times age_i + \theta_2 \times bmi_i \right], \text{ and} \tag{7.10}$$

$$\lambda_i[t] = \lambda_0[t] \exp\left[\sum_{h=2}^{7} \beta_h \times dbp_{ih} + \gamma \times male_i + \sum_{h=2}^{7} \delta_h \times dbp_{ih} \right.$$

$$\left. \times male_i + \theta_1 \times age_i + \theta_2 \times bmi_i + \theta_3 \times scl_i \right]. \tag{7.11}$$

Note that model (7.8) is nested within model (7.9), model (7.9) is nested within model (7.10), and model (7.10) is nested within model (7.11). Hence, we can derive the change in model deviance with each successive model to test whether each new term significantly improves the model fit. These tests show that age, body mass index, and serum cholesterol all substantially improve the model fit, and that the null hypotheses $\theta_1 = 0$, $\theta_2 = 0$, and $\theta_3 = 0$ may all be rejected with overwhelming statistical significance. These tests also show that these variables are important independent predictors of CHD. Table 7.4 shows the estimated relative risks of CHD associated with DBP and gender that are obtained from model (7.11).

7.5.5. Interpretation

Tables 7.2, 7.3, and 7.4 are all estimating similar relative risks from the same data set. It is therefore sobering to see how different these estimates are. It is very important to understand the implications of the models used to derive these tables. Men in DBP Group 1 have a lower risk in Table 7.2 than in Table 7.3 while the converse is true for men in DBP Group 7. This is because model (7.7) forces the relative risks in Table 7.2 to obey the multiplicative assumption while model (7.8) permits the effect of gender on CHD to diminish with increasing DBP.

Table 7.4. Effect of gender and baseline diastolic blood pressure (DBP) on coronary heart disease. The Framingham Heart Study data are analyzed using model (7.11). This model includes gender–DBP interaction terms and adjusts for age, body mass index and serum cholesterol.

Baseline diastolic blood pressure	Gender				
	Women		Men	
	Relative risk	95% confidence interval	Relative risk	95% confidence interval
≤60 mm Hg	1.0*		1.98	(0.79–5.0)
61–70 mm Hg	1.51	(0.76–3.0)	3.53	(1.8–7.0)
71–80 mm Hg	1.65	(0.85–3.2)	3.88	(2.0–7.6)
81–90 mm Hg	1.91	(0.98–3.7)	3.33	(1.7–6.5)
91–100 mm Hg	1.94	(0.97–3.9)	4.86	(2.5–9.5)
101–110 mm Hg	3.10	(1.5–6.3)	6.29	(3.1–13)
>110 mm Hg	5.27	(2.5–11)	6.40	(2.9–14)

*Denominator of relative risk
[†]Adjusted for age, body mass index, and serum cholesterol.

The relative risks in Table 7.4 are substantially smaller than those in Table 7.3. It is important to realize that the relative risks in Table 7.4 compare people of the same age, body mass index, and serum cholesterol while those of Table 7.3 compare people without regard to these three risk factors. Our analyses show that age, body mass index, and serum cholesterol are risk factors for CHD in their own right. Also, these risk factors are positively correlated with DBP. Hence, it is not surprising that the unadjusted risks of DBP and gender in Table 7.3 are inflated by confounding due to these other variables. In general, the decision as to which variables to include as confounding variables is affected by how the results are to be used and our knowledge of the etiology of the disease being studied. For example, since it is easier to measure blood pressure than serum cholesterol, it might be more clinically useful to know the effect of DBP on CHD without adjustment for serum cholesterol. If we are trying to establish a causal link between a risk factor and a disease, then it is important to avoid adjusting for any condition that may be an intermediate outcome between the initial cause and the final outcome.

7.5.6. Alternative Models

In model (7.11) we treat age, body mass index, and serum cholesterol as continuous variables while DBP is recoded into seven dichotomous variables involving six parameters. We could have treated these confounding variables in the same way as DBP. In our analysis of esophageal cancer in Chapter 5 we treated age in precisely this way. In general, it is best to recode those continuous variables that are of primary interest into several dichotomous variables in order to avoid assuming a linear relationship between these risk factors and the log relative risk. It may, however, be reasonable to treat confounding variables as continuous. The advantage of putting a continuous variable directly into the model is that it requires only one parameter. The cost of making the linear assumption may not be too important for a variable that is included in the model only because it is a confounder. A method for testing the adequacy of the linearity assumption using orthogonal polynomials is discussed in Hosmer and Lemeshow (1989).

7.6. Cox–Snell Generalized Residuals and Proportional Hazards Models

We need to be able to verify that the proportional hazards model is appropriate for our data (see Section 7.1). Let

$$\Lambda_i [t] = \int_0^t \lambda_i [u] \, du \qquad (7.12)$$

be the **cumulative hazard function** for the ith patient by time t. That is, $\Lambda_i[t]$ is the area under the curve $\lambda_i[u]$ between 0 and t. Let t_i and f_i be defined as in Section 7.1, and let $\varepsilon_i = \Lambda_i[t_i]$ be the total cumulative hazard for the ith patient at her exit time. It can be shown that if $f_i = 1$, then ε_i has a **unit exponential distribution** whose survival function is given by

$$S[\varepsilon_i] = \exp[-\varepsilon_i]. \qquad (7.13)$$

If $f_i = 0$, then ε_i is a censored observation from this distribution. A **Cox–Snell generalized residual** is an estimate $\hat{\varepsilon}_i$ of ε_i. To check the validity of the proportional hazards assumption, we can derive a Kaplan–Meier survival curve for the event of interest using the Cox–Snell residuals as the time variable. Figure 7.5 shows such a plot for model (7.11) applied to the Framingham Heart Study data. The black line on this plot is a Kaplan–Meier survival plot using this model's Cox–Snell residuals as the time variable. The

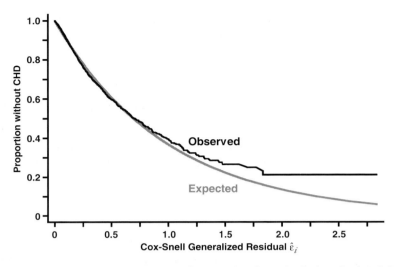

Figure 7.5   Observed and expected Cox–Snell generalized residual plots for model (7.11) applied to the Framingham Heart Study data. The black line is the observed Kaplan–Meier survival curve for coronary heart disease (CHD) using the Cox-Snell residual as the time variable. The gray line is the unit exponential distribution. If model (7.11) is correct, then the expected shape of the observed survival plot is given by the gray line.

gray line is equation (7.13). The Kaplan–Meier curve is in close agreement with the standard exponential distribution for most of these residuals (96% of the residuals are less than 1). There is, however, some evidence that some patients with large residuals are not suffering CHD at quite as high a rate as model (7.11) predicts they should. Nevertheless, the proportional hazards assumption of this model appears to be approximately correct. A patient can obtain a residual of a given size either by being at high risk for a short time or at lesser risk for a longer time. Since follow-up lasted for over 30 years, it is reasonable to assume that most patients with large residuals were followed for many years and were fairly old towards the end of their follow-up. In Section 7.9.2 we will consider evidence that the protective effects of female gender on CHD diminish after the menopause. It is likely that the mild evidence of departure from the proportional hazards assumption indicated by Figure 7.5 is due to the reduced risk of CHD in men relative to women after age 60. This departure, however, is not large enough to invalidate the inferences from this model.

There are a number of ways in which $\hat{\varepsilon}_i$ may be estimated. The approach that we will use was developed by Therneau et al. (1990) in the derivation of their martingale residual. The formula for this estimate is complicated but readily derived by the Stata software package.

Taking logarithms of both sides of equation (7.13) gives that $-\log[S[\varepsilon_i]] = \varepsilon_i$. Hence, if the model is correct, then the graph of $-\log[S[\hat{\varepsilon}_i]]$ against $\hat{\varepsilon}_i$ should approximate a straight line going through the origin that makes a 45° angle with the *x*-axis. This plot is the traditional way of presenting Cox–Snell residual analyses. I personally prefer to present them as in Figure 7.5 as it is easier in this figure to discern whether the deviation from the proportional hazards model is in the direction of too few events or too many.

7.7. Proportional Hazards Regression Analysis using Stata

The following log file and comments illustrate how to perform the analyses from the preceding sections using Stata.

```
. * 7.7.Framingham.log
. *
. * Proportional hazards regression analysis of the effect of gender and
. * baseline diastolic blood pressure (DBP) on coronary heart disease (CHD)
. * adjusted for age, body mass index (BMI) and serum cholesterol (SCL).
. *
. set memory 2000                                                      {1}
(2000k)

. use  C:\WDDtext\2.20.Framingham.dta, clear

. set textsize 120

. *
. * Univariate analysis of the effect of DBP on CHD
. *
. graph dbp, bin(50) freq xlabel(40,60 to 140) xtick(50,70 to 150)     {2}
> ylabel(0,100 to 600) ytick(50,100 to 550) gap (4)
```
                                                    {Graph omitted. See Figure 7.1}
```
. generate dbpgr = recode(dbp,60,70,80,90,100,110,111)                 {3}

. tabulate dbpgr chdfate                                               {4}
```

```
              |    Coronary Heart
              |        Disease
     dbpgr   |  Censored     CHD |  Total
   ---------+-------------------+-------
        60  |     132        18 |    150
        70  |     592       182 |    774
        80  |    1048       419 |   1467
        90  |     863       404 |   1267
       100  |     417       284 |    701
       110  |     125       110 |    235
       111  |      49        56 |    105
   ---------+-------------------+-------
     Total  |    3226      1473 |   4699
```

```
. label define dbp 60 "DBP<= 60" 70 "60<DBP70" 80 "70<DBP80" 90 "80<DBP90" 100
> "90DBP100" 110 "100BP110" 111 "110< DBP"

. label values  dbpgr dbp

. generate time = followup/365.25                                          {5}

. label variable time "Follow-up in Years"

. stset time, failure(chdfate)

    failure event:  chdfate ~= 0 & chdfate ~=.
obs. time interval:  (0, time]
 exit on or before:  failure

-----------------------------------------------------------------
    4699   total obs.
       0   exclusions
-----------------------------------------------------------------
    4699   obs. remaining, representing
    1473   failures in single record/single failure data
103710.1   total analysis time at risk, at risk from t =          0
                          earliest observed entry t =          0
                             last observed exit t =         32
. sts graph , by(dbpgr) xlabel(0,5 to 30) ylabel(0,.2 to 1)                {6}
> ytick(.1, .3 to .9) l1title(Proportion Without CHD) gap(6) noborder
```
{Graph omitted. See Figure 7.2}

```
        failure _d:  chdfate
analysis time _t:  time

. sts test dbpgr                                                           {7}
```

```
        failure _d:  chdfate
analysis time _t:  time

Log-rank test for equality of survivor functions
------------------------------------------------
          |  Events
dbpgr     |  observed      expected
----------+------------------------
DBP<= 60  |        18         53.63
60<DBP70  |       182        275.72
70<DBP80  |       419        489.41
80<DBP90  |       404        395.62
90DBP100  |       284        187.97
100BP110  |       110         52.73
110< DBP  |        56         17.94
----------+------------------------
Total     |      1473       1473.00

              chi2(6) =      259.71
              Pr>chi2 =     0.0000
```

. sts test *dbpgr* if *dbpgr* == *60* |*dbpgr* == *70*   {8}

```
failure _d:  chdfate
   analysis time _t:  time

Log-rank test for equality of survivor functions
------------------------------------------------
          |  Events
dbpgr     |  observed      expected
----------+------------------------
DBP<= 60  |        18         32.58
60<DBP70  |       182        167.42
----------+------------------------
Total     |       200        200.00

              chi2(1) =        7.80
              Pr>chi2 =     0.0052
```

. sts test *dbpgr* if *dbpgr* == *70* | *dbpgr* == *80*   {9}
              Pr>chi2 =   0.0028   {Output omitted}

. sts test *dbpgr* if *dbpgr* == *80* | *dbpgr* == *90*   {Output omitted}

```
            Pr>chi2 =        0.0090
```

`. sts test `*`dbpgr`*` if `*`dbpgr == 90 | dbpgr == 100`*   {Output omitted}
```
            Pr>chi2 =        0.0000
```

`. sts test `*`dbpgr`*` if `*`dbpgr == 100 | dbpgr == 110`*   {Output omitted}
```
            Pr>chi2 =        0.0053
```

`. sts test `*`dbpgr`*` if `*`dbpgr == 110 | dbpgr == 111`*   {Output omitted}
```
            Pr>chi2 =        0.0215
```

`. xi: stcox i.`*`dbpgr`*   {10}
```
i.dbpgr                 _Idbpgr_1-7      (_Idbpgr_1 for dbpgr==60 omitted)
        failure _d:    chdfate

   analysis time _t:    time
```
                                                          (Output omitted}
```
Cox regression -- Breslow method for ties

No. of subjects =         4699          Number of obs   =      4699
No. of failures =         1473
Time at risk    =     103710.0917

                                        LR chi2(6)      =    221.83
Log likelihood  =     -11723.942        Prob > chi2     =    0.0000   {11}

------------------------------------------------------------------------
      _t |
      _d | Haz. Ratio   Std. Err.     z     P>|z|   [95% Conf. Interval]
---------+--------------------------------------------------------------
_Idbpgr_2 |   1.968764    .486453    2.742   0.006    1.213037    3.195312  {12}
_Idbpgr_3 |   2.557839   .6157326    3.901   0.000    1.595764    4.099941
_Idbpgr_4 |   3.056073   .7362768    4.637   0.000    1.905856    4.900466
_Idbpgr_5 |    4.53703   1.103093    6.220   0.000    2.817203    7.306767
_Idbpgr_6 |   6.291702   1.600738    7.229   0.000    3.821246   10.35932
_Idbpgr_7 |   9.462228   2.566611    8.285   0.000    5.560408   16.10201
------------------------------------------------------------------------
```

`. *`
`. * `*`Univariate analysis of the effect of gender on CHD`*
`. *`
`. sts graph, by(`*`sex`*`) xlabel(`*`0,5,10,15,20,25,30`*`) ylabel(`*`0,.1,.2,.3,.4,.5`*`)` {13}
`> failure l1title("`*`Cumulative CHD Morbidity`*`")    gap(`*`3`*`) noborder`
                                              {Output omitted. See Figure 7.3}
```
        failure _d:   chdfate
analysis time _t:   time
```

```
. sts test sex                                                              {14}

      failure _d:  chdfate
analysis time _t:  time

Log-rank test for equality of survivor functions
------------------------------------------------
        | Events
sex     | observed          expected
--------+-------------------------------
Men     |      823            589.47
Women   |      650            883.53
--------+-------------------------------
Total   |     1473           1473.00

          chi2(1) =         154.57
          Pr>chi2 =         0.0000
. generate male = sex == 1                                                  {15}

. stcox male                                                                {16}
                                                             {Output omitted}

-----------------------------------------------------------------------
  _t |
  _d | Haz. Ratio    Std. Err.      z      P>|z|    [95% Conf. Interval]
-----+-----------------------------------------------------------------
male |   1.900412     .0998308   12.223    0.000    1.714482    2.106504
-----------------------------------------------------------------------

. *
. * Fit multiplicative model of DBP and gender on risk of CHD
. *
. xi: stcox  i.dbpgr male                                                   {17}
i.dbpgr           _Idbpgr_1-7       (_Idbpgr_1 for dbpgr==60 omitted)
                                                             {Output omitted}
Log likelihood  =  -11657.409              Prob > chi2    =     0.0000
-----------------------------------------------------------------------
       _t |
       _d | Haz. Ratio    Std. Err.      z     P>|z|    [95% Conf. Interval]
----------+------------------------------------------------------------
_Idbpgr_2 |   1.911621     .4723633    2.622   0.009    1.177793    3.102662
_Idbpgr_3 |   2.429787     .585021     3.687   0.000    1.515737    3.895044
_Idbpgr_4 |   2.778377     .6697835    4.239   0.000    1.732176    4.456464
```

```
_Idbpgr_5 |   4.060083    .9879333    5.758   0.000     2.520075    6.541184
_Idbpgr_6 |   5.960225    1.516627    7.015   0.000     3.619658    9.814262
_Idbpgr_7 |   9.181868    2.490468    8.174   0.000     5.395767    15.6246
    male |   1.833729    .0968002   11.486   0.000     1.653489    2.033616
----------------------------------------------------------------------------
```

. lincom _Idbpgr_2 + male, hr   {18}

(1)   _Idbpgr_2 + male = 0.0

```
---------------------------------------------------------------------------
  _t | Haz. Ratio   Std. Err.      z     P>|z|    [95% Conf. Interval]
------+--------------------------------------------------------------------
  (1) |   3.505395    .8837535    4.975   0.000     2.138644     5.7456
---------------------------------------------------------------------------
```

. lincom _Idbpgr_3 + male, hr

                                             {Output omitted. See Table 7.2}

. lincom _Idbpgr_4 + male, hr

                                             {Output omitted. See Table 7.2}

. lincom_Idbpgr_5 + male, hr

                                             {Output omitted. See Table 7.2}

. lincom _Idbpgr_6 + male, hr

                                             {Output omitted. See Table 7.2}

. lincom _Idbpgr_7 + male, hr

                                             {Output omitted. See Table 7.2}

. display 2*(11723.942 -11657.409)   {19}
133.066
. display chi2tail(1,133.066)   {20}
8.746e-31

. *
. * Fit model of DBP and gender on risk of CHD using interaction terms
. *
. xi: stcox i.dbpgr*i.male   {21}
i.dbpgr   _Idbpgr_1-7   (_Idbpgr_1 for dbpgr==60 omitted)
i.male   _Imale_0-1   (naturally coded; _Imale_0 omitted)
i.dbpgr*i.male   _IdbpXmal_#_#   (coded as above)
                                                        {Output omitted}

Log likelihood =   -11646.794   Prob > chi2   =   0.0000
```
```

```
--------------------------------------------------------------------------
        _t |
        _d |   Haz. Ratio    Std. Err.      z     P>|z|     [95% Conf. Interval]
-----------+--------------------------------------------------------------
  _Idbpgr_2 |    1.82731      .6428651    1.714    0.087     .9169625    3.64144
  _Idbpgr_3 |    2.428115     .8298216    2.596    0.009      1.2427     4.744299
  _Idbpgr_4 |    3.517929    1.201355     3.683    0.000     1.801384    6.870179
  _Idbpgr_5 |    4.693559    1.628053     4.458    0.000     2.378188    9.263141
  _Idbpgr_6 |    7.635131    2.736437     5.672    0.000     3.782205   15.41302
  _Idbpgr_7 |   13.62563     5.067901     7.023    0.000     6.572973   28.24565
    Imale_1 |    2.372645    1.118489     1.833    0.067     .9418198    5.977199
_IdbpXma~2_1 |   1.058632     .5235583    0.115    0.908     .4015814    2.79072
_IdbpXma~3_1 |    .9628061     .4637697   -0.079    0.937     .3745652    2.474858
_IdbpXma~4_1 |    .6324678     .3047828   -0.951    0.342     .2459512    1.626402
_IdbpXma~5_1 |    .7437487     .3621623   -0.608    0.543     .2863787    1.931576
_IdbpXma~6_1 |    .6015939     .3059896   -0.999    0.318     .2220014    1.630239
_IdbpXma~7_1 |    .401376      .2205419   -1.661    0.097     .1367245    1.178302
--------------------------------------------------------------------------
. display 2*(11657.409 -11646.794)
21.23
. display chi2tail(6, 21.23)                                              {22}
00166794
. lincom _Idbpgr_2 + Imale_1 + _IdbpXmal_2_1, hr                          {23}
( 1)   _Idbpgr_2 + Imale_1 + _IdbpXmal_2_1 = 0.0

---------------------------------------------------------------------
 _t |  Haz. Ratio    Std. Err.      z     P>|z|    [95% Conf. Interval]
----+----------------------------------------------------------------
(1) |   4.589761    1.595446     4.384    0.000    2.322223    9.071437
---------------------------------------------------------------------

. lincom _Idbpgr_3 + Imale_1 + _IdbpXmal_3_1, hr
```
{Output omitted. See Table 7.3}
```
. lincom _Idbpgr_4 + Imale_1 + _IdbpXmal_4_1, hr
```
{Output omitted. See Table 7.3}
```
. lincom _Idbpgr_5 + Imale_1 + _IdbpXmal_5_1, hr
```
{Output omitted. See Table 7.3}
```
. lincom _Idbpgr_6 + Imale_1 + _IdbpXmal_6_1, hr
```
{Output omitted. See Table 7.3}

```
. lincom _Idbpgr_7 + Imale_1 + _IdbpXmal_7_1, hr
```
{Output omitted. See Table 7.3}
```
. *
. * Adjust model for age, BMI and SCL
. *
. xi: stcox i.dbpgr*i.male  age                                              {24}
```
{Output omitted}
```
Log likelihood =   −11517.247           Prob > chi2     =    0.0000
```
{Output omitted}
```
. display   2*(11646.794 −11517.247)                                         {25}
259.094

. display chi2tail(1,259.094)
2.704e-58

. xi: stcox i.dbpgr*i.male age bmi                                           {26}
```
{Output omitted}
```
Log likelihood =     −11490.733          Prob > chi2     =    0.0000
```
{Output omitted}
```
. display   2*(11517.247 −11490.733)
53.028

. display chi2tail(1,53.028)
3.288e-13

. xi: stcox i.dbpgr*i.male age bmi scl, mgale(mg)                            {27}
```
{Output omitted}
```
Log likelihood =  −11382.132            Prob > chi2     =    0.0000
```

```
-------------------------------------------------------------------------
       _t |
       _d | Haz. Ratio   Std. Err.     z    P>|z|    [95% Conf. Interval]
----------+--------------------------------------------------------------
 _Idbpgr_2 |  1.514961    .5334695    1.180  0.238    .7597392    3.020916
 _Idbpgr_3 |  1.654264    .5669665    1.469  0.142    .8450299    3.238451
 _Idbpgr_4 |  1.911763    .6566924    1.887  0.059    .9750921    3.748199
 _Idbpgr_5 |  1.936029    .6796612    1.882  0.060    .9729479    3.852425
 _Idbpgr_6 |  3.097614    1.123672    3.117  0.002    1.521425    6.306727
 _Idbpgr_7 |  5.269096    1.988701    4.403  0.000    2.514603    11.04086
   Imale_1 |  1.984033    .9355668    1.453  0.146    .7873473    4.999554
_IdbpXma~2_1 |  1.173058    .5802796    0.323  0.747    4448907    3.09304
_IdbpXma~3_1 |   1.18152    .5693995    0.346  0.729    .4594405    3.038457
_IdbpXma~4_1 |  .8769476    .4230106   −0.272  0.785    .3407078    2.257175
```

```
_IdbpXma~5_1 |    1.265976    .6179759     0.483   0.629    .4863156    3.295585
_IdbpXma~6_1 |    1.023429    .5215766     0.045   0.964    .3769245    2.778823
_IdbpXma~7_1 |    .6125694    .3371363    -0.890   0.373    .2082976    1.801467
        age  |    1.04863     .003559     13.991   0.000    1.041677    1.055628
        bmi  |    1.038651    .0070125     5.617   0.000    1.024998    1.052487
        scl  |    1.005788    .0005883     9.866   0.000    1.004635    1.006941
------------------------------------------------------------------------------
```

. display 2*(11490.733 −11382.132)   {28}
217.202

. display chi2tail(1,217.202)
3.687e-49

. lincom _Idbpgr_2 + Imale_1 + _IdbpXmal_2_1, hr

{Output omitted. See Table 7.4}

. lincom _Idbpgr_3 + Imale_1 + _IdbpXmal_3_1, hr

{Output omitted. See Table 7.4}

. lincom _Idbpgr_4 + Imale_1 + _IdbpXmal_4_1, hr

{Output omitted. See Table 7.4}

. lincom _Idbpgr_5 + Imale_1 + _IdbpXmal_5_1, hr

{Output omitted. See Table 7.4}

. lincom _Idbpgr_6 + Imale_1 + _IdbpXmal_6_1, hr

{Output omitted. See Table 7.4}

. lincom _Idbpgr_7 + Imale_1 + _IdbpXmal_7_1, hr

{Output omitted. See Table 7.4}

. *
. * Perform Cox-Snell generalized residual analysis
. *
. predict cs, csnell   {29}
(41 missing values generated)

. stset cs, failure(chdfate)   {30}
     failure event: chdfate ~= 0 & chdfate ~=.
obs. time interval: (0, cs]
 exit on or before: failure

```
------------------------------------------------------------------------------
  4699  total obs.
    41  event time missing (cs==.)                    PROBABLE ERROR    {31}
------------------------------------------------------------------------------
  4658  obs. remaining, representing
  1465  failures in single record/single failure data
```

```
 1465   total analysis time at risk, at risk from t =          0
                      earliest observed entry t =          0
                          last observed exit t =   2.833814
```

`. sts generate km = s`   {32}

`. generate es = exp(-cs)`   {33}

`(41 missing values generated)`

`. sort cs`

`. graph km es cs, connect(ll) symbol(..) xlabel(0 .5 to 2.5)`

`> ylabel(0 .2 to 1.0) xtick(.25 .75 to 2.75) ytick(.1.2 to 1)`   {34}

{Graph omitted. See Figure 7.5}

Comments

1 By default, Stata reserves one megabyte of memory for its calculations. Calculating some statistics on large data sets may require more than this. The logrank test given below is an example of such a calculation. The *set memory* command specifies the memory size in kilobytes. This command may not be used when a data set is open.

2 This graph command draws a histogram of *dbp* with 50 bars (bins) that is similar to Figure 7.1.

3 Define *dbpgr* to be a categorical variable based on *dbp*. The *recode* function sets

$$dbpgr = \begin{cases} 60: & \text{if } dbp \leq 60 \\ 70: & \text{if } 60 < dbp \leq 70 \\ & \vdots \\ 110: & \text{if } 100 < dbp \leq 110 \\ 111: & \text{if } 110 < dbp. \end{cases}$$

4 This command tabulates *dbpgr* by *chdfate*. Note that the proportion of patients with subsequent CHD increases with increasing blood pressure. I recommend that you produce simple tabulations of your results frequently as a crosscheck on your more complicated statistics.

5 In order to make our graphs more intelligible we define *time* to be patient follow-up in years.

6 This command produces a Kaplan–Meier survival graph that is similar to Figure 7.2.

7 This *sts test* command performs a logrank test on the groups of patients defined by *dbpgr*. The highlighted *P* value for this test is $< 0.000\,05$.

8 This logrank test is restricted to patients with *dbpgr* equal to 60 or 70. In other words, this command tests whether the survival curves for patients with DBPs ≤60 and DBPs between 60 and 70 are equal. The *P* value associated with this test equals 0.0052.

9 The next five commands test the equality of the other adjacent pairs of survival curves in Figure 7.2.

10 The syntax of the *xi:* prefix for the *stcox* command works in exactly the same way as in logistic regression. See Sections 5.10 and 5.23 for a detailed explanation. This command performs the proportional hazards regression analysis specified by model (7.4). The variables *_Idbpgr_2*, *_Idbpgr_3*,..., *_Idbpgr_7* are dichotomous classification variables that are created by this command. In model (7.4) $dbp_{i2} = $ *_Idbpgr_2*, $dbp_{i3} = $ *_Idbpgr_3*, et cetera.

11 The maximum value of the log likelihood function is highlighted. We will use this statistic in calculating change in model deviance.

12 The column titled *Haz. Ratio* contains relative risks under the proportional hazards model. The relative risk estimates and 95% confidence intervals presented in Table 7.1 are highlighted. For example, $\exp[\beta_2] =$ 1.968 764, which is the relative risk of people in DBP Group 2 relative to DBP Group 1.

13 The *failure* option of the *sts graph* command produces a cumulative morbidity plot. The resulting graph is similar to Figure 7.3.

14 The logrank test of the CHD morbidity curves for men and women is of overwhelming statistical significance.

15 In the database, *sex* is coded as 1 for men and 2 for women. As men have the higher risk of CHD we will treat male sex as a positive risk factor. (Alternatively, we could have treated female sex as a protective risk factor.) To do this in Stata, we need to give men a higher code than women. The logical value *sex* == 1 is true (equals 1) when the subject is a man (*sex* = 1), and is false (equals 0) when she is a woman (*sex* = 2). Hence the effect of this *generate* command is to define the variable *male* as equaling 0 or 1 for women or men, respectively.

16 This command performs the simple proportional hazards regression specified by model (7.6). It estimates that men have 1.90 times the risk of CHD as women. The 95% confidence interval for this risk is also given.

17 This command performs the proportional hazards regression specified by model (7.7). In this command *male* specifies the covariate $male_i$ in model (7.7). The highlighted relative risks and confidence intervals are also given in Table 7.2. Note that since *male* is already dichotomous, it is not necessary to create a new variable using the *i.male* syntax.

18 The covariates _Idbpgr_2 and *male* equal dbp_{i2} and $male_i$, respectively in model (7.7). The coefficients associated with these covariates are β_2 and γ. The *hr* option of the *lincom* command has the same effect as the *or* option. That is, it exponentiates the desired expression and then calculates a confidence interval using equation (5.31). The only difference between the *or* and *hr* options is that in column heading of the resulting output "*Odds Ratio*" is replaced by "*Haz. Ratio*". This *lincom* command calculates $\exp[\hat{\beta}_2 + \hat{\gamma}] = \exp[\hat{\beta}_2] \times \exp[\hat{\gamma}] = 1.911\,621 \times 1.833\,729 = 3.505\,395$, which is the relative risk for a man in DBP Group 2 relative to women in DBP Group 1. (See Comment 6 of Section 5.20 for additional explanation.) This and the next five *lincom* commands provide the relative risks and confidence intervals needed to complete Table 7.2.

19 This command calculates the change in model deviance between model (7.4) and model (7.7), which equals 133.

20 The function *chi2tail*(*df, chi2*) calculates the probability that a chi-squared statistic with *df* degrees of freedom exceeds *chi2*. The probability that a chi-squared statistic with one degree of freedom exceeds 133 is 8.7×10^{-31}. This is the *P* value associated with the change in model deviance between models (7.4) and (7.7).

21 This command regresses CHD free survival against DBP and gender using model (7.8) See Section 5.23 for a detailed explanation of this syntax. The names of the dichotomous classification variables created by this command are indicated in the first three lines of output. For example, in model (7.8) dbp_{i2} equals _Idbpgr_2, $male_i$ equals _Imale_1, and $dbp_{i2} \times male_i$ equals _IdbpXmal_2_1. Note that the names of the interaction covariates are truncated to 12 characters in the table of hazard ratios. Hence, _IdbpXma~2_1 denotes _IdbpXmal_2_1, et cetera. The highlighted relative risks and confidence intervals are also given in Table 7.3.

22 These calculations allow us to reject the multiplicative model (7.7) with $P = 0.0017$.

23 This *lincom* command calculates $\exp[\hat{\beta}_2 + \hat{\gamma} + \hat{\delta}_2] = 4.589\,761$, which is the relative risk of men in DBP Group 2 relative to women from DBP Group 1 under model (7.8). This and the following five *lincom* commands calculate the relative risks needed to complete Table 7.3.

24 This command regresses CHD free survival against DBP and gender adjusted for age using model (7.9).

25 Adding *age* to the model greatly reduces the model deviance.

26 This command regresses CHD free survival against DBP and gender adjusted for age and BMI using model (7.10). The model deviance is again significantly reduced by adding BMI to the model.

27 This command regresses CHD free survival against DBP and gender adjusted for age, BMI, and SCL using model (7.11). The highlighted relative risks and confidence intervals are entered into Table 7.4. The subsequent *lincom* commands are used to complete this table. The option *mgale(mg)* creates a variable *mg* that contains the martingale residuals for this model. These residuals are used by the subsequent *predict* command that calculates Cox–Snell residuals.

28 The change in model deviance between models (7.8), (7.9), (7.10), and (7.11) indicate a marked improvement in model fit with each successive model.

29 The *csnell* option of this *predict* command calculates Cox–Snell residuals for the preceding Cox hazard regression. Martingale residuals must have been calculated for this regression.

30 This *stset* command redefines the time variable to be the Cox–Snell residual *cs*. The failure variable *chdfate* is not changed.

31 There are 41 patients who are missing at least one covariate from model (7.11). These patients are excluded from the hazard regression analysis. Consequently no value of *cs* is derived for these patients.

32 This *sts generate* command defines *km* to be the Kaplan–Meier CHD free survival curve using *cs* as the time variable.

33 This command defines *es* to be the expected survival function for a unit exponential distribution using *cs* as the time variable.

34 This command graphs *km* and *es* against *cs*. The resulting plot is similar to Figure 7.5.

7.8. Stratified Proportional Hazards Models

In Section 7.1, we defined the hazard for the ith patient at time t by equation (7.1). This hazard function obeys the proportional hazards assumption. One way to weaken this assumption is to subdivide the patients into $j = 1, \ldots, J$ stratum defined by the patient's covariates. We then define the hazard for the ith patient from the jth stratum at time t to be

$$\lambda_{ij}[t] = \lambda_{0j}[t] \exp[\beta_1 x_{ij1} + \beta_2 x_{ij2} + \cdots + \beta_q x_{ijq}], \qquad (7.14)$$

where $x_{ij1}, x_{ij2}, \ldots, x_{ijq}$, are the covariate values for this patient, and $\lambda_{0j}[t]$ is the baseline hazard for patients from the jth stratum. Model (7.14) makes no assumptions about the shapes of the J baseline hazard functions. Within each stratum the proportional hazards assumption applies. However, patients from different strata need not have proportional hazards.

For example, suppose that we were interested in the risk of CHD due to smoking in women and men. We might stratify the patients by gender, letting $j = 1$ or 2 designate men or women, respectively. Let

$$x_{ij} = \begin{cases} 1: \text{if } i^{\text{th}} \text{ patient from } j^{\text{th}} \text{ stratum smokes} \\ 0: \text{otherwise, and} \end{cases}$$

$\lambda_{ij}[t]$ be the CHD hazard for the ith patient from the jth stratum. Then model (7.14) reduces to

$$\lambda_{ij}[t] = \lambda_{0j}[t] \exp[\beta x_{ij}]. \tag{7.15}$$

In this model, $\lambda_{01}[t]$ and $\lambda_{02}[t]$ represent the CHD hazard for men and women who do not smoke, while $\lambda_{01}[t]\,e^{\beta}$ and $\lambda_{02}[t]\,e^{\beta}$ represents this hazard for men and women who do. By an argument similar to that given in Section 7.2, the within-strata relative risk of CHD in smokers relative to non-smokers is e^{β}. That is, smoking women have e^{β} times the CHD risk of non-smoking women while smoking men have e^{β} times the CHD risk of non-smoking men. Model (7.15) makes no assumptions about how CHD risk varies with time among non-smoking men or women. It does, however, imply that the relative CHD risk of smoking is the same among men as it is among women.

In Stata, a stratified proportional hazards model is indicated by the *strata(varnames)* option of the *stcox* command. Model (7.15) might be implemented by a command such as

```
stcox smoke, strata(sex)
```

where *smoke* equals 1 or 0 for patients who did or did not smoke, respectively.

7.9. Survival Analysis with Ragged Study Entry

Usually the time variable in a survival analysis measures follow-up time from some event. This event may be recruitment into a cohort, diagnosis of cancer, et cetera. In such studies everyone is at risk at time zero, when they enter the cohort. Sometimes, however, we may wish to use the patient's age as the time variable rather than follow-up time. Both Kaplan–Meier survival curves and hazard regression analyses can be easily adapted to this situation. The key difference is that when age is the time variable, patients are not observed to fail until after they reach the age when they enter the cohort. Hence, it is possible that no one will enter the study at age zero, and that subjects will enter the analysis at different "times" when they reach their age at recruitment. These analyses must be interpreted as the effect of age and other covariates on the risk of failure conditioned on the fact that each patient had not failed prior to her age of recruitment.

7.9.1. Kaplan–Meier Survival Curve and the Logrank Test with Ragged Entry

In Section 6.3, we defined the Kaplan–Meier survival curve $\hat{S}(t)$ to be a product of probabilities p_i on each death day prior to time t. Each probability $p_i = (n_i - d_i) / n_i$, where n_i are the number of patients at risk at the beginning of the ith death day and d_i are the number of deaths on this day. In a traditional survival curve, n_i must decrease with increasing i since the entire cohort is at risk at time 0 and death or censoring can only decrease this number with time. With ragged entry, $\hat{S}(t)$ is calculated in the same way only now the number of patients at risk can increase as well as decrease; n_i equals the total number of people to be recruited before time t minus the total number of people who die or are censored prior to this time. The cumulative mortality curve is $\hat{D}[t] = 1 - \hat{S}[t]$ as was the case in Section 6.3.

The logrank test is performed in exactly the same way as in Section 6.8. The only difference is that now the number of patients at risk at the beginning of each death day equals the number of patients recruited prior to that day minus the number of patients who have previously died or been censored.

7.9.2. Age, Sex, and CHD in the Framingham Heart Study

Figure 7.4 shows that the distribution of age at entry in the Framingham Heart Study was very wide. This means that at any specific follow-up time in Figure 7.3, we are comparing men and women with a wide variation in ages. Figure 7.6 shows the cumulative CHD mortality in men and women as a function of age rather than years since recruitment. This figure reveals an aspect of CHD epidemiology that is missed in Figure 7.3. The morbidity curves for men and women diverge most rapidly prior to age sixty. Thereafter, they remain relatively parallel. This indicates that the protective effects of female gender on CHD are greatest in the pre- and perimenopausal ages, and that this protective effect is largely lost a decade or more after the menopause. This interaction between age and sex on CHD is not apparent

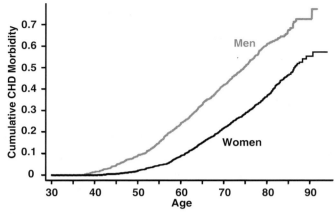

Figure 7.6　Cumulative coronary heart disease (CHD) morbidity with increasing age among men and women from the Framingham Heart Study (Levy et al., 1999).

in the Kaplan–Meier curves in Figure 7.3 that were plotted as a function of time since recruitment.

7.9.3. Proportional Hazards Regression Analysis with Ragged Entry

Proportional hazards regression analysis also focuses on the number of patients at risk and the number of deaths on each death day. For this reason, they are easily adapted for analyses of data with ragged study entry. A simple example of such a proportional hazards model is

$$\lambda_i[age] = \lambda_0[age] \exp[\beta \times male_i], \tag{7.16}$$

where *age* is a specific age for the ith subject, $\lambda_0[age]$ is the CHD hazard for women at this age, $male_i$ equals 1 if the ith subject is a man and equals 0 if she is a woman, and $\lambda_i[age]$ is the CHD hazard for the ith study subject at the indicated age. Model (7.16) differs from model (7.6) only in that in model (7.6) t represents time since entry while in model (7.16) *age* represents the subject's age. Under model (7.16), a man's hazard is $\lambda_0[age]\exp[\beta]$. Hence, the age-adjusted relative risk of CHD in men compared to women is $\exp[\beta]$. Applying model (7.16) to the Framingham Heart Study data gives this relative risk of CHD for men to be 2.01 with a 95% confidence interval of (1.8–2.2). Note, however, that model (7.16) assumes that the relative risk of CHD between men and women remains constant with age. This assumption is rather unsatisfactory in view of the evidence from Figure 7.6 that this relative risk diminishes after age 60.

7.9.4. Survival Analysis with Ragged Entry using Stata

The following log file and comments illustrate how to perform the analyses discussed above using Stata.

```
. * 7.9.4.Framingham.log
. *
. * Plot Kaplan-Meier cumulative CHD morbidity curves as a function of age.
. * Patients from the Framingham Heart Study enter the analysis when they
. * reach the age of their baseline exam.
. *
. set memory 2000
(2000k)

. use C:\WDDtext\2.20.Framingham.dta, clear

. set textsize 120

. graph age, bin(39) xlabel(30,35 to 65) ylabel(0,.01 to .04) gap(3)
```
{Graph omitted. See Figure 7.4}
```
. generate time = followup/365.25

. label variable time "Follow-up in Years"

. generate exitage =  age + time                                            {1}

. stset  exitage, enter(time age) failure(chdfate)                          {2}

        failure event:   chdfate ~= 0 & chdfate ~=.
   obs. time interval:   (0, exitage]
   enter on or after:    time age
   exit on or before:    failure

---------------------------------------------------------------
    4699   total obs.
       0   exclusions
---------------------------------------------------------------
    4699   obs. remaining, representing
    1473   failures in single record/single failure data
103710.1   total analysis time at risk, at risk from t =        0
                           earliest observed entry t =         30
                              last observed exit t =           94

. sts graph , by(sex) tmin(30) xlabel(30 40 to 90) ylabel(0, .1 to .8) failure
> l1title("Cumulative CHD Morbidity") gap(3) noborder                       {3}
```

```
        failure _d:  chdfate
 analysis time _t:  exitage
enter on or after:  time age

. *
. *  Calculate the logrank test corresponding to these morbidity functions
. *
. sts test sex                                                          {4}
        failure _d:  chdfate
 analysis time _t:  exitage
enter on or after:  time age

Log-rank test for equality of survivor functions
----------------------------------------------------
        |   Events
sex     |  observed    expected
------+----------------------
Men     |      823       571.08
Women   |      650       901.92
------+----------------------
Total   |     1473      1473.00

            chi2(1) =    182.91
            Pr>chi2 =    0.0000
. *
. *  Calculate the relative risk of CHD for men relative to women using age as
. *  the time variable.
. *
. generate male = sex == 1

. stcox male                                                            {5}
        failure _d:  chdfate
 analysis time _t:  exitage
enter on or after:  time age

                                                        {Output omitted}
Cox regression -- Breslow method for ties
No. of subjects =         4699          Number of obs   =      4699
No. of failures =         1473
Time at risk    = 103710.0914
                                        LR chi2(1)      =    177.15
Log likelihood  =   −11218.785          Prob > chi2     =    0.0000
```

```
-----------------------------------------------------------------------
  _t |
  _d | Haz. Ratio    Std. Err.      z      P>|z|      [95% Conf. Interval]
-----+-----------------------------------------------------------------
male |   2.011662    .1060464    13.259   0.000      1.814192    2.230626
-----------------------------------------------------------------------
```

Comments

1 We define *exitage* to be the patient's age at exit. This is the age when she either suffered CHD or was censored.

2 This command specifies the survival-time and fate variables for the subsequent survival commands. It defines *exitage* to be the time (age) when the subject's follow-up ends, *age* to be the time (age) when she is recruited into the cohort, and *chdfate* to be her fate at exit. Recall that *age* is the patient's age at her baseline exam and that she was free of CHD at that time (see Section 3.10).

3 This command plots cumulative CHD morbidity as a function of age for men and women. Strictly speaking, these plots are for people who are free of CHD at age 30, since this is the earliest age at recruitment. However, since CHD is rare before age 30, these plots closely approximate the cumulative morbidity curves from birth.

4 The logrank text is performed in exactly the same way as in Section 7.7. Changing the survival-time variable from years of follow-up to age increases the statistical significance of this test.

5 This command performs the proportional hazards regression defined by model (7.16).

7.10. Hazard Regression Models with Time-Dependent Covariates

Sometimes the relative risk between two groups varies appreciably with time. In this case, the proportional hazards assumption is invalid. We can weaken this assumption by using **time-dependent covariates**. That is, we assume that the ith patient has q covariates $x_{i1}[t], x_{i2}[t], \ldots, x_{iq}[t]$ that are themselves functions of time t. The hazard function for this patient is

$$\lambda_i[t] = \lambda_0[t] \exp[x_{i1}[t]\beta_1 + x_{i2}[t]\beta_2 + \cdots + x_{iq}[t]\beta_q]. \tag{7.17}$$

The simplest time-dependent covariates are **step-functions**. For example, in Figure 7.6 we saw strong evidence that the protective effect for a woman against CHD was greatest prior to her menopause. Moreover, it appears that the divergence of the morbidity curves diminishes at about age 57. To estimate how the relative risk of being male varies with age we could define the following covariate step functions:

$$male_{i1}[age] = \begin{cases} 1: i^{th} \text{ patient is a man} \leq age\ 57 \\ 0: \text{otherwise, and} \end{cases}$$

$$male_{i2}[age] = \begin{cases} 1: i^{th} \text{ patient is a man age} > 57 \\ 0: \text{otherwise.} \end{cases}$$

They are called step-functions because they equal 1 on one age interval and then step down to 0 for ages outside this interval. The boundary between these intervals (age 57) is called a **cut point**. The hazard model is then

$$\lambda_i[age] = \lambda_0[age]\ \exp[male_{i1}[age]\beta_1 + male_{i2}[age]\beta_2]. \tag{7.18}$$

The functions $male_{i1}[age]$ and $male_{i2}[age]$ are associated with two parameters β_1 and β_2 that assess the effect of male gender on CHD risk before and after age 57. Note that β_1 has no effect on CHD hazard after age 57 since, for $age > 57$, $x_{i1}[age] = 0$ regardless of the patient's sex. Similarly, β_2 has no effect on CHD hazard before time age 57. Hence, the hazard for men is $\lambda_0[age]\exp[\beta_1]$ prior to age 57 and $\lambda_0[age]\exp[\beta_2]$ thereafter. The hazard for women at any age is $\lambda_0[age]$. Therefore, the age-adjusted relative risk of CHD in men compared to women is $\exp[\beta_1]$ before age 57 and $\exp[\beta_2]$ afterwards. (If $\beta_1 = \beta_2 = \beta$ then the hazard for men at any age is $\lambda_0[age]\exp[\beta]$ and the proportional hazards assumption holds.) Of course, the true hazard undoubtedly is a continuous function of age. However, hazard functions with step-function covariates are often useful approximations that have the advantage of providing relevant relative risk estimates.

Applying model (7.18) to the Framingham data set gives estimates of $\hat{\beta}_1 = 1.291$ and $\hat{\beta}_2 = 0.541$. The standard errors of these estimates are $se[\hat{\beta}_1] = 0.1226$ and $se[\hat{\beta}_2] = 0.059\ 66$. Hence, among people ≤ 57 years old the age-adjusted relative risk of CHD for men relative to women is $\exp[1.291] = 3.64$, with a 95% confidence interval of $(3.64 \times \exp[-1.96 \times 0.1226],\ 3.64 \times \exp[1.96 \times 0.1226]) = (2.9–4.6)$. For people older than 57, this relative risk is reduced to $\exp[0.541] = 1.72$, with a 95% confidence interval of $(1.72 \times \exp[-1.96 \times 0.059\ 66],\ 1.72 \times \exp[1.96 \times 0.059\ 66]) = (1.5–1.9)$.

7.10.1. Cox–Snell Residuals for Models with Time-Dependent Covariates

The validity of survival models with time-dependent covariates may also be assessed using Cox–Snell residuals. This is done in the same way as in Section 7.6. When calculating these residuals with Stata you should use the *ccsnell* option rather than the *csnell* option of the *predict* post-estimation command. Stata handles time-dependent covariates by using multiple records per patient in the data set (see Section 7.11). The *ccsnell* option writes the Cox–Snell residual in the last record of each patient.

7.10.2. Testing the Proportional Hazards Assumption

If the proportional hazards assumption is true, then β_1 will equal β_2 in model (7.18). That is, if $\beta_1 = \beta_2 = \beta$, then model (7.18) reduces to the proportional hazards model (7.16). Hence, we can test the proportional hazards assumption by testing the null hypothesis that $\beta_1 - \beta_2 = 0$. In the Framingham study, this test yields a z statistic of 5.5 with $P < 10^{-7}$. Thus, the Framingham data set provides compelling evidence that the protection women enjoy against CHD diminishes after the menopause.

7.10.3. Alternative Models

There are, of course, many ways that we might choose to model the data using time-dependent covariates. For example, we could have several age groups with a separate time-dependent covariate for each group. We must also choose the cut points for our step functions. We could have chosen a round number such as age 60 to mark the boundary between the two age groups. I chose age 57, in part, by inspection of Figure 7.6. However, this age also minimizes the model deviance among models similar to model (7.18) only with other integer-valued ages for the cut point. Looking at the effect of cut points on model deviance is a good systematic way of selecting these values.

7.11. Modeling Time-Dependent Covariates with Stata

Stata can analyze hazard regression models with time-dependent covariates that are step-functions. To do this, we must first define multiple data records per patient in such a way that the covariate functions for the patient are constant for the period covered by each record. This is best explained

Table 7.5. Reformatting of the data for Framingham patient 18 needed to analyze model (7.18). For time-dependent hazard regression models the data must be split into multiple records per patient in such a way that the covariates remain constant over the time period covered by each record (see text).

id	male1	male2	enter	exit	fate
18	1	0	42	57	0
18	0	1	57	63	1

by an example. Suppose that we wished to analyze model (7.18). In the Framingham data set, patient 18 is a man who entered the study at age 42 and exits with CHD at age 63. For this patient $id = 18$, $age = 42$, $exitage = 63$, and $chdfate = 1$. We replace the record for this patient with two records. The first of these records describes his covariates from age 42 to age 57 while the other describes his covariates from age 57 to age 63. We define new variables $male1$, $male2$, $enter$, $exit$ and $fate$ whose values are shown in Table 7.5. The variable $enter$ equals his true entry age (42) in the first record and equals 57 in the second; $exit$ equals 57 in the first record and equals his true exit age (63) in the second. The variable $fate$ denotes his CHD status at the age given by $exit$. In the first record, $fate = 0$ indicating that he had not developed CHD by age 57. In the second record, $fate = 1$ indicating that he did develop CHD at age 63. The variable $male1$ equals the age dependent covariate $male_{i1}(age)$. In the first record $male1 = 1$ since $male_{i1}(age) = 1$ from entry until age 57. In the second record $male1 = 0$ since $male_{i1}(age) = 0$ after age 57 even though patient 18 is a man. Similarly $male2$ equals $male_{i2}(age)$, which equals 0 before age 57 and 1 afterwards.

We need two records only for patients whose follow-up spans age 57. Patients who exit the study before age 57 or enter after age 57 will have a single record. In this case, $enter$ will equal the patient's entry age and $exit$ will equal his or her age at the end of follow-up; $fate$ will equal $chdfate$ and $male1$ and $male2$ will be defined according to the patient's gender and age during follow-up. Time-dependent analyses must have an identification variable that allows Stata to keep track of which records belong to which patients. In this example, this variable is id.

The only tricky part of a time-dependent hazard regression analysis is defining the data records as described above. Once this is done, the analysis is straightforward. We illustrate how to modify the data file and do this analysis below. The log file *7.9.4.Framingham.log* continues as follows.

```
. *
. * Perform hazard regression with time dependent covariates for sex
. *
. tabulate chdfate male                                              {1}
```

```
Coronary |
   Heart |           male
 Disease |         0               1 |      Total
---------+--------------------------+----------
Censored |      2000            1226 |       3226
     CHD |       650             823 |       1473
---------+--------------------------+----------
   Total |      2650            2049 |       4699
```

```
. generate records = 1
```

```
. replace records = 2 if age < 57 & exitage > 57                     {2}
(3331 real changes made)
```

```
. expand records                                                     {3}
(3331 observations created)
```

```
. sort id                                                            {4}
```

```
. generate enter = age
```

```
. replace enter = 57 if id == id[_n-1]                               {5}
(3331 real changes made)
```

```
. generate exit = exitage
```

```
. replace exit = 57 if id == id[_n+1]                                {6}
(3331 real changes made)
```

```
. generate fate = chdfate
```

```
. replace fate = 0 if id == id[_n+1]                                 {7}
(855 real changes made)
```

```
. tabulate fate male                                                 {8}
         |           male
    fate |         0               1 |      Total
---------+--------------------------+----------
       0 |      3946            2611 |       6557
       1 |       650             823 |       1473
---------+--------------------------+----------
   Total |      4596            3434 |       8030
```

```
. generate male1 = male*(enter < 57)                              {9}

. generate male2= male*(exit > 57)                                {10}

. tabulate male1 male2                                            {11}

           |            male2
    male1  |         0            1 |      Total
-----------+------------------------+----------
        0  |      4596         1672 |       6268
        1  |      1762            0 |       1762
-----------+------------------------+----------
    Total  |      6358         1672 |       8030
```

```
. stset exit, id(id) enter(time enter) failure(fate)              {12}

                  id:  id
      failure event:  fate ~= 0 & fate ~=.
obs. time interval:  (exit[_n-1], exit]
 enter on or after:  time enter
 exit on or before:  failure
------------------------------------------------------
    8030  total obs.
       0  exclusions
------------------------------------------------------
    8030  obs. remaining, representing
    4699  subjects
    1473  failures in single failure-per-subject data
103710.1  total analysis time at risk, at risk from t =      0
                        earliest observed entry t =     30
                          last observed exit t =     94
```

```
. stcox male1 male2                                               {13}

      failure _d:  fate
 analysis time _t:  exit
enter on or after:  time enter
              id:  id
```

                                                          {Output omitted}

```
Cox regression -- Breslow method for ties

No. of subjects =         4699        Number of obs    =        8030
No. of failures =         1473
Time at risk    =  103710.0914
```

```
                                    LR chi2(2)      =      209.41
Log likelihood  =  -11202.652       Prob > chi2     =      0.0000

-----------------------------------------------------------------
    _t |
    _d |   Haz. Ratio   Std. Err.     z      P>|z|    [95% Conf. Interval]
-------+---------------------------------------------------------
 male1 |    3.636365    .4457209   10.532   0.000    2.859782    4.623831
 male2 |    1.718114    .1024969    9.072   0.000    1.528523    1.93122
-----------------------------------------------------------------

. lincom male1 - male2                                              {14}

(1)  male1 - male2 = 0.0
-----------------------------------------------------------------
    _t |     Coef.    Std. Err.     z    P>|z|    [95% Conf. Interval]
-------+---------------------------------------------------------
   (1) |   .7497575   .1363198    5.500  0.000   .4825755    1.01694
-----------------------------------------------------------------
```

Comments

1 The next few commands will create the multiple records that we need. It is prudent to be cautious doing this and to create before and after tables to confirm that we have done what we intended to do.

2 We define *records* to equal the number of records needed for each patient. This is either 1 or 2. Two records are needed only if the subject is recruited before age 57 and exits after age 57.

3 The *expand* command creates identical copies of records in the active data set. It creates one fewer new copy of each record than the value of the variable *records*. Hence, after this command has been executed there will be either 1 or 2 records in the file for each patient depending on whether *records* equals 1 or 2. The new records are appended to the bottom of the data set.

4 The *2.20.Framingham.dta* data set contains a patient identification variable called *id*. Sorting by *id* brings all of the records on each patient together. It is prudent to open the Stata editor frequently during data manipulations to make sure that your commands are having the desired effect. You should also make sure that you have a back-up copy of your original data as it is all too easy to replace the original file with one that has been modified.

5 Stata allows us to refer to the values of records adjacent to the current record. The value $\_n$ always equals the record number of the current record; $id[\_n-1]$ equals the value of id in the record preceding the current record, while $id[\_n+1]$ equals the value of id in the record following the current record.

If $id == id[\_n-1]$ is true then we are at the second of two records for the current patient. The previous command defined *enter* to equal *age*. This command replaces *enter* with the value 57 whenever we are at a patient's second record. Hence *enter* equals the patients entry age in the first record for each patient, and equals 57 in the second. If there is only one record for the patient, then *enter* equals the patient's entry age.

6 Similarly *exit* is set equal to *exitage* unless we are at the first of two records for the same patient, in which case *exit* equals 57.

7 The variable *fate* equals *chdfate* unless we are at the first of two records for the same patient. If a second record exists, then the first record must be for the first age interval and her follow-up must extend beyond age 57. Hence, the patient must not have developed CHD by age 57. For this reason we set *fate* = 0 whenever we encounter the first of two records for the same patient.

8 This table shows that there are 650 records for women showing CHD and 823 such records for men. This is the same as the number of women and men who had CHD. Thus, we have not added or removed any CHD events by the previous manipulations.

9 We set *male1* = 1 if and only if the subject is male and the record describes a patient in the first age interval. Otherwise, *male1* = 0. (Note that if *enter* <57 then we must have that *exit* ≤57.)

10 Similarly, *male2* = 1 if and only if the subject is male and the record describes a patient in the second age interval.

11 No records have both *male1* and *male2* equal to 1. There are 4596 records of women with both *male1* and *male2* equal 0, which agrees with the preceding table.

12 We define *exit* to be the exit time, *id* to be the patient identification variable, *enter* to be the entry time, and *fate* to be the fate indicator. The *stset* command also checks the data for errors or inconsistencies in the definition of these variables. Note that the total number of subjects has not been changed by our data manipulation.

13 Finally, we perform a hazard regression analysis with the time-dependent covariates *male1* and *male2*. The age-adjusted relative risks of CHD for men prior to, and after, age 57 are highlighted and agree with those given in Section 7.10.

14 This *lincom* statement tests the null hypothesis that $\beta_1 = \beta_2$ in model (7.18) (see Section 7.10.2).

7.12. Additional Reading

See Section 6.18 for some standard references on hazard regression analysis.

Fleming and Harrington (1991) is an advanced text on survival methods with an extensive discussion of residual analysis.

Cox and Snell (1968) is the original reference on Cox–Snell generalized residuals.

Kay (1977) applied the concept of Cox–Snell residuals to the analysis of censored survival data.

Therneau et al. (1990) is the original reference on martingale residuals. These residuals are used by Stata to calculate the Cox–Snell residuals discussed in this text.

7.13. Exercises

1 Using model (7.8) estimate the risk of CHD of men in each DBP group relative to women in the same group. Calculate 95% confidence intervals for these relative risks.

2 Fit a multiplicative model similar to model (7.11) but without the interaction terms for sex and blood pressure. Do the interaction terms in model (7.11) significantly improve the model fit over the multiplicative model that you have just created? How does your answer affect which model you would use if you were publishing these results?

3 The relative risk obtained from model (7.16) is age-adjusted while the relative risk derived from model (7.6) is not. Explain why this is so.

The following questions concern the *6.ex.breast.dta* data set introduced in the exercises for Chapter 6.

4 Calculate the relative risks of breast cancer among women with AH and PDWA compared to women without PD. Adjust for age by including age at entry biopsy as a covariate in your model. Calculate the 95% confidence intervals for these risks. Does this model give a better estimate of these risks than the model used in Question 4 in Chapter 6? If so, why?

5 Repeat Question 4 only this time adjust for age using a categorical variable that groups age at biopsy as follows: ≤ 30, 31–40, 41–50, 51–60, >60. Compare your answers to these questions. What are the strengths and weaknesses of these methods of age adjustment?

6 Build a proportional hazards model of the effects of entry biopsy diagnosis and family history on the risk of breast cancer. Adjust for age at biopsy by including *entage* as a covariate in your model. Treat PD and FH as categorical variables and include appropriate interaction terms. Fill in the following table. What is the risk of women with both AH and FH relative to women with FH but without PD? What is a 95% confidence interval for this risk?

	First degree family history of breast cancer			
	No		Yes	
Entry histology	Relative risk	95% confidence interval	Relative risk	95% confidence interval
No PD	1.0*			
PDWA				
AH				

*Denominator of relative risk

7 Plot the observed and expected breast cancer free survivorship curve against the Cox–Snell residuals from the model you used in Question 6. Does this graph provide any evidence that the proportional hazards assumption is invalid for this model? When assessing the overall appropriateness of the model, you should pay attention to the region of the graph that involves the vast majority of the residuals. What is the 95 percentile for these residuals?

8 What are the relative risks of AH and PDWA compared to No PD in the first ten years after biopsy? What are these risks after ten years for women who remain free of breast cancer for the first ten years following biopsy? To answer this question, build the following hazard regression model with time-dependent covariates. Define two step functions: the first should equal 1 on the interval 0–10 and 0 elsewhere; the second should equal 0 on the interval 0–10 and 1 elsewhere. Adjust for age at biopsy by including *entage* as a covariate in the model. Include two parameters to model the risk of AH in the first ten years and thereafter. Include another two parameters to model these risks for PDWA (reference: Dupont and Page, 1989).

9 Use your model for Question 8 to test the proportional hazards assumption for the model used in Question 6. Is this assumption reasonable?

8

Introduction to Poisson Regression: Inferences on Morbidity and Mortality Rates

In previous chapters the basic unit of observation has been the individual patient. Sometimes, however, it makes more sense to analyze events per person-year of observation. This may be either because the data comes to us in this form or because survival methods using suitable models are too complex and numerically intensive. For example, analyzing large cohorts with hazard regression models that have many time-dependent covariates can require substantial computation time. In this situation, converting the data to events per person-year of observation can greatly simplify the analysis. If the event rate per unit of time is low, then an excellent approach to consider is Poisson regression. We will introduce this technique in the next two chapters.

8.1. Elementary Statistics Involving Rates

The **incidence** I of an event is the expected number of events during 100 000 person-years of follow-up. Suppose that we observe d independent events during n person-years of observation, where d is small compared to n. Then the **observed incidence** of the event is $\hat{I} = 100\,000 \times d/n$, which is the observed number of events per 100 000 of patient-years of follow-up. For example, Table 8.1 is derived from the 4699 patients in the didactic data set from the Framingham Heart Study (Levy, 1999). This data set contains a total of 104 461 person-years of follow-up. Let d_i be the number of CHD events observed in n_i person-years of follow-up among men ($i = 1$) and women ($i = 0$), respectively. The observed incidence of coronary heart disease (CHD) in men is $\hat{I}_1 = 100\,000 \times d_1/n_1 = 100\,000 \times 823/42\,688 = 1927.9$, while the corresponding incidence in women is $\hat{I}_0 = 100\,000 \times d_0/n_0 = 100\,000 \times 650/61\,773 = 1052.2$. Incidence rates are always expressed as the observed or expected number of events in a specified number of patients during a specified interval of time. For example, an incidence rate might also

Table 8.1. Coronary heart disease and patient-years of follow-up in the Framingham Heart Study (Levy, 1999).

	Men		Women		Total
Cases of coronary heart disease	$d_1 =$	823	$d_0 =$	650	1 473
Person-years of follow-up	$n_1 = 42\,688$		$n_0 = 61\,773$		104 461

be expressed as the expected number of events per thousand person-months of observation.

Suppose that the incidences of some event are I_0 and I_1 in patients from Groups 0 and 1, respectively. Then the **relative risk** of the event in Group 1 compared to Group 0 is

$$R = I_1/I_0, \tag{8.1}$$

which is the ratio of the incidence rates in the two groups. We estimate this relative risk by $\hat{R} = \hat{I}_1/\hat{I}_0$. For example, the estimated relative risk of CHD in men compared to women in Table 8.1 is $\hat{R} = \hat{I}_1/\hat{I}_0 = 1927.9/1052.2 = 1.832$.

The logarithm of $\hat{R}$ has an approximately normal distribution whose variance is estimated by

$$s^2_{\log(\hat{R})} = \frac{1}{d_0} + \frac{1}{d_1}. \tag{8.2}$$

Hence, a 95% confidence interval for R is

$$\hat{R} \, \exp[\pm 1.96 s_{\log(\hat{R})}]. \tag{8.3}$$

For the patients from the Framingham Heart Study, $s^2_{\log(\hat{R})} = \frac{1}{823} + \frac{1}{650} = 0.002\,754$. Hence, a 95% confidence interval for the risk of CHD in men relative to women is

$$\hat{R} = (1.832 \exp[-1.96 \times \sqrt{0.002\,754}], \, 1.832 \exp[1.96 \times \sqrt{0.002\,754}])$$

$$= (1.65, 2.03).$$

8.2. Calculating Relative Risks from Incidence Data using Stata

The following log file and comments illustrate how to calculate relative risks from incidence data using Stata.

```
. * 8.2.Framingham.log

. *

. * Estimate the crude (unadjusted) relative risk of
```

```
. * coronary heart disease in men compared to women using
. * person-year data from the Framingham Heart Study.
. *
. iri 823 650 42688 61773                                                    {1}

                  | Exposed    Unexposed |     Total
------------------+----------------------+----------
          Cases  |    823          650   |     1473
    Person-time  |  42688        61773   |   104461
------------------+----------------------+----------
                  |                      |
  Incidence Rate  | .0192794    .0105224 |    .014101
                  |                      |
                  |  Point estimate      | [95% Conf. Interval]
                  |----------------------+----------------------
  Inc. rate diff. |       .008757        | .0072113    .0103028
  Inc. rate ratio |      1.832227        | 1.651129    2.033851   (exact)
  Attr. frac. ex. |      .4542162        | .3943538    .5083219   (exact)
  Attr. frac. pop |      .2537814        |
                  +-------------------------------------------------
                     (midp)   Pr(k>=823) =                0.0000   (exact)
                     (midp) 2*Pr(k>=823) =                0.0000   (exact)
```

Comment

1 The *ir* command is used for incidence rate data. Shown here is the immediate version of this command, called *iri*, which analyses the four data values
   given in the command line. These data are the number of exposed and
   unexposed cases together with the person-years of follow-up of exposed
   and unexposed subjects. In this example, "exposed" patients are male and
   "unexposed" patients are female. Cases are people who develop CHD. The
   arguments of the *iri* command are the number of men with CHD (exposed cases), the number of women with CHD (unexposed cases), and
   the number of person-years of follow-up in men and women, respectively.
   The relative risk of CHD in men compared to women is labeled "Inc. rate
   ratio". This relative risk, together with its 95% confidence interval, have
   been highlighted. They agree with equations (8.1) and (8.3) to three significant figures. Stata uses an exact confidence interval that has a more
   complicated formula than equation (8.3) and provides slightly wider
   intervals.

8.3. The Binomial and Poisson Distributions

Suppose that d unrelated deaths are observed among n patients. Let π be the probability that any individual patient dies. Then d has a binomial distribution with parameters n and π. The probability of observing d deaths is

$$\Pr[d \text{ deaths}] = \frac{n!}{(n-d)!d!}\pi^d(1-\pi)^{(n-d)}. \tag{8.4}$$

In equation (8.4) d can take any integer value between 0 and n. The expected number of deaths is $\mathrm{E}[d_i] = n\pi$, and the variance of d is $\mathrm{var}[d_i] = n\pi(1-\pi)$ (see Section 4.4). Poisson (1781–1849) showed that when n is large and π is small the distribution of d is closely approximated by a **Poisson distribution**. If $n\pi$ approaches λ as n gets very large then the distribution of d approaches

$$\Pr[d \text{ deaths}] = \frac{e^{-\lambda}(\lambda)^d}{d!}, \tag{8.5}$$

where d can be any non-negative integer. Under a Poisson distribution the expected value and variance of d both equal λ. Although it is not obvious from these formulas, the convergence of the binomial distribution to the Poisson is quite rapid. Figure 8.1 shows a Poisson distribution with expected

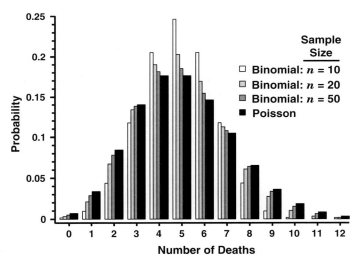

Figure 8.1   This graph illustrates the convergence of the binomial distribution to the Poisson distribution with increasing sample size (*n*) but constant expected value. The depicted distributions all have expected value five. By the time $n = 50$, the binomial distribution closely approximates the Poisson distribution with the same expected value.

value $\lambda = 5$. Binomial distributions are also shown with expected value $n\pi = 5$ for $n = 10, 20$, and 50. Note that the binomial distribution with $n = 50$ and $\pi = 0.1$ is very similar to the Poisson distribution with $\lambda = 5$.

8.4. Simple Poisson Regression for 2 × 2 Tables

Suppose that we have two groups of subjects who either are, or are not, exposed to some risk factor of interest. Let

n_i be the number of patients or patient-years of observation of subjects who are ($i = 1$) or are not ($i = 0$) exposed,

d_i be the number of deaths among exposed ($i = 1$) and unexposed ($i = 0$) subjects,

π_i be the true death rate in exposed ($i = 1$) and unexposed ($i = 0$) people, and

$x_i = 1$ or 0 be a covariate that indicates patients who are ($i = 1$) or are not ($i = 0$) exposed.

Then

$R = \pi_1/\pi_0$ is the relative risk of death associated with exposure, and

$\hat{\pi}_i = d_i/n_i$ is the estimated death rate in exposed ($i = 1$) or unexposed ($i = 0$) people.

The expected number of deaths in Group i is $\mathrm{E}[d_i \mid x_i] = n_i\pi_i$. Also $\mathrm{E}[\hat{\pi}_i \mid x_i] = \mathrm{E}[(d_i/n_i) \mid x_i] = \mathrm{E}[d_i \mid x_i]/n_i = \pi_i$, which implies that $\log[\pi_0] = \log[\mathrm{E}[d_0|x_0]] - \log[n_0]$ and $\log[\pi_1] = \log[\mathrm{E}[d_1|x_i]] - \log[n_1]$. Now since $R = \pi_1/\pi_0$, we also have that $\log[\pi_1] = \log[R] + \log[\pi_0]$. Hence,

$\log[\mathrm{E}[d_0 \mid x_0]] = \log[n_0] + \log[\pi_0]$ and
$\log[\mathrm{E}[d_1 \mid x_0]] = \log[n_1] + \log[\pi_0] + \log[R]$.

Let $\alpha = \log[\pi_0]$ and $\beta = \log[R]$. Then

$$\log[\mathrm{E}[d_i \mid x_i]] = \log[n_i] + \alpha + x_i\beta \tag{8.6}$$

for $i = 0$ or 1. If π_i is small we assume that d_i has a Poisson distribution. We estimate the mean and variance of this distribution by d_i. Equation (8.6) defines the simplest example of a **Poisson regression model.**

Our primary interest in model (8.6) is in β, which equals the log relative risk for exposed patients compared to unexposed patients. We will use the method of maximum likelihood to obtain an estimate $\hat{\beta}$ of β. We then estimate the risk of exposed subjects relative to unexposed subjects by

$$\hat{R} = e^{\hat{\beta}}. \tag{8.7}$$

The maximum likelihood technique also provides us with an estimate of the standard error of $\hat{\beta}$ which we will denote se$[\hat{R}]$. A 95% confidence interval for $\hat{R}$ is therefore

$$(\hat{R} \times \exp[-1.96 \mathrm{se}[\hat{\beta}]], \quad \hat{R} \times \exp[1.96 \mathrm{se}[\hat{\beta}]]). \tag{8.8}$$

The α coefficient in model (8.6) is called a **nuisance parameter**. This is one that is required by the model but is not used to calculate interesting statistics. An **offset** is a known quantity that must be included in a model. The term $\log[n_i]$ in model (8.6) is an example of an offset.

Let us apply model (8.6) to the Framingham Heart Study data in Table 8.1. Let $x_0 = 0$ and $x_1 = 1$ for person-years of follow-up in women and men, respectively. Regressing CHD against gender with this model gives estimates $\hat{\beta} = 0.6055$ and se$[\hat{\beta}] = 0.052\,47$. Applying equations (8.7) and (8.8) to these values gives a relative risk estimate of CHD in men relative to women to be $\hat{R} = 1.832$. The 95% confidence interval for this risk is $(1.65, 2.03)$. This relative risk and confidence interval are identical to the classical estimates obtained in Section 8.1.

8.5. Poisson Regression and the Generalized Linear Model

Poisson regression is another example of a generalized linear model. Recall that any generalized linear model is characterized by a random component, a linear predictor, and a link function (see Section 4.6). In Poisson regression the random component is the number of events d_i in the ith group of n_i patients or patient-years of observation. The linear predictor is $\log[n_i] + \alpha + x_i\beta$. The expected number of deaths in Group i, $\mathrm{E}[d_i \mid x_i]$, is related to the linear predictor through a logarithmic link function.

8.6. Contrast Between Poisson, Logistic, and Linear Regression

The models for simple linear, logistic, and Poisson regression are as follows:

$\mathrm{E}[y_i \mid x_i] = \alpha + \beta x_i$ for $i = 1, 2, \ldots, n$ defines the linear model;

$\mathrm{logit}[\mathrm{E}[d_i \mid x_i]/n_i] = \alpha + \beta x_i$ for $i = 1, 2, \ldots, n$ defines the logistic model; and

$\log[\mathrm{E}[d_i \mid x_i]] = \log[n_i] + \alpha + \beta x_i$ for $i = 0$ or 1 defines the Poisson model.

In linear regression, the random component is y_i, which has a normal distribution. The standard deviation of y_i given x_i is σ. The linear predictor is $\alpha + \beta x_i$ and the link function is the identity function $I[x] = x$. The sample size n must be fairly large since we must estimate σ before we can estimate α or β. In logistic regression, the random component is d_i events observed in n_i trials. This random component has a binomial distribution. The linear predictor is $\alpha + \beta x_i$ and the model has a logit link function. In Poisson regression, the random component is also d_i events observed in n_i trials or person-years of observation. This random component has a Poisson distribution. The linear predictor is $\log(n_i) + \alpha + \beta x_i$ and the model has a logarithmic link function. In the simple Poisson regression i takes only two values. This may also be the case for simple logistic regression. It is possible to estimate β in these situations since we have reasonable estimates of the mean and variance of d_i given x_i for both of these models.

8.7. Simple Poisson Regression with Stata

We apply a simple Poisson regression model to the data in Table 8.1 as follows.

```
. * 8.7.Framingham.log
. *
. * Simple Poisson regression analysis of the effect of gender on
. * coronary heart disease in the Framingham Heart Study.
. *
. use C:\WDDtext\8.7.Framingham.dta, clear
. list                                                              {1}
         chd           per_yrs           male
1.       650            61773              0
2.       823            42688              1
. glm chd male, family(poisson) link(log) lnoffset(per_yrs)         {2}
                                                        {Output omitted}
-----------------------------------------------------------------------

   chd |      Coef.   Std. Err.       z    P>|z|    [95% Conf. Interval]
-------+---------------------------------------------------------------
  male |   .6055324    .052474    11.540  0.000     .5026852    .7083796
 _cons |  -4.554249   .0392232  -116.111  0.000    -4.631125   -4.477373
per_yrs |  (exposure)
-----------------------------------------------------------------------
```

```
. lincom male, irr                                                    {3}
          (1)   [chd]male = 0.0
------------------------------------------------------------------
chd  |       IRR    Std. Err.      z      P>|z|  [95% Conf. Interval]
-----+------------------------------------------------------------
(1)  |   1.832227    .0961444   11.540   0.000  1.653154     2.030698
------------------------------------------------------------------
```

Comments

1 The data in Table 8.1 is stored in two records of *8.7.Framingham.dta*. These records contain the number of patient-years of follow-up in women (*male* = 0) and men (*male* = 1), respectively. The variable *chd* records the number of cases of coronary heart disease observed during follow-up.

2 This *glm* command regresses *chd* against *male* using model (8.6). The *family(poisson)* and *link(log)* options specify that *chd* has a Poisson distribution and that a logarithmic link function is to be used. The *lnoffset(per_yrs)* option specifies that the logarithm of *per_yrs* is to be included as an offset in the model.

3 The *irr* option of this *lincom* command has the same effect as the *or* and *hr* options. That is, it exponentiates the coefficient associated with *male* to obtain the estimated relative risk of CHD in men relative to women (see Section 5.20). It differs only in that it labels the second column of output IRR, which stands for incidence rate ratio. This rate ratio is our estimated relative risk. It and its associated confidence interval are in exact agreement with those obtained from equations (8.7) and (8.8).

8.8. Poisson Regression and Survival Analysis

For large data sets, Poisson regression is much faster than hazard regression analysis with time dependent covariates. If we have reason to believe that the proportional hazards assumption is false, it makes sense to do our exploratory analyses using Poisson regression. Before we can do this we must first convert the data from survival format to person-year format.

8.8.1. Recoding Survival Data on Patients as Patient-Year Data

Table 8.2 shows a survival data set consisting of entry age, exit age, treatment, and fate on five patients. The conversion of this survival data set to a patient-year data set is illustrated in Figure 8.2. Individual patients

8.8. Poisson regression and survival analysis

Table 8.2. This table shows survival data for five hypothetical patients. Each patient contributes person-years of follow-up to several strata defined by age and treatment. The conversion of this data set into a person-year data set for Poisson regression analysis is depicted in Figure 8.2.

Patient ID	Entry age	Exit age	Treatment	Fate
A	1	4	1	Alive
B	3	5	1	Dead
C	3	6	2	Alive
D	2	3	2	Dead
E	1	3	2	Dead

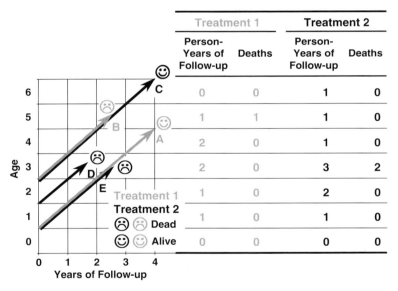

	Treatment 1		Treatment 2	
	Person-Years of Follow-up	Deaths	Person-Years of Follow-up	Deaths
	0	0	1	0
	1	1	1	0
	2	0	1	0
	2	0	3	2
	1	0	2	0
	1	0	1	0
	0	0	0	0

Figure 8.2   The survival data from Table 8.2 is depicted in the graph on the left of this figure. As the study subjects age during follow-up, they contribute person-years of observation to strata defined by age and treatment. Before performing Poisson regression, the survival data must be converted into a table of person-year data such as that given on the right of this figure. For example, three patients (B, C, and A) contribute follow-up to four-year-old patients. Two of them (B and A) are in Treatment 1 and one (C) is in Treatment 2. No deaths were observed at this age. Patients D and E do not contribute to this age because they died at age three.

contribute person-years of follow-up to a number of different ages. For example, Patient B enters the study at age 3 and dies at age 5. She contributes one year of follow-up at age 3, one at age 4, and one at age 5. To create the corresponding person-year data set we need to determine the number of patient-years of follow-up and number of deaths for each age in each treatment. This is done by summing across the rows of Figure 8.2. For example, consider age 3. There are three person-years of follow-up in Treatment 2 at this age that are contributed by patients C, D, and E. Deaths occur in two of these patient-years (Patients D and E). In Treatment 1 there are two person-years of follow-up for age 3 and no deaths (Patients B and A). The remainder of the table on the right side of Figure 8.2 is completed in a similar fashion. Note that the five patient survival records are converted into 14 records in the person-year file.

8.8.2. Converting Survival Records to Person-Years of Follow-Up using Stata

The following program may be used as a template to convert survival records on individual patients into records giving person-years of follow-up. It also demonstrates many of the ways in which data may be manipulated with Stata.

```
. * 8.8.2.Survival_to_Person-Years.log
. *
. * Convert survival data to person-year data.
. * The survival data set must have the following variables:
. *      id       = patient id,
. *      age_in   = age at start of follow-up,
. *      age_out  = age at end of follow-up,
. *      fate     = fate at exit: censored = 0, dead = 1,
. *      treat    = treatment variable.
. *
. * The person-year data set created below will contain one
. * record per unique combination of treatment and age.
. *
. * Variables in the person-year data set that must not be in the
. * original survival data set are
. *      age_now = an age of people in the cohort,
. *      pt_yrs  = number of patient-years of observations of people
. *                who are age_now years old,
. *      deaths  = number of events (fate=1) occurring in pt_yrs of
. *                follow-up for this group of patients.
. *
```

```
. use C:\WDDtext\8.8.2.Survival.dta, clear

. list

         id    age_in   age_out    treat      fate
  1.      A        1         4        1         0
  2.      B        3         5        1         1
  3.      C        3         6        2         0
  4.      D        2         3        2         1
  5.      E        1         3        2         1
```

```
. expand age_out - age_in + 1                                       {1}
(11 observations created)

. sort id                                                           {2}

. list if id == "B"                                                 {3}

         id    age_in   age_out    treat      fate
  5.      B        3         5        1         1
  6.      B        3         5        1         1
  7.      B        3         5        1         1
```

```
. generate  first = id[_n] ~= id[_n-1]                              {4}

. generate age_now = age_in

. replace age_now = age_now[_n-1]+1 if ~first                       {5}
(11 real changes made)

. generate last = id[_n] ~= id[_n+1]                                {6}

. generate observed = fate*last                                     {7}

. generate one = 1                                                  {8}

. list id age_in age_out first age_now if id == "B"                 {9}

         id    age_in   age_out    first     age_now
  5.      B        3         5        1         3
  6.      B        3         5        0         4
  7.      B        3         5        0         5
```

```
. list   id treat fate last observed one if id == "B"              {10}

         id    treat     fate     last    observed     one
  5.      B       1        1        0          0         1
  6.      B       1        1        0          0         1
  7.      B       1        1        1          1         1
```

```
. sort treat age_now                                               {11}

. collapse (sum) pt_yrs = one deaths = observed, by(treat age_now) {12}

. list treat age_now pt_yrs deaths                                 {13}
```

	treat	age_now	pt_yrs	deaths
1.	1	1	1	0
2.	1	2	1	0
3.	1	3	2	0
4.	1	4	2	0
5.	1	5	1	1
6.	2	1	1	0
7.	2	2	2	0
8.	2	3	3	2
9.	2	4	1	0
10.	2	5	1	0
11.	2	6	1	0

```
. save C:\WDDtext\8.8.2.Person-Years.dta, replace                    {14}
file C:\WDDtext\8.8.2.Person-years.dta saved
```

Comments

1 We expand the number of records per patient so that each patient has as many records as years of follow-up.

2 The file is sorted by *id* to make all records on the same patient contiguous.

3 For example, patient B enters the study at age 3 and exits at age 5. Therefore we create three records for this patient corresponding to ages 3, 4, and 5.

4 The variable *first* is set equal to 1 on the first record for each patient and equals zero on subsequent records. This is done by setting *first* = TRUE if the value of *id* in the preceding record is not equal to its value in the current record; *first* = FALSE otherwise. Recall that the numeric values for TRUE and FALSE are 1 and 0, respectively.

5 Increment the value of *age_now* by 1 for all but the first record of each patient. In the ith record for each patient, *age_now* equals the patient's age in her i^{th} year of follow-up.

6 The variable *last* = 1 in the last record for each patient; *last* = 0 otherwise.

7 The variable *observed* = 1 if the patient dies during the current year; *observed* = 0 otherwise. Since the patient must have survived the current year if she has an additional record, *observed* = 1 if and only if the patient dies in her last year of follow-up (*fate* = 1) and we have reached her last year (*last* = 1).

8 We will use the variable *one* = 1 to count patient-years of follow-up.

9 For example, patient *B* is followed for three years. Her age in these years is recorded in *age_now*, which is 3, 4, and 5 years, respectively.

10 Patient *B* dies in her fifth year of life. She was alive at the end of her third

and fourth year. Hence, *observed* equals 0 in her first two records and equals 1 in her last.

11 We now sort by *treat* and *age_now* to make all records of patients with the same treatment and age contiguous.

12 This statement collapses all records with identical values of *treat* and *age_now* into a single record. The variable *pt_yrs* is set equal to the number of records collapsed (the sum of *one* over these records) and *deaths* is set equal to the number of deaths (the sum of *observed* over these records). All variables are deleted from memory except *treat, age_now, pt_yrs,* and *deaths*.

13 The data set now corresponds to the right-hand side of Figure 8.2. Note, however, that the program only creates records for which there is at least one person-year of follow-up. The reason why there are 11 rather than 14 records in the file is that there are no person-years of follow-up for 6 year-old patients on treatment 1 or for patients on either treatment in their first year of life.

14 The data set is saved for future Poisson regression analysis.

N.B. If you are working on a large data set with many covariates, you can reduce the computing time by keeping only those covariates that you will need in your model(s) before you start to convert to patient-year data. It is a good idea to check that you have not changed the number of deaths or number of years of follow-up in your program. See the *8.9.Framingham.log* file in the next section for an example of how this can be done.

8.9. Converting the Framingham Survival Data Set to Person-Time Data

The following Stata log file and comments illustrate how to convert a real survival data set for Poisson regression analysis.

```
. * 8.9.Framingham.log
. *
. * Convert Framingham survival data set to person-year data for
. * Poisson regression analysis.
. *
. set memory 11000                                                    {1}
(11000k)

. use C:\WDDtext\2.20.Framingham.dta, clear
. *
. * Convert bmi, scl and dbp into categorical variables that subdivide
. * the data set into quartiles for each of these variables.
```

```
. *
. centile bmi dbp scl, centile(25,50,75)                                    {2}

                                  -- Binom. Interp. --
Variable |    Obs   Percentile   Centile   [95% Conf. Interval]
---------+-----------------------------------------------------
    bmi |   4690          25      22.8      22.7           23
        |                 50      25.2      25.1      25.36161
        |                 75        28      27.9         28.1
    dbp |   4699          25        74        74           74
        |                 50        80        80           82
        |                 75        90        90           90
    scl |   4666          25       197       196          199
        |                 50       225       222          225
        |                 75       255       252          256
```

```
. generate bmi_gr = recode(bmi, 22.8, 25.2, 28, 29)
(9 missing values generated)

. generate dbp_gr = recode(dbp, 74,80,90,91)

. generate scl_gr = recode(scl, 197, 225, 255, 256)
(33 missing values generated)

. *
. * Calculate years of follow-up for each patient.
. * Round to nearest year for censored patients.
. * Round up to next year when patients exit with CHD
. *
. generate years = int(followup/365.25) + 1 if chdfate              {3}
(3226 missing values generated)

. replace years = round(followup/365.25, 1) if ~chdfate             {4}
(3226 real changes made)

. table sex dbp_gr, contents(sum years) row col                     {5}
```

```
-------+---------------------------------------
       |              dbp_gr
  Sex |     74      80      90      91    Total
-------+---------------------------------------
  Men |  10663   10405   12795    8825    42688
Women |  21176   14680   15348   10569    61773
       |
Total |  31839   25085   28143   19394   104461
-------+---------------------------------------
```

```
. table sex dbp_gr, contents(sum chdfate) row col                   {6}
```

```
-------+-----------------------------------
       |                dbp_gr
  Sex  |    74     80     90     91    Total
-------+-----------------------------------
  Men  |   161    194    222    246      823
Women  |   128    136    182    204      650
       |
Total  |   289    330    404    450     1473
-------+-----------------------------------
```

. generate *age_in = age*

. generate *age_out = age + years - 1*

. generate *age_now = age*

. *

. * *Transform data set so that there is one record per patient-year of*

. * *follow-up. Define age_now to be the patient's age in each record.*

. * *Define fate = 1 for the last record of each patient who develops CHD,*

. *   *= 0 otherwise.*

. *

. expand *years*
(99762 observations created)

. sort *id*

. generate *first = id[_n] ~= id[_n-1]*

. replace *age_now = age_now[_n-1]+1 if ~first*
(99762 real changes made)

. generate *last = id[_n] ~= id[_n+1]*

. generate *fate = chdfate*last*

. generate *one = 1*

. list *id age_in age_out age_now first last chdfate fate in 20/26*, nodisplay   {7}

	id	age_in	age_out	age_now	first	last	chdfate	fate
20.	1	60	79	79	0	1	Censored	0
21.	2	46	50	46	1	0	CHD	0
22.	2	46	50	47	0	0	CHD	0
23.	2	46	50	48	0	0	CHD	0
24.	2	46	50	49	0	0	CHD	0
25.	2	46	50	50	0	1	CHD	1
26.	3	49	80	49	1	0	Censored	0

. generate *age_gr = recode(age_now, 45,50,55,60,65,70,75,80,81)*   {8}

```
. label define age 45 "<= 45" 50 "45-50" 55 "50-55" 60 "55-60" 65 "60-65" 70
> "65-70" 75 "70-75" 80 "75-80" 81 "> 80"

. label values age_gr age

. sort sex bmi_gr scl_gr dbp_gr age_gr

. *
. * Combine records with identical values of
. * sex bmi_gr scl_gr dbp_gr and age_gr.
. *
. collapse (sum) pt_yrs=one chd_cnt=fate, by(sex bmi_gr scl_gr dbp_gr age_gr)   {9}

. list sex bmi_gr scl_gr dbp_gr age_gr pt_yrs chd_cnt in 310/315, nodisplay

         sex    bmi_gr    scl_gr    dbp_gr    age_gr     pt_yrs    chd_cnt
310.     Men        28       197        90     45-50        124          0
311.     Men        28       197        90     50-55        150          1
312.     Men        28       197        90     55-60        158          2
313.     Men        28       197        90     60-65        161          4
314.     Men        28       197        90     65-70        100          2
315.     Men        28       197        90     70-75         55          1
```

```
. table sex dbp_gr, contents(sum pt_yrs) row col                                {10}

---------+---------------------------------------------
         |                    dbp_gr
   Sex   |      74        80        90        91     Total
---------+---------------------------------------------
   Men   |   10663     10405     12795      8825     42688
 Women   |   21176     14680     15348     10569     61773
         |
 Total   |   31839     25085     28143     19394    104461
---------+---------------------------------------------
```

```
. table sex dbp_gr, contents(sum chd_cnt) row col                               {11}


---------+---------------------------------------------
         |                    dbp_gr
   Sex   |      74        80        90        91     Total
---------+---------------------------------------------
   Men   |     161       194       222       246       823
 Women   |     128       136       182       204       650
         |
 Total   |     289       330       404       450      1473
---------+---------------------------------------------
```

```
. generate male = sex == 1                                          {12}

. display _N                                                        {13}
1267

. save C:\WDDtext\8.12.Framingham.dta                               {14}
file C:\WDDtext\8.12.Framingham.dta saved
```

Comments

1 The Framingham data set requires 11 megabytes for these calculations.

2 The *centile* command gives percentiles for the indicated variables. The *centile* option specifies the percentiles of these variables that are to be listed, which in this example are the 25th, 50th, and 75th. These are then used as arguments in the *recode* function to define the categorical variables *bmi_gr*, *dbp_gr*, and *scl_gr*.

   In the next chapter we will consider body mass index, serum cholesterol, and diastolic blood pressure as confounding variables in our analyses. We convert these data into categorical variables grouped by quartiles.

3 The last follow-up interval for most patients is a fraction of a year. If the patient's follow-up was terminated because of a CHD event, we include the patient's entire last year as part of her follow-up. The *int* function facilitates this by truncating follow-up in years to a whole integer. We then add 1 to this number to include the entire last year of follow-up.

4 If the patient is censored at the end to follow-up, we round this number to the nearest integer using the *round* function; $round(x, 1)$ rounds x to the nearest integer.

5 So far, we haven't added any records or modified any of the original variables. Before doing this it is a good idea to tabulate the number of person-years of follow-up and CHD events in the data set. At the end of the transformation we can recalculate these tables to ensure that we have not lost or added any spurious years of follow-up or CHD events. This tables show these data cross tabulated by *sex* and *dbp_gr*. The *contents*(*sum years*) option causes *years* to be summed over every unique combination of values of *sex* and *dbp_gr* and displayed in the table. For example, the sum of the *years* variable for men with *dbp_gr* = 90 is 12 795. This means that there are 12 795 person-years of follow-up for men with baseline diastolic blood pressures between 80 and 90 mm Hg.

6 This table shows the number of CHD events by sex and DBP group.

7 The expansion of the data set, and the definitions of *age_now*, *fate*, and *one* are done in the same way as in Section 8.8.2. This *list* command

shows the effects of these transformations. Note that patient 2 enters the study at age 46 and exits at age 50 with CHD. The expanded data set contains one record for each of these years; *age_now* increases from 46 to 50 in these records, and *fate* equals 1 only in the final record for this patient.

8 Recode *age_now* into 5-year age groups.

9 Collapse records with identical values of *sex*, *bmi_gr*, *scl_gr*, *dbp_gr*, and *age_gr*. The variable *pt_yrs* records the number of patient-years of follow-up associated with each record while *chd_cnt* records the corresponding number of CHD events. For example, the subsequent listing shows that there were 161 patient-years of follow-up in men aged 61 to 65 with body mass indexes between 25.3 and 28, serum cholesterols less than or equal to 197, and diastolic blood pressures between 81 and 90 on their baseline exams. Four CHD events occurred in these patients during these years of follow-up.

10 This table shows total person-years of follow-up cross-tabulated by *sex* and *dbp_gr*. Note that this table is identical to the one produced before the data transformation.

11 This table shows CHD events of follow-up cross-tabulated by *sex* and *dbp_gr*. This table is also identical to its pre-transformation version and provides evidence that we have successfully transformed the data in the way we intended.

12 Define *male* to equal 1 for men and 0 for women. In later analyses male gender will be treated as a risk factor for coronary heart disease.

13 We have created a data set with 1267 records. There is one record for each unique combination of covariate values for the variables *sex*, *bmi_gr*, *scl_gr*, *dbp_gr*, and *age_gr*.

14 The person-year data set is stored away for future analysis. We will use this data set in Section 8.12 and in Chapter 9.

N.B. It is very important that you specify a new name for the transformed data set. If you use the original name, you will lose the original data set. It is also a very good idea to always keep back-up copies of your original data sets in case you accidentally destroy the copy that you are working with.

8.10. Simple Poisson Regression with Multiple Data Records

In Section 8.9, we created a data set from the Framingham Heart Study with 1267 records. Each of these records describes a number of person-years of follow-up and number of CHD events associated with study subjects with a specific value for each of the covariates. Suppose that we wanted to repeat the analysis of the effect of gender on CHD from Section 8.4 using this data set. The model for this analysis is

$$\log[\mathrm{E}[d_i \mid x_i]] = \log[n_i] + \alpha + x_i\beta, \tag{8.9}$$

where where α and β are model parameters,

n_i is the number of person-years of follow-up in the ith record of this data set,

d_i is the number of CHD events observed in these n_i person-years of follow-up, and

$$x_i = \begin{cases} 1: & \text{if the } i^{\text{th}} \text{ record describes follow-up of men} \\ 0: & \text{if the } i^{\text{th}} \text{ record describes follow-up of women.} \end{cases}$$

Note that models (8.9) and (8.6) are almost identical. In model (8.6) there are only two records and n_0 and n_1 equal the total number of person-years of follow-up in women and men, respectively. In model (8.9) there are 1267 records and n_i equals the total number of person-years of follow-up in the ith record. The person-years of follow-up and CHD events in women and men from model (8.6) have been distributed over a much larger number of records in model (8.9). This difference in data organization has no effect on our estimate of the relative risk of CHD in men compared to women. Regressing CHD against gender using model (8.9) gives a relative risk estimate of $\hat{R} = 1.832$, with a 95% confidence interval of $(1.65, 2.03)$. This estimate and confidence interval are identical to those obtained from model (8.6) in Section 8.4. Model (8.9) will work as long as the division of person-years of follow-up is done in such a way that each record describes follow-up in a subgroup of men or a subgroup of women (but not of both genders combined).

8.11. Poisson Regression with a Classification Variable

Suppose that we wished to determine the crude relative risks of CHD among subjects whose body mass index (BMI) is in the second, third, and fourth quartiles relative to subjects in the first BMI quartile. We do this in much the same way as we did for logistic regression (see Section 5.11). Suppose that the data are organized so that each record describes person-years of follow-up and CHD events in subjects whose BMIs are in the same quartile. Consider the model

$$\log[\mathrm{E}[d_i \mid ij]] = \log[n_i] + \alpha + \beta_2 \times bmi_{i2} + \beta_3 \times bmi_{i3} + \beta_4 \times bmi_{i4}, \tag{8.10}$$

where n_i and d_i describe the number of person-years of follow-up and CHD events in the ith record,

j is the BMI quartile of patients from the ith record,

$$bmi_{ih} = \begin{cases} 1: & \text{if patients from the } i^{th} \text{ record are in the } h^{th} \text{ BMI quartile} \\ 0: & \text{otherwise.} \end{cases}$$

Let π_j be the CHD event rate of patients in the jth BMI quartile, and let $R_j = \pi_j/\pi_1$ be the relative risk of people in the jth quartile compared to the first. Then for records describing patients in the first BMI quartile, model (8.10) reduces to

$$\log[E[d_i \mid i1]] = \log[n_i] + \alpha. \tag{8.11}$$

Subtracting $\log[n_i]$ from both sides of equation (8.11) gives us

$$\log[E[d_i \mid i1]] - \log[n_i] = \log[E[d_i/n_i \mid i1]] = \log[\pi_1] = \alpha. \tag{8.12}$$

For records of patients from the fourth BMI quartile model (8.10) reduces to

$$\log[E[d_i \mid i4]] = \log[n_i] + \alpha + \beta_4. \tag{8.13}$$

Subtracting $\log[n_i]$ from both sides of equation (8.13) gives us

$$\log[E[d_i \mid i4]] - \log[n_i] = \log[E[d_i/n_i \mid i4]] = \log[\pi_4] = \alpha + \beta_4. \tag{8.14}$$

Subtracting equation (8.12) from equation (8.14) gives us

$$\log[\pi_4] - \log[\pi_1] = \log[\pi_4/\pi_1] = \log[R_4] = \beta_4.$$

Hence, β_4 is the log relative risk of CHD for people in the fourth BMI quartile relative to people in the first BMI quartile. By a similar argument, β_2 and β_3 estimate the log relative risks of people in the second and third BMI quartiles,

Table 8.3. Effect of baseline body mass index on coronary heart disease. The Framingham Heart Study data were analyzed using model (8.10).

Baseline body mass index		Person-years of follow-up	Patients with coronary heart disease	Relative risk	95% confidence interval
Quartile	Range				
1	≤ 22.8 kg/m^2	27 924	239	1*	
2	22.8–25.2 kg/m^2	26 696	337	1.47	(1.2–1.7)
3	25.2–28 kg/m^2	26 729	443	1.94	(1.7–2.3)
4	> 28 kg/m^2	22 977	453	2.30	(2.0–2.7)
Total		104 326	1472		

* Denominator of relative risk

respectively. Applying model (8.10) to the Framingham Heart Study data reformatted in Section 8.9 gives the relative risk estimates and confidence intervals presented in Table 8.3.

8.12. Applying Simple Poisson Regression to the Framingham Data

The following log file and comments illustrate how to perform the analysis of models (8.9) and (8.10) using Stata.

```
. * 8.12.Framingham.do
. *
. * Analysis of the effects of gender and body mass index
. * on coronary heart disease using person-year data from the
. * Framingham Heart Study.
. *
. use C:\WDDtext\8.12.Framingham.dta, clear

. *
. * Regress CHD against gender using model 8.9.
. *
. glm chd_cnt male, family(poisson) link(log) lnoffset(pt_yrs) eform          {1}
                                                              {Output omitted}
-------------------------------------------------------------------------------
chd_cnt |         IRR    Std. Err.      z      P> |z|    [95% Conf. Interval]
--------+----------------------------------------------------------------------
   male |    1.832227    .0961442   11.540    0.000    1.653154    2.030698
 pt_yrs |   (exposure)
-------------------------------------------------------------------------------

. table bmi_gr, contents(sum pt_yrs) row                                        {2}

--------+------------
 bmi_gr | sum(pt_yrs)
--------+------------
   22.8 |       27924
   25.2 |       26696
     28 |       26729
     29 |       22977
        |
  Total |      104326
--------+------------

. table bmi_gr, contents(sum chd_cnt) row                                       {3}
```

```
---------+--------------
 bmi_gr  |  sum(chd_cnt)
---------+--------------
   22.8  |           239
   25.2  |           337
     28  |           443
     29  |           453
         |
  Total  |          1472
---------+--------------
```

```
. *
. * Regress CHD against BMI using model 8.10.
. *
. xi: glm chd_cnt i.bmi_gr, family(poisson) link(log) lnoffset(pt_yrs) eform  {4}
i.bmi_gr    _Ibmi_gr_1-4    (_Ibmi_gr_1 for bmi~r==22.79999923706054 omitted)
```
                                                                    {Output omitted}
```
-------------------------------------------------------------------------
  chd_cnt |       IRR   Std. Err.     z     P>|z|   [95% Conf. Interval]
----------+--------------------------------------------------------------
_Ibmi_gr_2 |   1.474903   .1247271   4.595   0.000   1.249627     1.74079   {5}
_Ibmi_gr_3 |   1.936425   .1554147   8.234   0.000   1.654568    2.266298
_Ibmi_gr_4 |   2.303481   .1841576  10.437   0.000   1.969396    2.694239
    pt_yrs |  (exposure)
-------------------------------------------------------------------------
```

Comments

1 See Comment 2 of Section 8.7 for an explanation of the syntax of this command. The number of CHD events in each record, *chd_cnt*, is regressed against *male* using model (8.9). The variable *pt_yrs* gives the number of patient-years of follow-up per record. The *eform* option specifies that the estimate of the model coefficient for the covariate *male* is to be exponentiated. This gives an estimate of the relative risk of CHD in men without having to use a *lincom* command. The heading IRR stands for incidence rate ratio, which is a synonym for relative risk. The highlighted relative risk and confidence interval are identical to those obtained in Section 8.7 from model (8.6).

2 Create a table of the number of patient-years of follow-up among patients in each quartile of BMI. A separate row of the table is generated for each distinct value of *bmi_gr*. The *contents(sum pt_yrs)* option sums and lists

the value of *pt_yrs* over all records with the same value of *bmi_gr*. The *row* option provides the total number of patient-years of follow-up among patients whose BMI is known. This total is less than that given in Table 8.1 because some patients have missing BMIs.

3   This table sums the total number of CHD events observed among patients in each BMI quartile. The output from this and the preceding table is entered in Table 8.3.

4   The *xi* prefix works exactly the same way for the *glm* command as for the *logistic* command. The term *i.bmi_gr* creates separate indicator variables for all but the first value of the classification variable *bmi_gr*. In Section 8.9, we defined *dbp_gr* to take the values 22.8, 25.2, 28, and 29 for patients whose BMI was in the first, second, third, and fourth quartile, respectively. The indicator variables that are generated are called *_Ibmi_gr_2*, *_Ibmi_gr_3*, and *_Ibmi_gr_4*. *_Ibmi_gr_2* equals 1 for patients whose BMI is in the second quartile and equals 0 otherwise. *_Ibmi_gr_3* and *_Ibmi_gr_4* are similarly defined for patients whose BMIs are in the third and fourth quartiles, respectively. These covariates are entered into the model. In other words, *i.bmi_gr* enters the terms $\beta_2 \times bmi_{i2} + \beta_3 \times bmi_{i3} + \beta_4 \times bmi_{i4}$ from model (8.10). Thus, the entire command regresses CHD against BMI using model (8.10).

5   The highlighted relative risks and confidence intervals were used to create Table 8.3.

8.13. Additional Reading

Rothman and Greenland (1998) discuss classical methods of estimating relative risks from incidence data.

Breslow and Day (1987) provides an excellent discussion of Poisson regression. I recommend this text to readers who are interested in the mathematical underpinnings of this technique.

McCullagh and Nelder (1989) is a standard reference that discusses Poisson regression within the framework of the generalized linear model.

8.14. Exercises

Scholer et al. (1997) studied a large cohort of children from Tennessee with known risk factors for injuries (see also the exercises from Chapter 5). Children were followed until their fifth birthday. Data from a subset of this study is posted on my web site in a file called *8.ex.InjuryDeath.dta*. There is one record in this data file for each distinct combination of the following covariates from the original file. These covariates are defined as follows:

age   Child's age in years

age_mom   Mother's age in years when her child was born, categorized as
               19:   age < 20
               24:   $20 \leq$ age ≤ 24
               29:   $25 \leq$ age ≤ 29
               30:   age > 29

lbw   Birth weight, categorized as
               0:    ≥ 2500 gm
               1:    < 2500 gm

educ_mom   Mother's years of education, categorized as
               11:   < 12 years
               12:   12 years
               15:   13–15 years
               16:   >15 years

income   Maternal neighborhood's average income, categorized by quintiles

illegit   Maternal marital status at time of birth, categorized as
               0:    Married
               1:    Single

oth_chld   Number of other children, categorized as
               0:    No siblings
               1:    1 sibling
               2:    2 siblings
               3:    3 siblings
               4:    4 or more siblings

race_mom   Race of mother, categorized as
               0:    White
               1:    Black

pnclate   Late or absent prenatal care, categorized as
               0:    Care in first 4 months of pregnancy
               1:    No care in first 4 months of pregnancy

Also included in each record is

childyrs   The number of child-years of observation among children with the specified covariate values

inj_dth   The number of injury deaths observed in these child-years of observation

1 Using the *8.ex.InjuryDeath.dta* data set, fill in the following table of person-years of follow-up in the Tennessee Children's Cohort, subdivided by the mother's marital status and injury deaths in the first five years of life.

	Marital status of mother		
	Not married	Married	Total
Injury deaths			
Child-years of follow-up			

2 Using classical methods, estimate the risk of injury deaths in children born to unmarried mothers relative to children born to married mothers. Calculate a 95% confidence interval for this relative risk. How does your answer differ from the relative risk for illegitimacy that you calculated in Question 4 of Chapter 5? Explain any differences you observe.

3 Use Poisson regression to complete the following table. How does your estimate of the relative risk of injury death associated with illegitimacy compare to your answer to Question 2?

Numerator of relative risk	Denominator of relative risk	Crude relative risk*	95% confidence interval
Maternal age 25–29	Maternal age > 29		
Maternal age 20–24	Maternal age > 29		
Maternal age < 20	Maternal age > 29		
Birth weight < 2500 gm	Birth weight ≥ 2500 gm		
Mother's education. 13–15 yrs.	Mother's ed. > 15 yrs.		
Mother's education = 12 yrs.	Mother's ed. > 15 yrs.		
Mothers education < 12 yrs.	Mother's ed. > 15 yrs.		
Income in lowest quintile	Income in highest quintile		
Income in 2nd quintile	Income in highest quintile		
Income in 3rd quintile	Income in highest quintile		
Income in 4th quintile	Income in highest quintile		
Unmarried mother	Married mother		

One sibling	No siblings
Two siblings	No siblings
Three siblings	No siblings
> 3 siblings	No siblings
Black mother	White mother
Late/no prenatal care	Adequate prenatal care
1st year of life	3 year old
1 year old	3 year old
2 year old	3 year old
4 year old	3 year old

* Unadjusted for other covariates

9

Multiple Poisson Regression

Simple Poisson regression generalizes to multiple Poisson regression in the same way that simple logistic regression generalizes to multiple logistic regression. The response variable is a number of events observed in a given number of person-years of observation. We regress this response variable against several covariates, using the logarithm of the number of person-years of observation as an offset in the model. This allows us to estimate event rates that are adjusted for confounding variables or to determine how specific variables interact to affect these rates. We can add interaction terms to our model in exactly the same way as in the other regression techniques discussed in this text.

The methods used in this chapter are very similar to those used in Chapter 5 for multiple logistic regression. You will find this chapter easier to read if you have read Chapter 5 first.

9.1. Multiple Poisson Regression Model

Suppose that data on patient-years of follow-up can be logically grouped into J strata based on age or other factors, and that there are K exposure categories that affect morbidity or mortality in the population. For $j = 1, \ldots, J$ and $k = 1, \ldots, K$ let

n_{jk} be the number of person-years of follow-up observed among patients in the jth stratum who are in the kth exposure category,

d_{jk} be the number of morbid or mortal events observed in these n_{jk} person-years of follow-up,

$x_{jk1}, x_{jk2}, \cdots, x_{jkq}$ be explanatory variables that describe the kth exposure group of patients in stratum j, and

$\mathbf{x}_{jk} = (x_{jk1}, x_{jk2}, \cdots, x_{jkq})$ denote the values of all of the covariates for patients in the jth stratum and k^{th} exposure category.

Then the **multiple Poisson regression** model assumes that

$$\log[\text{E}[d_{jk} \mid \mathbf{x}_{jk}]] = \log[n_{jk}] + \alpha_j + \beta_1 x_{jk1} + \beta_2 x_{jk2} + \cdots + \beta_q x_{jkq}, \quad (9.1)$$

where

$\alpha_1, \ldots, \alpha_J$ are unknown nuisance parameters, and
$\beta_1, \beta_2, \ldots, \beta_q$ are unknown parameters of interest.

For example, suppose that there are $J = 5$ age strata, and that patients are classified as light or heavy drinkers and light or heavy smokers in each stratum. Then there are $K = 4$ exposure categories (two drinking categories times two smoking categories). We might choose $q = 2$ and let

$$x_{jk1} = \begin{cases} 1: \text{for patients who are heavy drinkers} \\ 0: \text{for patients who are light drinkers,} \end{cases}$$

$$x_{jk2} = \begin{cases} 1: \text{for patients who are heavy smokers} \\ 0: \text{for patients who are light smokers.} \end{cases}$$

Then model (9.1) reduces to

$$\log[E[d_{jk}|\mathbf{x}_{jk}]] = \log[n_{jk}] + \alpha_j + \beta_1 x_{jk1} + \beta_2 x_{jk2}. \tag{9.2}$$

The relationship between the age strata, exposure categories, and covariates of this model is clarified in Table 9.1.

Let $\lambda_{jk} = E[d_{jk}/n_{jk} \mid \mathbf{x}_{jk}]$ be the expected morbidity incidence rate for people from stratum j who are in exposure category k. If we subtract $\log(n_{jk})$ from both sides of model (9.1) we get

$$\log[E[d_{jk} \mid \mathbf{x}_{jk}]/n_{jk}] = \log[E[d_{jk}/n_{jk} \mid \mathbf{x}_{jk}]] =$$

$$\log[\lambda_{jk}] = \alpha_j + \beta_1 x_{jk1} + \beta_2 x_{jk2} + \cdots + \beta_q x_{jkq}. \tag{9.3}$$

Table 9.1. This table shows the relationships between the age strata, the exposure categories and the covariates of model (9.2).

		Exposure Category			
		$k = 1$	$k = 2$	$k = 3$	$k = 4$
	$K = 4$	Light drinker	Light drinker	Heavy drinker	Heavy drinker
	$J = 5$	light smoker	heavy smoker	light smoker	heavy smoker
	$p = 2$	$x_{j11} = 0, x_{j12} = 0$	$x_{j21} = 0, x_{j22} = 1$	$x_{j31} = 1, x_{j32} = 0$	$x_{j41} = 1, x_{j42} = 1$
Age Stratum	$j = 1$	$x_{111} = 0, x_{112} = 0$	$x_{121} = 0, x_{122} = 1$	$x_{131} = 1, x_{132} = 0$	$x_{141} = 1, x_{142} = 1$
	$j = 2$	$x_{211} = 0, x_{212} = 0$	$x_{221} = 0, x_{222} = 1$	$x_{231} = 1, x_{232} = 0$	$x_{241} = 1, x_{242} = 1$
	$j = 3$	$x_{311} = 0, x_{312} = 0$	$x_{321} = 0, x_{322} = 1$	$x_{331} = 1, x_{332} = 0$	$x_{341} = 1, x_{342} = 1$
	$j = 4$	$x_{411} = 0, x_{412} = 0$	$x_{421} = 0, x_{422} = 1$	$x_{431} = 1, x_{432} = 0$	$x_{441} = 1, x_{442} = 1$
	$j = 5$	$x_{511} = 0, x_{512} = 0$	$x_{521} = 0, x_{522} = 1$	$x_{531} = 1, x_{532} = 0$	$x_{541} = 1, x_{542} = 1$

In other words, model (9.1) imposes a log linear relationship between the expected morbidity rates and the model covariates. Note that this model permits people in the same exposure category to have different morbidity rates in different strata. This is one of the more powerful features of Poisson regression in that it makes it easy to model incidence rates that vary with time.

Suppose that two groups of patients from the jth stratum have been subject to exposure categories f and g. Then the relative risk of an event for patients in category f compared to category g is $\lambda_{jf}/\lambda_{jg}$. Equation (9.3) gives us that

$$\log[\lambda_{jf}] = \alpha_j + x_{jf1}\beta_1 + x_{jf2}\beta_2 + \cdots + x_{jfq}\beta_q, \text{ and} \tag{9.4}$$

$$\log[\lambda_{jg}] = \alpha_j + x_{jg1}\beta_1 + x_{jg2}\beta_2 + \cdots + x_{jgq}\beta_q. \tag{9.5}$$

Subtracting equation (9.5) from equation (9.4) gives that the within-stratum log relative risk of group f subjects relative to group g subjects is

$$\log[\lambda_{jf}/\lambda_{jg}] = (x_{jf1} - x_{jg1})\beta_1 + (x_{jf2} - x_{jg2})\beta_2 + \cdots + (x_{jfq} - x_{jgq})\beta_q. \tag{9.6}$$

Thus, we can estimate log relative risks in Poisson regression models in precisely the same way that we estimated log odds ratios in logistic regression. Indeed, the only difference is that in logistic regression weighted sums of model coefficients are interpreted as log odds ratios while in Poisson regression they are interpreted as log relative risks. An important feature of equation (9.6) is that the relative risk $\lambda_{jf}/\lambda_{jg}$ may vary between the different strata.

The nuisance parameters $\alpha_1, \alpha_2, \ldots, \alpha_J$ are handled in the same way that we handle any parameters associated with a categorical variable. That is, for any two values of j and h between 1 and J we let

$$strata_{jh} = \begin{cases} 1: \text{if } j = h \\ 0: \text{otherwise}. \end{cases}$$

Then model (9.1) can be rewritten as

$$\log[\text{E}[d_{jk} \mid \mathbf{x}_{jk}]] = \log[n_{jk}] + \sum_{h=1}^{J} \alpha_h \times strata_{jh}$$

$$+ \beta_1 x_{jk1} + \beta_2 x_{jk2} + \cdots + \beta_q x_{jkq}. \tag{9.7}$$

Models (9.1) and (9.7) are algebraically identical. We usually write the simpler form (9.1) when the strata are defined by confounding variables that are not of primary interest. However, in Stata these models are always specified in a way that is analogous to equation (9.7).

We derive maximum likelihood estimates $\hat{\alpha}_j$ for α_j and $\hat{\beta}_1, \ldots, \hat{\beta}_q$ for $\beta_1, \ldots, \beta_q$. Inferences about these parameter estimates are made in the same way as in Section 5.13 through 5.15. Again the only difference is that in Section 5.14 weighted sums of parameter estimates were interpreted as estimates of log odds ratios, while here they are interpreted as log relative risks. Suppose that f is a weighted sum of parameters that corresponds to a log relative risk of interest, $\hat{f}$ is the corresponding weighted sum of parameter estimates from a large study, and s_f is the estimated standard error of $\hat{f}$. Then under the null hypothesis that the relative risk $\exp[f] = 1$, the test statistic

$$z = \hat{f}/s_f \tag{9.8}$$

will have an approximately standard normal distribution if the sample size is large. A 95% confidence interval for this relative risk is given by

$$(\exp[\hat{f} - 1.96s_f], \ \exp[\hat{f} + 1.96s_f]). \tag{9.9}$$

9.2. An Example: The Framingham Heart Study

In Section 8.9 we created a person-year data set from the Framingham Heart Study for Poisson regression analysis. Patients were divided into strata based on age, body mass index, serum cholesterol, and baseline diastolic blood pressure. Age was classified into nine strata. The first and last consisted of people ≤ 45 years of age, and people older than eighty years, respectively. The inner strata consisted of people 46–50, 51–55, $\ldots$, and 76–80 years of age. The values of the other variables were divided into strata defined by quartiles. Each record in this data set consists of a number of person-years of follow-up of people of the same gender who are in the same strata for age, body mass index, serum cholesterol, and diastolic blood pressure. Let n_k be the number of person-years of follow-up in the kth record of this file and let d_k be the number of cases of coronary heart disease observed during these n_k person-years of follow-up. Let

$$male_k = \begin{cases} 1: & \text{if record } k \text{ describes men} \\ 0: & \text{if it describes women,} \end{cases}$$

$$age_{jk} = \begin{cases} 1: & \text{if record } k \text{ describes people from the } j^{\text{th}} \text{ age stratum} \\ 0: & \text{otherwise,} \end{cases}$$

$$bmi_{jk} = \begin{cases} 1: & \text{if record } k \text{ describes people from the } j^{\text{th}} \text{ BMI quartile} \\ 0: & \text{otherwise,} \end{cases}$$

$$scl_{jk} = \begin{cases} 1: & \text{if record } k \text{ describes people from the } j^{\text{th}} \text{ SCL quartile} \\ 0: & \text{otherwise, and} \end{cases}$$

$$dbp_{jk} = \begin{cases} 1: & \text{if record } k \text{ describes people from the } j^{\text{th}} \text{ DBP quartile} \\ 0: & \text{otherwise.} \end{cases}$$

For any model that we will consider let

$\mathbf{x}_k = (x_{jk1}, x_{jk2}, \ldots, x_{jkq})$ denote the values of all of the covariates of people in the kth record that are included in the model,

$\lambda_k = \mathrm{E}[d_k/n_k \mid \mathbf{x}_k]$ be the expected CHD incidence rate for people in the kth record given their covariates $\mathbf{x}_k$. We will now build several models with these data.

9.2.1. A Multiplicative Model of Gender, Age and Coronary Heart Disease

Consider the model

$$\log[\mathrm{E}[d_k \mid \mathbf{x}_k]] = \log[n_k] + \alpha + \sum_{j=2}^{9} \beta_j \times age_{jk} + \gamma \times male_k, \tag{9.10}$$

where $\alpha, \beta_2, \beta_3, \ldots, \beta_9$ and γ are parameters in the model. Subtracting $\log[n_k]$ from both sides of equation (9.10) gives that

$$\log[\lambda_k] = \alpha + \sum_{j=2}^{9} \beta_j \times age_{jk} + \gamma \times male_k. \tag{9.11}$$

If record f describes women from the first age stratum then equation (9.11) reduces to

$$\log[\lambda_f] = \alpha. \tag{9.12}$$

If record g describes men from the first stratum then equation (9.11) reduces to

$$\log[\lambda_g] = \alpha + \gamma. \tag{9.13}$$

Subtracting equation (9.12) from equation (9.13) gives that

$$\log[\lambda_g] - \log[\lambda_f] = \log[\lambda_g/\lambda_f] = (\alpha + \gamma) - \alpha = \gamma.$$

In other words, γ is the log relative risk of CHD for men compared to women within the first age stratum. Similarly, if records f and g now describe women and men, respectively, from the jth age stratum with $j > 1$ then

$$\log[\lambda_f] = \alpha + \beta_j \text{ and} \tag{9.14}$$

$$\log[\lambda_g] = \alpha + \beta_j + \gamma. \tag{9.15}$$

Subtracting equation (9.14) from (9.15) again yields that

$$\log[\lambda_g/\lambda_f] = \gamma.$$

Hence, γ is the within-stratum (i.e., age-adjusted) log relative risk of CHD for men compared to women for all age strata. We have gone through virtually identical arguments many times in previous chapters. By subtracting appropriate pairs of log incidence rates you should also be able to show that β_j is the sex-adjusted log relative risk of CHD for people from the jth age stratum compared to the first, and that $\beta_j + \gamma$ is the log relative risk of CHD for men from the jth stratum compared to women from the first. Hence, the age-adjusted risk for men relative to women is $\exp[\gamma]$, the sex-adjusted risk of people from the jth age stratum relative to the first is $\exp[\beta_j]$, and the risk for men from the jth age stratum relative to women from the first is $\exp[\gamma] \times \exp[\beta_j]$. Model (9.10) is called a multiplicative model because this latter relative risk equals the risk for men relative to women times the risk for people from the jth stratum relative to people from the first.

The maximum likelihood estimate of γ in (9.10) is $\hat{\gamma} = 0.6912$. Hence, the age-adjusted estimate of the relative risk of CHD in men compared to women from this model is $\exp[0.6912] = 2.00$. The standard error of $\hat{\gamma}$ is 0.0527. Therefore, from equation (9.9), the 95% confidence interval for this relative risk is $(\exp[0.6912 - 1.96 \times 0.0527], \exp[0.6912 + 1.96 \times 0.0527]) = (1.8, 2.2)$. This risk estimate is virtually identical to the estimate we obtained from model (7.16), which was a proportional hazards model with ragged entry.

Model (9.10) is not of great practical interest because we know from Chapter 7 that the risk of CHD in men relative to women is greater for premenopausal ages than for postmenopausal ages. The incidence of CHD in women in the jth stratum is the sum of all CHD events in women from this stratum divided by the total number of women-years of follow-up in this strata. That is, this incidence is

$$\hat{I}_{0j} = \sum_{\{k: \, male_k = 0, \, age_{jk} = 1\}} d_k \Bigg/ \sum_{\{k: \, male_k = 0, \, age_{jk} = 1\}} n_k. \tag{9.16}$$

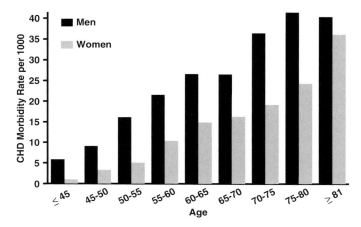

Figure 9.1   Age–sex specific incidence of coronary heart disease (CHD) in people from the Framingham Heart Study (Levy, 1999).

Similarly, the incidence of CHD in men from the jth age stratum can be estimated by

$$\hat{I}_{1j} = \sum_{\{k:\ male_k = 1,\ age_{jk} = 1\}} d_k \bigg/ \sum_{\{k:\ male_k = 1,\ age_{jk} = 1\}} n_k. \tag{9.17}$$

Equations (9.16) and (9.17) are used in Figure 9.1 to plot the age-specific incidence of CHD in men and women from the Framingham Heart Study. This figure shows dramatic differences in CHD rates between men and women; the ratio of these rates at each age diminishes as people grow older. To model these rates effectively we need to add interaction terms into our model.

9.2.2. A Model of Age, Gender and CHD with Interaction Terms

Let us expand model (9.10) as follows:

$$\log[E[d_k \mid \mathbf{x}_k]] = \log[n_k] + \alpha + \sum_{j=2}^{9} \beta_j \times age_{jk} + \gamma \times male_k$$

$$+ \sum_{j=2}^{9} \delta_j \times age_{jk} \times male_k. \tag{9.18}$$

If record f describes women from the jth age stratum with $j > 1$ then model (9.18) reduces to

$$\log[\lambda_f] = \alpha + \beta_j. \tag{9.19}$$

Table 9.2. Age-specific relative risks of coronary heart disease (CHD) in men compared to women from the Framingham Heart Study (Levy, 1999). These relative risk estimates were obtained from model (9.18). Five-year age intervals are used. Similar relative risks from contiguous age strata have been highlighted.

Age	Patient-years of follow-up		CHD events		Relative risk	95% confidence interval
	Men	Women	Men	Women		
≤45	7370	9205	43	9	5.97	2.9–12
46–50	5835	7595	53	25	2.76	1.7–4.4
51–55	6814	9113	110	46	3.20	2.3–4.5
56–60	7184	10 139	155	105	2.08	1.6–2.7
61–65	6678	9946	178	148	1.79	1.4–2.2
66–70	4557	7385	121	120	1.63	1.3–2.1
71–75	2575	4579	94	88	1.90	1.4–2.5
76–80	1205	2428	50	59	1.71	1.2–2.5
≥81	470	1383	19	50	1.12	0.66–1.9

If record g describes men from the same age stratum then model (9.18) reduces to

$$\log[\lambda_g] = \alpha + \beta_j + \gamma + \delta_j. \tag{9.20}$$

Subtracting equation (9.19) from equation (9.20) gives the log relative risk of CHD for men versus women in the jth age stratum to be

$$\log[\lambda_g/\lambda_f] = \gamma + \delta_j. \tag{9.21}$$

Hence, we estimate this relative risk by

$$\exp[\hat{\gamma} + \hat{\delta}_j]. \tag{9.22}$$

A similar argument gives that the estimated relative risk of men compared to women in the first age stratum is

$$\exp[\hat{\gamma}]. \tag{9.23}$$

Equations (9.22) and (9.23) are used in Table 9.2 to estimate the age-specific relative risks of CHD in men versus women. Ninety-five percent confidence intervals are calculated for these estimates using equation (9.9).

When models (9.10) and (9.18) are fitted to the Framingham Heart data they produce model deviances of 1391.3 and 1361.6, respectively. Note that model (9.10) is nested within model (9.18) (see Section 5.24). Hence, under the null hypothesis that the multiplicative model (9.10) is correct, the change

Table 9.3. Age-specific relative risks of coronary heart disease (CHD) in men compared to women from the Framingham Heart Study (Levy, 1999). Age intervals from Table 9.2 that had similar relative risks have been combined in this figure giving age intervals with variable widths.

Age	Patient-years of follow-up		CHD events		Relative risk	95% confidence interval
	Men	Women	Men	Women		
≤45	7370	9205	43	9	5.97	2.9–12
46–55	12 649	16 708	163	71	3.03	2.3–4.0
56–60	7184	10 139	155	105	2.08	1.6–2.7
61–80	15 015	24 338	443	415	1.73	1.5–2.0
≥81	470	1383	19	50	1.12	0.66–1.9

in deviance will have a chi-squared distribution with as many degrees of freedom as there are extra parameters in model (9.18). As there are eight more parameters in model (9.18) than model (9.10) this chi-squared statistic will have eight degrees of freedom. The probability that this statistic will exceed $1391.3 - 1361.6 = 29.7$ is $P = 0.0002$. Hence, these data allow us to reject the multiplicative model with a high level of statistical significance.

Table 9.2 shows a marked drop in the risk of CHD in men relative to women with increasing age. Note, however, that the relative risks for ages 46–50 and ages 51–55 are similar, as are the relative risks for ages 61–65 through 76–80. Hence, we can reduce the number of age strata from nine to five with little loss in explanatory power by lumping ages 46–55 into one stratum and ages 61–80 into another. This reduces the number of parameters in model (9.18) by eight (four age parameters plus four interaction parameters). Refitting model (9.18) with only these five condensed age strata rather than the original nine gives the results presented in Table 9.3. Note that the age-specific relative risk of men verses women in this table diminishes with age but remains significantly different from one for all ages less than 80. Gender does not have a significant influence on the risk of CHD in people older than 80. These data are consistent with the hypothesis that endogenous sex hormones play a cardioprotective role in premenopausal women.

9.2.3. Adding Confounding Variables to the Model

Let us now consider the effect of possibly confounding variables on our estimates in Table 9.3. The variables that we will consider are body mass index, serum cholesterol, and diastolic blood pressure. We will add these variables one at a time in order to gauge their influence on the model deviance. As we will see in Section 9.3, all of these variables have an overwhelmingly significant effect on the change in model deviance. The final model that we will consider is

$$\log[E[d_k \mid \mathbf{x}_k]] = \log[n_k] + \alpha + \sum_{j=2}^{5} \beta_j \times age_{jk} + \gamma \times male_k$$

$$+ \sum_{j=2}^{5} \delta_j \times age_{jk} \times male_k + \sum_{f=2}^{4} \theta_f \times bmi_{fk}$$

$$+ \sum_{g=2}^{4} \phi_g \times scl_{gk} + \sum_{h=2}^{4} \psi_h \times dbp_{hk}, \qquad (9.24)$$

where the age strata are those given in Table 9.3 rather than those given at the beginning of Section 9.2. Recall that bmi_{fk}, scl_{gk}, and dbp_{hk} are indicator covariates corresponding to the four quartiles of body mass index, serum cholesterol, and diastolic blood pressure, respectively. By the usual argument, the age-specific CHD risk for men relative to women adjusted for body mass index, serum cholesterol, and diastolic blood pressure is either

$$\exp[\gamma] \qquad (9.25)$$

for the first age stratum or

$$\exp[\gamma + \delta_j] \qquad (9.26)$$

for the other age strata. Substituting the maximum likelihood estimates of γ and δ_j into equations (9.25) and (9.26) gives the adjusted relative risk estimates presented in Table 9.4. Comparing these results with those of

Table 9.4. Age-specific relative risks of coronary heart disease (CHD) in men compared to women adjusted for body mass index, serum cholesterol, and baseline diastolic blood pressure (Levy, 1999). These risks were derived using model (9.24). They should be compared with those from Table 9.3.

Age	Adjusted relative risk	95% confidence interval
≤ 45	4.64	2.3–9.5
46–55	2.60	2.0–3.4
56–60	1.96	1.5–2.5
61–80	1.79	1.6–2.0
≥ 81	1.25	0.73–2.1

Table 9.3 indicates that adjusting for body mass index, serum cholesterol, and diastolic blood pressure does reduce the age-specific relative risk of CHD in men versus women who are less than 56 years of age.

9.3. Using Stata to Perform Poisson Regression

The following log file and comments illustrate how to perform the Poisson regressions of the Framingham Heart Study data that were described in Section 9.2. You should be familiar with how to use the *glm* and *logistic* commands to perform logistic regression before reading this section (see Chapter 5).

```
. * 9.3.Framingham.log

. *

. * Estimate the effect of age and gender on coronary heart disease (CHD)
. * using several Poisson regression models

. *

. * use C:\WDDtext\8.12.Framingham.dta, clear

. *

. * Fit a multiplicative model of the effect of gender and age on CHD
. *

. xi: glm chd_cnt i.age_gr male, family(poisson) link(log)
> lnoffset(pt_yrs) eform                                                    {1}
  i.age_gr          _Iage_gr_45-81      (naturally coded; _Iage_gr_45 omitted)
                                                                {Output omitted}
Generalized linear models                   No. of obs    =        1267
                                                                {Output omitted}
Deviance         =   1391.341888           (1/df) Deviance =    1.106875
                                                                {Output omitted}
```

```
---------------------------------------------------------------------------
     chd_cnt |        IRR    Std. Err.     z    P>|z|    [95% Conf. Interval]
-------------+-------------------------------------------------------------
 _Iage_gr_50 |   1.864355    .3337745    3.48   0.001    1.312618    2.648005
 _Iage_gr_55 |   3.158729    .5058088    7.18   0.000    2.307858    4.323303
 _Iage_gr_60 |   4.885053    .7421312   10.44   0.000    3.627069    6.579347
 _Iage_gr_65 |    6.44168    .9620181   12.47   0.000    4.807047    8.632168
 _Iage_gr_70 |   6.725369   1.028591    12.46   0.000    4.983469    9.076127
 _Iage_gr_75 |   8.612712   1.354852    13.69   0.000    6.327596    11.72306
 _Iage_gr_80 |   10.37219   1.749287    13.87   0.000    7.452702    14.43534
```

```
  _Iage_gr_81 |  13.67189   2.515296  14.22   0.000   9.532967   19.60781
         male |  1.996012   .1051841  13.12   0.000   1.800144   2.213192  {2}
       pt_yrs | (exposure)
```

```
. *
. * Tabulate patient-years of follow-up and number of
. * CHD events by sex and age group.
. *
. table sex, contents(sum pt_yrs sum chd_cnt) by(age_gr)                 {3}
```

```
------------------------------------------
age_gr       |
and Sex      |  sum(pt_yrs)   sum(chd_cnt)
-------------+----------------------------
<= 45        |
        Men  |        7370             43
      Women  |        9205              9
-------------+----------------------------
45-50        |
        Men  |        5835             53
      Women  |        7595             25
-------------+----------------------------
```
　　　　　　　　　　　　　　　　　　　　　　{Output omitted. See Table 9.2}
```
75-80        |
        Men  |        1205             50
      Women  |        2428             59
-------------+----------------------------
> 80         |
        Men  |         470             19
      Women  |        1383             50
------------------------------------------
```

```
. *
. * Calculate age-sex specific incidence of CHD
. *
. collapse (sum) patients = pt_yrs chd = chd_cnt, by(age_gr sex)
. generate rate = 1000* chd/patients                                     {4}
. generate men = rate if male == 1                                       {5}
(9 missing values generated)
. generate women = rate if male == 0
(9 missing values generated)
```

```
. set textsize 120

. graph men women, bar by(age_gr) ylabel(0 5 to 40) gap(3)              {6}
> l1title(CHD Morbidity Rate per 1000) title(Age)
```
{Graph omitted. See Figure 9.1}
```
. use C:\WDDtext\8.12.Framingham.dta, clear                             {7}

. *

. * Add interaction terms to the model

. *

. xi: glm chd_cnt i.age_gr*male, family(poisson) link(log) lnoffset(pt_yrs) {8}
i.age_gr        _Iage_gr_45-81      (naturally coded; _Iage_gr_45 omitted)
i.age_gr*male   _IageXmale_#        (coded as above)
```
{Output omitted}
```
Generalized linear models                        No. of obs  =      1267
```
{Output omitted}
```
Deviance      = 1361.574107              (1/df) Deviance  =   1.090131
```
{Output omitted}
```
------------------------------------------------------------------------------
     chd_cnt |      Coef.   Std. Err.      z     P>|z|     [95% Conf. Interval]
-------------+----------------------------------------------------------------
 _Iage_gr_50 |   1.213908   .3887301     3.12   0.002     .4520112    1.975805
 _Iage_gr_55 |   1.641462   .3644863     4.50   0.000     .9270817    2.355842
 _Iage_gr_60 |   2.360093   .3473254     6.80   0.000     1.679348    3.040838
 _Iage_gr_65 |   2.722564   .3433189     7.93   0.000     2.049671    3.395457
 _Iage_gr_70 |   2.810563   .3456074     8.13   0.000     2.133185    3.487941
 _Iage_gr_75 |   2.978378   .3499639     8.51   0.000     2.292462    3.664295
 _Iage_gr_80 |   3.212992   .3578551     8.98   0.000     2.511609    3.914375
 _Iage_gr_81 |    3.61029   .3620927     9.97   0.000     2.900602    4.319979
        male |   1.786305   .3665609     4.87   0.000     1.067858    2.504751
_IageXmal~50 |   -.771273   .4395848    -1.75   0.079    -1.632843    .0902975
_IageXmal~55 |   -.623743   .4064443    -1.53   0.125    -1.420359    .1728731
_IageXmal~60 |  -1.052307   .3877401    -2.71   0.007    -1.812263   -.2923503
_IageXmal~65 |  -1.203381   .3830687    -3.14   0.002    -1.954182   -.4525805
_IageXmal~70 |  -1.295219   .3885418    -3.33   0.001    -2.056747   -.5336915
_IageXmal~75 |  -1.144716    .395435    -2.89   0.004    -1.919754   -.3696772
_IageXmal~80 |  -1.251231   .4139035    -3.02   0.003    -2.062467   -.4399949
_IageXmal~81 |  -1.674611   .4549709    -3.68   0.000    -2.566338   -.7828845
       _cons |  -6.930278   .3333333   -20.79   0.000    -7.583599   -6.276956
      pt_yrs |  (exposure)
------------------------------------------------------------------------------
```

```
. lincom male, irr
  (1)  [chd_cnt]male = 0.0

------------------------------------------------------------------------------
   chd_cnt |      IRR    Std. Err.      z    P>|z|     [95% Conf. Interval]
-----------+------------------------------------------------------------------
       (1) |   5.96736    2.187401    4.87   0.000     2.909143    12.24051
------------------------------------------------------------------------------
```

```
. lincom male + _IageXmale_50, irr                                        {9}
  (1)  [chd_cnt]male + [chd_cnt]_IageXmale_50 = 0.0

------------------------------------------------------------------------------
   chd_cnt |      IRR    Std. Err.      z    P>|z|     [95% Conf. Interval]
-----------+------------------------------------------------------------------
       (1) |  2.759451   .6695176    4.18   0.000     1.715134    4.439635
------------------------------------------------------------------------------
```

```
. lincom male + _IageXmale_55, irr
```
                                          {Output omitted. See Table 9.2}
```
. lincom male + _IageXmale_60, irr
```
                                          {Output omitted. See Table 9.2}
```
. lincom male + _IageXmale_65, irr
```
                                          {Output omitted. See Table 9.2}
```
. lincom male + _IageXmale_70, irr
```
                                          {Output omitted. See Table 9.2}
```
. lincom male + _IageXmale_75, irr
```
                                          {Output omitted. See Table 9.2}
```
. lincom male + _IageXmale_80, irr
```
                                          {Output omitted. See Table 9.2}
```
. lincom male + _IageXmale_81, irr
  (1)  [chd_cnt]male + [chd_cnt]_IageXmale_81 = 0.0

------------------------------------------------------------------------------
   chd_cnt |      IRR    Std. Err.      z    P>|z|     [95% Conf. Interval]
-----------+------------------------------------------------------------------
       (1) |   1.11817   .3013496    0.41   0.679     .6593363    1.896308
------------------------------------------------------------------------------
```

```
. display chi2tail(8, 1391.341888 - 1361.574107)                          {10}
.00023231

. *

. * Refit model with interaction terms using fewer parameters.

. *
```

```
. generate age_gr2 = recode(age_gr, 45,55,60,80,81)

. xi: glm chd_cnt i.age_gr2*male, family(poisson) link(log)          {11}
> lnoffset(pt_yrs) eform
i.age_gr2          _Iage_gr2_45-81   (naturally coded; _Iage_gr2_45 omitted)
i.age_gr2*male     _IageXmale_#      (coded as above)
                                                         {Output omitted}
Generalized linear models              No. of obs    =      1267
                                                         {Output omitted}
Deviance         =   1400.582451      (1/df) Deviance =   1.114226
                                                         {Output omitted}
------------------------------------------------------------------------
       chd_cnt |      IRR    Std. Err.     z    P>|z|   [95% Conf. Interval]
-------------+----------------------------------------------------------
 _Iage_gr2_55 |  4.346255   1.537835    4.15   0.000    2.172374   8.695524
 _Iage_gr2_60 |  10.59194   3.678849    6.80   0.000    5.362059   20.92278
 _Iage_gr2_80 |  17.43992   5.876004    8.48   0.000    9.010534   33.75503
 _Iage_gr2_81 |  36.97678   13.38902    9.97   0.000    18.18508   75.18703
         male |  5.96736    2.187401    4.87   0.000    2.909143   12.24051
 _IageXmal~55 |  .5081773   .1998025   -1.72   0.085    .2351496   1.098212
 _IageXmal~60 |  .3491314   .1353722   -2.71   0.007    .1632841   .746507
 _IageXmal~80 |  .2899566   .1081168   -3.32   0.001    .1396186   .6021748
 _IageXmal~81 |  .1873811   .0852529   -3.68   0.000    .0768164   .4570857
       pt_yrs |  (exposure)
-------------+----------------------------------------------------------
. lincom male + _IageXmale_55, irr                                  {12}
(1) [chd_cnt]male + [chd_cnt]_IageXmale_55 = 0.0

------------------------------------------------------------------------
       chd_cnt |      IRR    Std. Err.     z    P>|z|   [95% Conf. Interval]
----------+-------------------------------------------------------------
        (1) |  3.032477   .4312037    7.80   0.000    2.294884   4.007138
------------------------------------------------------------------------

. lincom male + _IageXmale_60, irr
                                           {Output omitted. See Table 9.3}

. lincom male + _IageXmale_80, irr
                                           {Output omitted. See Table 9.3}

. lincom male + _IageXmale_81, irr
                                           {Output omitted. See Table 9.3}

. *

. * Adjust analysis for body mass index (BMI)
```

```
. *
. xi: glm chd_cnt i.age_gr2*male i.bmi_gr, family(poisson) link(log)          {13}
> lnoffset(pt_yrs)
i.age_gr2        _Iage_gr2_45-81   (naturally coded; _Iage_gr2_45 omitted)
i.age_gr2*male   _IageXmale_#      (coded as above)
i.bmi_gr         _Ibmi_gr_1-4      (_Ibmi_gr_1 for bmi~r==22.7999992370 omitted)
```
{Output omitted.}
```
Generalized linear models                    No. of obs      =        1234
```
{Output omitted.}
```
Deviance           =    1327.64597        (1/df) Deviance   =    1.087343
```
{Output omitted.}
```
------------------------------------------------------------------------------
    chd_cnt |     Coef.    Std. Err.      z     P>|z|     [95% Conf. Interval]
------------------------------------------------------------------------------
_Iage_gr2_55 |   1.426595    .3538794     4.03   0.000    .7330038    2.120185
_Iage_gr2_60 |   2.293218    .3474423     6.60   0.000    1.612244    2.974192
_Iage_gr2_80 |   2.768015    .3371378     8.21   0.000    2.107237    3.428793
_Iage_gr2_81 |   3.473889    .3625129     9.58   0.000    2.763377    4.184401
       male |   1.665895    .3669203     4.54   0.000    .9467445    2.385046
_IageXmal~55 |  -.6387422    .3932103    -1.62   0.104   -1.40942     .1319358
_IageXmal~60 |  -.9880222    .3878331    -2.55   0.011   -1.748161   -.2278834
_IageXmal~80 |  -1.147882    .3730498    -3.08   0.002   -1.879046   -.4167177
_IageXmal~81 |  -1.585361    .4584836    -3.46   0.001   -2.483972   -.6867492
  _Ibmi_gr_2 |    .231835    .08482       2.73   0.006    .0655909    .3980791
  _Ibmi_gr_3 |   .4071791    .0810946     5.02   0.000    .2482366    .5661216
  _Ibmi_gr_4 |   .6120817    .0803788     7.61   0.000    .4545421    .7696213
       _cons |  -7.165097    .3365738   -21.29   0.000   -7.824769   -6.505424
     pt_yrs |  (exposure)
------------------------------------------------------------------------------

. display chi2tail(3,1400.582451 - 1327.64597)
1.003e-15

. *
. * Adjust estimates for BMI and serum cholesterol
. *
. xi: glm chd_cnt i.age_gr2*male i.bmi_gr i.scl_gr, family(poisson)          {14}
> link(log) lnoffset(pt_yrs)
i.age_gr2        _Iage_gr2_45-81   (naturally coded; _Iage_gr2_45  omitted)
i.age_gr2*male   _IageXmale_#      (coded as above)
i.bmi_gr         _Ibmi_gr_1-4      (_Ibmi_gr_1 for bmi~r==22.7999992370 omitted)
```

```
i.scl_gr          _Iscl_gr_1-4      (_Iscl_gr_1 for scl_gr==197 omitted)
                                                        {Output omitted.}
Generalized linear models                 No. of obs      =        1134
                                                        {Output omitted.}
Deviance         =    1207.974985         (1/df) Deviance =    1.080479
                                                        {Output omitted.}
------------------------------------------------------------------------
      chd_cnt |     Coef.    Std. Err.     z    P>|z|    [95% Conf. Interval]
--------------+---------------------------------------------------------
 _Iage_gr2_55 |   1.355072   .3539895    3.83   0.000    .6612658   2.048879
 _Iage_gr2_60 |   2.177981   .3477145    6.26   0.000    1.496473   2.859489
 _Iage_gr2_80 |   2.606272   .3376428    7.72   0.000    1.944504    3.26804
 _Iage_gr2_81 |   3.254865   .3634043    8.96   0.000    2.542605   3.967124
         male |   1.569236   .3671219    4.27   0.000    .8496906   2.288782
_IageXmal~55 |  -.5924132   .3933748   -1.51   0.132   -1.363414    .1785873
_IageXmal~60 |  -.8886722   .3881045   -2.29   0.022   -1.649343   -.1280013
_IageXmal~80 |  -.9948713   .3734882   -2.66   0.008   -1.726895   -.2628478
_IageXmal~81 |  -1.400993   .4590465   -3.05   0.002   -2.300708   -.5012786
  _Ibmi_gr_2 |   .1929941   .0849164    2.27   0.023    .0265609    .3594273
  _Ibmi_gr_3 |    .334175   .0814824    4.10   0.000    .1744724    .4938776
  _Ibmi_gr_4 |   .5230984   .0809496    6.46   0.000    .3644401    .6817566
  _Iscl_gr_2 |    .192923   .0843228    2.29   0.022    .0276532    .3581927
  _Iscl_gr_3 |   .5262667   .0810581    6.49   0.000    .3673957    .6851377
  _Iscl_gr_4 |   .6128653   .0814661    7.52   0.000    .4531947    .7725359
        _cons |  -7.340659   .3392167  -21.64   0.000   -8.005512   -6.675807
       pt_yrs |  (exposure)
------------------------------------------------------------------------

. display chi2tail(3,1327.64597 - 1207.974985)
9.084e-26

. *
. * Adjust estimates for BMI, serum cholesterol and
. * diastolic blood pressure
. *
. xi: glm chd_cnt i.age_gr2*male i.bmi_gr i.scl_gr i.dbp_gr, family(poisson)  {15}
> link(log) lnoffset(pt_yrs) eform
i.age_gr2       _Iage_gr2_45-81   (naturally coded; _Iage_gr2_45 omitted)
i.age_gr2*male  _IageXmale_#      (coded as above)
i.bmi_gr        _Ibmi_gr_1-4      (_Ibmi_gr_1 for bmi~r==22.7999992370 omitted)
i.scl_gr        _Iscl_gr_1-4      (_Iscl_gr_1 for scl_gr==197 omitted)
```

```
i.dbp_gr        _Idbp_gr_74-91   (naturally coded; _Idbp_gr_74 omitted
```
{Output omitted.}
```
Generalized linear models                    No. of obs    =    1134
```
{Output omitted.}
```
Deviance      =   1161.091086          (1/df) Deviance = 1.041337
```
{Output omitted.}

```
------------------------------------------------------------------------
    chd_cnt |       IRR    Std. Err.      z    P>|z|    [95% Conf. Interval]
------------+-----------------------------------------------------------
_Iage_gr2_55 |  3.757544   1.330347    3.74   0.000    1.877322   7.520891
_Iage_gr2_60 |  8.411826   2.926018    6.12   0.000    4.254059   16.63325
_Iage_gr2_80 |  12.78983   4.320508    7.54   0.000    6.596628   24.79748
_Iage_gr2_81 |  23.92787   8.701246    8.73   0.000    11.73192   48.80217
       male |  4.637662   1.703034    4.18   0.000    2.257991   9.525239
_IageXmal~55 |  .5610101   .2207001   -1.47   0.142    .2594836   1.212210
_IageXmal~60 |  .4230946   .1642325   -2.22   0.027    .1977092   .9054158
_IageXmal~80 |  .3851572   .1438922   -2.55   0.011    .1851974   .8010161
_IageXmal~81 |  .2688892   .1234925   -2.86   0.004    .1093058   .6614603
  _Ibmi_gr_2 |  1.159495   .0991218    1.73   0.083    .9806235   1.370994
  _Ibmi_gr_3 |  1.298532   .1077862    3.15   0.002    1.103564   1.527944
  _Ibmi_gr_4 |  1.479603   .1251218    4.63   0.000    1.253614   1.746332
  _Iscl_gr_2 |  1.189835   .1004557    2.06   0.040    1.008374   1.403952
  _Iscl_gr_3 |  1.649807   .1339827    6.16   0.000    1.407039   1.934462
  _Iscl_gr_4 |  1.793581   .1466507    7.15   0.000    1.527999   2.105323
  _Idbp_gr_80 |  1.18517   .0962869    2.09   0.037    1.010709   1.389744
  _Idbp_gr_90 |  1.122983  .0892217    1.46   0.144    .9610473   1.312205
  _Idbp_gr_91 |  1.638383  .1302205    6.21   0.000    1.402041   1.914564
     pt_yrs |  (exposure)
------------------------------------------------------------------------
```

```
. lincom male + _IageXmale_55, irr                                    {16}
```

```
(1)  [chd_cnt]male + [chd_cnt]_IageXmale_55 = 0.0
------------------------------------------------------------------------
    chd_cnt |      IRR    Std. Err.     z     P>|z|     [95% Conf. Interval]
----------+-------------------------------------------------------------
       (1) |  2.601775   .3722797    6.68    0.000     1.965505   3.444019
------------------------------------------------------------------------
```

```
. lincom male + _IageXmale_60, irr
```
{Output omitted. See Table 9.4}

```
. lincom male + _IageXmale_80, irr
```
{Output omitted. See Table 9.4}

```
. lincom male + _IageXmale_81, irr
```
{Output omitted. See Table 9.4}

```
. display chi2tail(3,1207.974985 - 1161.091086)
3.679e-10
```

Comments

1. This *glm* command analyzes model (9.10). The *family(poisson)* and *link(log)* options specify that a Poisson regression model is to be analyzed. The variables *chd_cnt*, *male*, and *pt_yrs* give the values of d_k, $male_k$ and n_k, respectively. The syntax of *i.age_gr* is explained in Section 5.10 and generates the indicator variables age_{jk} in model (9.10). These variables are called *_Iage_gr_50*, *_Iage_gr_55*, ..., and *_Iage_gr_81* by Stata.

2. The *eform* option in the *glm* command dictates that the estimates of the model coefficients are to be exponentiated. The highlighted value in this column equals $\exp[\hat{\gamma}]$, which is the estimated age-adjusted CHD risk for men relative to women. The other values in this column are sex-adjusted risks of CHD in people of the indicated age strata relative to people from the first age strata. The 95% confidence interval for the age-adjusted relative risk for men is also highlighted.

3. This *table* command sums the number of patient-years of follow-up and CHD events in groups of people defined by sex and age strata. The values tabulated in this table are the denominators and numerators of equations (9.16) and (9.17). They are also given in Table 9.2. The output for ages 51–55, 56–60, 61–65, 66–70 and 71–75 have been deleted from this log file.

4. This *generate* command calculates the age-gender-specific CHD incidence rates using equations (9.16) and (9.17). They are expressed as rates per thousand person-years of follow-up.

5. The variable *men* is missing for records that describe women.

6. This command produces a grouped bar chart similar to Figure 9.1. The *bar* and *by(age_gr)* options specify that a bar chart is to be drawn with separate bars for each value of *age_gr*. The length of the bars is proportional to the sum of the values of the variables *men* and *women* in records with the same value of *age_gr*. However, the preceding *collapse* and *generate* commands have ensured that there is only one non-missing value of *men* and *women* for each age stratum. It is the lengths of these values that are plotted. The *title(age)* option adds a title to the *x*-axis.

7 The previous collapse command altered the data set. We reload the *8.12.-Framingham.dta* data set before proceeding with additional analyses.

8 This *glm* command specifies model (9.18). The syntax of *i.age_gr*male* is analogous to that used for the logistic command in Section 5.23. This term specifies the covariates and parameters to the right of the offset term in equation (9.18). Note that since *male* is already a zero–one indicator variable, it is not necessary to write *i.age_gr*i.male* to specify this part of the model. This latter syntax would, however, have generated the same model.

In this command I did not specify the *eform* option in order to output the parameter estimates. Note that the interaction terms become increasingly more negative with increasing age. This has the effect of reducing the age-specific relative risk of CHD in men versus women as their age increases.

9 This *lincom* statement calculates the CHD risk for men relative to women from the second age stratum (ages 46–50) using equation (9.21). The following *lincom* commands calculate this relative risk for the other age strata. The output from these commands has been omitted here but has been entered into Table 9.2.

10 This command calculates the *P* value associated with the change in model deviance between models (9.10) and (9.18).

11 This command analyzes the model used to produce Table 9.3. It differs from model (9.18) only in that it uses five age strata rather than nine. These five age strata are specified by *age_gr2*. The highlighted relative risk estimate and confidence interval is also given for the first stratum in Table 9.3.

12 This and subsequent *lincom* commands provide the remaining relative risk estimates in Table 9.3.

13 The term *i.bmi_gr* adds

$$\sum_{f=2}^{4} \theta_f \times bmi_{fk}$$

to our model. It adjusts our risk estimates for the effect of body mass index as a confounding variable.

14 The term *i.scl_gr* adds

$$\sum_{g=2}^{4} \phi_g \times scl_{gk}$$

to our model. It adjusts our risk estimates for the effect of serum cholesterol as a confounding variable.

15 This *glm* command implements model (9.24). The term *i.dbp_gr* adds

$$\sum_{h=2}^{4} \psi_h \times dbp_{hk}$$

to the preceding model. The highlighted relative risk in the output is that for men versus women from the first stratum adjusted for body mass index, serum cholesterol, and diastolic blood pressure. This risk and its confidence interval are also given in Table 9.4.

16 This *lincom* command calculates the CHD risk for men relative to women from the second age stratum adjusted for body mass index, serum cholesterol, and diastolic blood pressure. The highlighted output is also given in Table 9.4. The output from the subsequent *lincom* commands complete this table.

9.4. Residual Analyses for Poisson Regression Models

A good way to check the adequacy of a Poisson regression model is to graph a scatterplot of standardized residuals against estimated expected incidence rates. As with logistic regression, such plots can identify covariate patterns that fit the model poorly. In order to best identify outlying covariate patterns, you should always condense your data set so that there is only one record per covariate pattern. That is, you should sum the values of d_k and n_k over all records for which the covariate patterns from your model are identical. We will let d_i and n_i denote the number of observed events and person-years of follow-up associated with the ith distinct covariate pattern in the model

9.4.1. Deviance Residuals

An excellent residual for use with either Poisson or logistic regression is the deviance residual. The model deviance can be written in the form $D = \sum_i c_i$, where c_i is a non-negative value that represents the contribution to the deviance of the ith group of patients with identical covariate values (see Section 5.24). Let

$$r_i = \text{sign}[d_i / n_i - \hat{\lambda}_i] \sqrt{c_i} = \begin{cases} \sqrt{c_i} : \text{if } d_i / n_i \geq \hat{\lambda}_i \\ -\sqrt{c_i} : \text{if } d_i / n_i < \hat{\lambda}_i, \end{cases} \tag{9.27}$$

where $\hat{\lambda}_i$ is the estimated incidence rate for people with the ith covariate pattern under the model. Then r_i is the **deviance residual** for this covariate pattern and

$$D = \sum_i r_i^2.$$

If the model is correct then the overwhelming majority of these residuals should fall between ±2. The magnitude of r_i increases as d_i / n_i diverges from $\hat{\lambda}_i$, and a large value of r_i indicates a poor fit of the associated group of patients to the model.

As with Pearson residuals, deviance residuals are affected by varying degrees of leverage associated with the different covariate patterns (see Section 5.28). This leverage tends to shorten the residual by pulling the estimate of λ_i in the direction of d_i / n_i. We can adjust for this shrinkage by calculating the **standardized deviance residual** for the ith covariate pattern, which is

$$d_{sj} = d_i / \sqrt{1 - h_i}. \tag{9.28}$$

In equation (9.28), h_i is the leverage of the ith covariate pattern. If the model is correct, roughly 95% of these residuals should lie between ±2. A residual plot provides evidence of poor model fit if substantially more than 5% of the residuals have an absolute value greater than two or if the average residual value varies with the estimated incidence of the disease.

Figure 9.2 shows a plot of standardized deviance residuals against expected CHD incidence from model (9.24). A lowess regression curve of this residual versus CHD incidence is also plotted in this figure. If the model is correct, this curve should be flat and near zero for the great majority of residuals. In Figure 9.2 the lowess regression curve is very close to zero for incidence

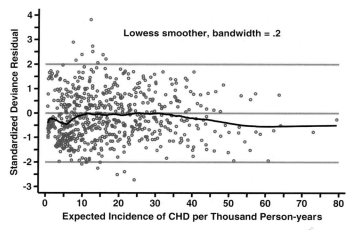

Figure 9.2   Plot of standardized deviance residuals against expected incidence of coronary heart disease (CHD) from model (9.24). The lowess regression line of these residuals versus expected incidence of CHD is also plotted. This graph indicates a good fit for these data. If model (9.24) is correct, we would expect that roughly 95% of the standardized deviance residuals would lie between ±2; the lowess regression line should be flat and lie near zero.

rates that range from about 10 to 35, and is never too far from zero outside of this range. This figure indicates a good fit for this model to the Framingham Heart Study data.

9.5. Residual Analysis of Poisson Regression Models using Stata

A residual analysis of model (9.24) is illustrated below. The Stata log file *9.3.Framingham.log* continues as follows.

```
. *
. * Compress data set for residual plot
. *
. sort male bmi_gr scl_gr dbp_gr age_gr2
. collapse (sum) pt_yrs = pt_yrs chd_cnt = chd_cnt, by          {1}
> (male bmi_gr scl_gr dbp_gr age_gr2)
. *
. * Re-analyze model (9.24)
. *
. xi: glm chd_cnt i.age_gr2*male i.bmi_gr i.scl_gr i.dbp_gr,    {2}
> family(poisson) link(log) lnoffset(pt_yrs)
```
{Output omitted. See previous analysis of this model}
```
. *
. * Estimate the expected number of CHD events and the
. * standardized deviance residual for each record in the data set.
. *
. predict e_chd, mu                                             {3}
(82 missing values generated)

. predict dev, standardized deviance                            {4}
(82 missing values generated)

. generate e_rate = 1000*e_chd/pt_yrs                           {5}
(82 missing values generated)

. label variable e_rate "Incidence of CHD per Thousand"

. *
. * Draw scatterplot of the standardized deviance residual versus the
. * incidence of CHD. Include lowess regression curve on this plot
. *
. ksm dev e_rate, lowess bwidth(.2) xlabel(0,10 to 80) ylabel(-3,-2 to 4)  {6}
> xtick(5, 15 to 75) ytick(-2.5, -1.5 to 3.5) gap(3) yline(-2,0,2)
```

Comments

1 This *collapse* command produces one record for each unique combination of the values of the covariates from model (9.24).

2 We need to repeat the analysis of this model in order to calculate the standardized deviance residuals from the compressed data set. The parameter estimates from this model are identical to those of the previous *glm* command.

3 This *predict* command calculates *e_chd* to equal $\hat{E}[d_i \mid \mathbf{x}_i]$, which is the estimated expected number of CHD events in people with the ith combination of covariate values.

4 This command sets *dev* equal to the standardized deviance residual for each combination of covariate values.

5 This command calculates *e_rate* to be the estimated incidence of CHD per thousand person-years among patients with the ith combination of covariate values.

6 This command produces a scatter plot with a lowess regression curve that is similar to Figure 9.2.

9.6. Additional Reading

Breslow and Day (1987) is an excellent reference on Poisson regression that I highly recommend to readers with at least an intermediate level background in biostatistics. These authors provide an extensive theoretical and practical discussion of this topic.

McCullagh and Nelder (1989) is a more theoretical reference that discusses Poisson regression in the context of the generalized linear model. This text also discusses deviance residuals.

Hosmer and Lemeshow (1989) also provide an excellent discussion of deviance residuals in the context of logistic regression.

Levy (1999) provides a thorough description of the Framingham Heart Study.

9.7. Exercises

The following exercises are concerned with the child injury death data set *8.ex.InjuryDeath.dta* from Chapter 8.

1 Fit a multiplicative Poisson regression model that includes the covariates, maternal age, birth weight, mother's education, income, mother's marital status at time of birth, number of siblings, mother's race, late or absent prenatal care, and age of child. Complete the following table; each relative risk should be adjusted for all of the other risk factors in your model.

Numerator of relative risk	Denominator of relative risk	Adjusted relative risk	95% confidence interval
Maternal age 25–29	Maternal age > 29		
Maternal age 20–24	Maternal age > 29		
Maternal age < 20	Maternal age > 29		
Birth weight < 2500 gm	Birth weight ≥ 2500 gm		
Mom's ed. 13–15 yrs.	Mom's education > 15 yrs.		
Mom's ed. = 12 yrs.	Mom's education > 15 yrs.		
Mom's ed. < 12 yrs.	Mom's education > 15 yrs.		
Income in lowest quintile	Income in highest quintile		
Income in 2nd quintile	Income in highest quintile		
Income in 3rd quintile	Income in highest quintile		
Income in 4th quintile	Income in highest quintile		
Unmarried mom	Married mom		
One sibling	No siblings		
Two siblings	No siblings		
Three siblings	No siblings		
> 3 siblings	No siblings		
Black mom	White mom		
Late/no prenatal care	Adequate prenatal care		
1st year of life	3 year old		
1 year old	3 year old		
2 year old	3 year old		
4 year old	3 year old		

2 Contrast your answers to those of question 4 in Chapter 8. In particular, what can you say about the relationship between race, prenatal care and the risk of injury death?

3 Graph a scatterplot of the standardized deviance residuals against the corresponding expected incidence of injury deaths from your model. Plot the lowess regression curve of the deviance residuals against the expected incidence of mortal injuries on this graph. What proportion of the residuals have an absolute value greater than two? List the standardized deviance residual, expected incidence of injury deaths, observed number of injury deaths, and number of child-years of follow-up for all records with a deviance residual greater than two and at least two child injury deaths. Comment on the adequacy of the model. What might you do to improve the fit?

10

Fixed Effects Analysis of Variance

The term **analysis of variance** refers to a very large body of statistical methods for regressing a dependent variable against one or more classification variables. Much of the literature on this topic is concerned with sophisticated study designs that could be evaluated using the electric calculators of the last century. Today, these designs are of limited utility in medical statistics. This is, in part, because the enormous computational power of modern computers makes the computational simplicity of these methods irrelevant, but also, because we are often unable to exert the level of experimental control over human subjects that is needed by these methods. As a consequence, regression methods using classification variables have replaced classical analyses of variance in many medical experiments today.

In this chapter we introduce traditional analysis of variance from a regression perspective. In these methods, each patient is observed only once. As a result, it is reasonable to assume that the model errors for different patients are mutually independent. These techniques are called **fixed-effects** methods because each observation is assumed to equal the sum of a fixed expected value and an independent error term. Each of these expected values is a function of fixed population parameters and the patient's covariates. In Chapter 11, we will discuss more complex designs in which multiple observations are made on each patient, and it is no longer reasonable to assume that different error terms for the same patient are independent.

10.1. One-Way Analysis of Variance

A **one-way analysis of variance** is a generalization of the independent t test. Suppose that patients are divided into k groups on the basis of some classification variable. Let n_i be the number of subjects in the ith group, $n = \sum n_i$ be the total number of study subjects, and y_{ij} be a continuous response variable on the jth patient from the ith group. We assume for $i = 1, 2, \ldots, k$; $j = 1, 2, \ldots, n_i$ that

$$y_{ij} = \beta_i + \varepsilon_{ij}, \tag{10.1}$$

where

$\beta_1, \beta_2, \ldots, \beta_k$ are unknown parameters, and

ε_{ij} are mutually independent, normally distributed error terms with mean 0 and standard deviation σ.

Under this model, the expected value of y_{ij} is $E[y_{ij}|i] = \beta_i$. Models like (10.1) are called **fixed-effects** models because the parameters $\beta_1, \beta_2, \ldots, \beta_k$ are fixed constants that are attributes of the underlying population. The response y_{ij} differs from β_i only because of the error term ε_{ij}. Let

$b_1, b_2, \ldots, b_k$ be the least squares estimates of $\beta_1, \beta_2, \ldots, \beta_k$, respectively,

$\bar{y}_i = \sum_{j=1}^{n_i} y_{ij}/n_i$ be the sample mean for the ith group, and

$$s^2 = \sum_{i=1}^{k} \sum_{j=1}^{n_i} (y_{ij} - \bar{y}_i)^2/(n-k) \tag{10.2}$$

be the mean squared error (MSE) estimate of σ^2. Equation (10.2) is analogous to equation (3.5). We estimate σ by s, which is called the root MSE. It can be shown that $E[y_{ij}|i] = b_i = \bar{y}_i$, and $E[s^2] = \sigma^2$. A 95% confidence interval for β_i is given by

$$\bar{y}_i \pm t_{n-k,0.025}(s/\sqrt{n_i}). \tag{10.3}$$

Note that model (10.1) assumes that the standard deviation of ε_{ij} is the same for all groups. If it appears that there is appreciable variation in this standard deviation among groups then the 95% confidence interval for β_i should be estimated by

$$\bar{y}_i \pm t_{n_i-1,0.025}(s_i/\sqrt{n_i}), \tag{10.4}$$

where s_i is the sample standard deviation of y_{ij} within the ith group.

We wish to test the null hypothesis that the expected response is the same in all groups. That is, we wish to test whether

$$\beta_1 = \beta_2 = \ldots = \beta_k. \tag{10.5}$$

We can calculate a statistic that has an **F distribution** with $k-1$ and $n-k$ degrees of freedom when this null hypothesis is true. The F distribution is another family of standard distributions like the chi-squared family. However, while a chi-squared distribution is determined by a single variable that gives its degrees of freedom, an F distribution is uniquely characterized by two separate degrees of freedom. These are called the numerator and denominator degrees of freedom, respectively. We reject the null hypothesis in favor of a multisided alternative hypothesis when the F statistic is sufficiently large. The P value associated with this test is the probability that this statistic exceeds the observed value when this null hypothesis is true.

When there are just two groups, the F statistic will have 1 and $n - 2$ degrees of freedom. In this case, the one-way analysis of variance is equivalent to an independent t test. The square root of this F statistic equals the absolute value of the t statistic given by equation (1.7). The square of a t statistic with n degrees of freedom equals an F statistic with numerator and denominator degrees of freedom of 1 and n, respectively.

A test due to Bartlett (1937) can be performed to test the assumption that the standard deviation of ε_{ij} is constant within each group. If this test is significant, or if there is considerable variation in the values of s_i, then you should use equation (10.4) rather than equation (10.3) to calculate confidence intervals for the group means. Armitage and Berry (1994) provide additional details about Bartlett's test.

10.2. Multiple Comparisons

In a one-way analysis of variance we are not only interested in knowing if the group means are all equal, but also which means are different. For example, we may wish to separately test whether $\beta_1 = \beta_2$, $\beta_2 = \beta_3$, ..., or $\beta_{k-1} = \beta_k$. For any individual test, a P value of 0.05 means that we have a 5% probability of false rejection of the null hypothesis. However, if we have multiple tests, the probability of false rejection of at least one test will be greater than 0.05. A mindless data dredging exercise that calculates many P values is likely to produce some tests of spurious significance. Various methods are available that adjust the P values of an experiment in such a way that the probably of false rejection of one or more of the associated null hypotheses is not greater than 0.05. Such P values are said to be adjusted for **multiple comparisons**. Discussion of these methods can be found in Armitage and Berry (1994), and Steel and Torrie (1980). An alternative approach, which we will use, is known as **Fisher's protected LSD procedure**. (Here, LSD stands for "least significant difference" rather than Fisher's favorite psychotropic medicine – see Steel and Torrie, 1980.) This approach proceeds as follows: first, we perform a one-way analysis of variance to test if all of the means are equal. If this test is not significant, we say that there is not sufficient statistical evidence to claim that there are any differences in the group means. If, however, the analysis of variance F

statistic is significant, then we have evidence from a single test that at least some of these means must differ from some others. We can use this evidence as justification for looking at pair-wise differences between the group means without adjusting for multiple comparisons. Comparisons between any two groups are performed by calculating a t statistic. If the standard deviations within the k groups appear similar we can increase the power of the test that $\beta_i = \beta_j$ by using the formula

$$t_{n-k} = (\bar{y}_i - \bar{y}_j) / \left(s \sqrt{\frac{1}{n_i} + \frac{1}{n_j}} \right), \tag{10.6}$$

where s is the root MSE estimate of σ obtained from the analysis of variance. Under the null hypothesis that $\beta_i = \beta_j$, equation (10.6) will have a t distribution with $n - k$ degrees of freedom. This test is more powerful than the independent t test because it uses all of the data to estimate σ (see Section 1.4.12). On the other hand, the independent t test is more robust than equation (10.6) since it makes no assumptions about the homogeneity of the standard deviations of groups other than i and j.

A 95% confidence interval for the difference in population means between groups i and j is

$$\bar{y}_i - \bar{y}_j \pm t_{n-k,0.025} \left(s \sqrt{\frac{1}{n_i} + \frac{1}{n_j}} \right). \tag{10.7}$$

Alternatively, a confidence interval based on the independent t test may be used if it appears unreasonable to assume a uniform standard deviation in all groups (see equations (1.8) and (1.11)).

There is considerable controversy about the best way to deal with multiple comparisons. Fisher's protected LSD approach works best when the hypothesized differences between the groups are predicted before the experiment is performed, when the number of groups is fairly small, or when there is some natural ordering of the groups. It should be noted, however, that if we are comparing groups receiving k unrelated treatments, then there are $k(k-1)$ possible contrasts between pairs of treatments. If k is large then the chance of false rejection of at least some of these null hypotheses may be much greater than 0.05 even when the overall F statistic is significant. In this situation, it is prudent to make a multiple comparisons adjustment to these P values.

A problem with multiple comparisons adjustment relates to how P values are used in medical science. Although a P value is, by definition, a probability, we use it as a measure of strength of evidence. That is, suppose we have two completely unrelated experiments comparing, say, survival among breast cancer patients and blood pressure reduction among hypertensive patients. If the logrank and t test P values from these two studies are equal, then we would like to conclude that the evidence against their respective null hypotheses is similar. In a large clinical study, we typically have a small number of primary hypotheses that are stipulated in advance. Such studies are very expensive and it makes sense to perform careful exploratory analyses to learn as much as possible about the treatments under study. This typically involves many sub-analyses. If we performed multiple comparisons adjustments on all of these analyses we would greatly reduce or eliminate the statistical significance of our tests of the primary hypotheses of interest. Moreover, these adjusted P values would not be comparable with P values of similar magnitude from experiments with fewer comparisons. In my opinion, it is usually best to report unadjusted P values and confidence intervals, but to make it very clear which hypotheses were specified in advance and which are the result of exploratory analyses. The latter results will need to be confirmed by other studies but may be of great value in suggesting the direction of future research. Also, investigators need to use good judgment and common sense in deciding which sub-analyses to report. Investigators are in no way obligated to report an implausible finding merely because its unadjusted P value is less than 0.05.

Classical methods of statistical inference almost always lead to sensible conclusions when applied with some common sense. There are, however, some fundamental problems with the philosophical foundations of classical statistical inference. An excellent review of these problems is given by Royall (1997), who discusses multiple comparisons in the context of the deeper problems of classical statistical inference. Dupont (1983) and Dupont (1986) give two examples of how classical inference can lead to unsatisfactory conclusions.

10.3. Reformulating Analysis of Variance as a Linear Regression Model

A one-way analysis of variance is, in fact, a special case of the multiple regression model we considered in Chapter 3. Let

y_h denote the response from the hth study subject, $h = 1, 2, \ldots, n$, and let

$$x_{hi} = \begin{cases} 1: & \text{if the } h^{\text{th}} \text{ patient is in the } i^{\text{th}} \text{ group} \\ 0: & \text{otherwise.} \end{cases}$$

Then model (10.1) can be rewritten

$$y_h = \alpha + \beta_2 x_{h2} + \beta_3 x_{h3} + \cdots + \beta_k x_{hk} + \varepsilon_h, \tag{10.8}$$

where ε_h are mutually independent, normally distributed error terms with mean 0 and standard deviation σ. Note that model (10.8) is a special case of model (3.1). Thus, this analysis of variance is also a regression analysis in which all of the covariates are zero–one indicator variables. Also,

$$E[y_h | x_{hi}] = \begin{cases} \alpha & \text{if the } h^{\text{th}} \text{ patient is from group 1} \\ \alpha + \beta_i & \text{if the } h^{\text{th}} \text{ patient is from group } i > 1. \end{cases}$$

Thus, α is the expected response of patients in the first group and β_i is the expected difference in the response of patients in the ith and first groups. The least squares estimates of α and β_i are $\bar{y}_1$ and $\bar{y}_i - \bar{y}_1$, respectively. We can use any multiple linear regression program to perform a one-way analysis of variance, although most software packages have a separate procedure for this task.

10.4. Non-parametric Methods

The methods that we have considered in this text so far assume a specific form for the distribution of the response variable that is determined by one or more parameters. These techniques are called **parametric methods**. For example, in model (10.1) we assume that y_{ij} is normally distributed with mean β_i and standard deviation σ. Our inferences are not greatly affected by minor violations of these distributional assumptions. However, if the true model differs radically from the one that we have chosen our conclusions may be misleading. In Section 2.17 we discussed transforming the dependent and independent variables in order to achieve a better model fit. Another approach is to use a method that avoids making any assumptions about the distribution of the response variable. These are called **non-parametric** methods. They tend to be less powerful than their parametric counterparts and are not useful for estimating attributes of the population of interest. They do, however, lead to robust tests of statistical significance when the distributional assumptions of the analogous parametric methods are wrong. They are particularly useful when there are extreme outliers in some of the groups or when the within-group distribution of the response variable is highly skewed.

10.5. Kruskal–Wallis Test

The **Kruskal–Wallis** test is the non-parametric analog of the one-way analysis of variance (Kruskal and Wallis, 1952). Model (10.1) assumes that the ε_{ij} terms are normally distributed and have the same standard deviation. If either of these assumptions is badly violated then the Kruskal–Wallis test should be used. Suppose that patients are divided into k groups as in model (10.1) and that y_{ij} is a continuous response variable on the jth patient from the ith group. The null hypothesis of this test is that the distributions of the response variables are the same in each group. Let n_i be the number of subjects in the ith group, and $n = \sum n_i$ be the total number of study subjects. We rank the values of y_{ij} from lowest to highest and let R_i be the sum of the ranks for the patients from the ith group. If all of the values of y_{ij} are distinct (no ties) then the Kruskal–Wallis test statistic is

$$H = \frac{12}{n(n+1)} \left(\sum \frac{R_i^2}{n_i} \right) - 3(n+1). \tag{10.9}$$

When there are ties a slightly more complicated formula is used (see Steel and Torrie, 1980). Under the null hypothesis, H will have a chi-squared distribution with $k-1$ degrees of freedom as long as the number of patients in each group is reasonably large. Note that the value of H will be the same for any two data sets in which the data values have the same ranks. Increasing the largest observation or decreasing the smallest observation will have no effect on H. Hence, extreme outliers will not unduly affect this test. The non-parametric analog of the independent t-test is the **Wilcoxon–Mann–Whitney rank-sum test**. This rank-sum test and the Kruskal–Wallis test are equivalent when there are only two groups of patients.

10.6. Example: A Polymorphism in the Estrogen Receptor Gene

The human estrogen receptor gene contains a two-allele restriction fragment length polymorphism that can be detected by Southern blots of DNA digested with the PuvII restriction endonuclease. Bands at 1.6 kb and/or 0.7 kb identify the genotype for these alleles. Parl et al. (1989) studied the relationship between this genotype and age of diagnosis among 59 breast cancer patients. Table 10.1 shows the average age of breast cancer diagnosis among these patients subdivided by genotype. The average age of diagnosis for patients who are homozygous for the 0.7 kb pattern allele was about 14 years younger than that of patients who were homozygous for the 1.6 kb pattern allele or who were heterozygous. To test the null hypothesis that the

10.6. Example: A polymorphism in the estrogen receptor gene

Table 10.1. Effect of estrogen receptor genotype on age at diagnosis among 59 breast cancer patients (Parl et al., 1989).

	Genotype*			
	1.6/1.6	1.6/0.7	0.7/0.7	Total
Number of patients	14	29	16	59
Age at breast cancer diagnosis				
Mean	64.643	64.379	50.375	60.644
Standard deviation	11.18	13.26	10.64	13.49
95% confidence interval				
Equation (10.3)	(58.1–71.1)	(59.9–68.9)	(44.3–56.5)	
Equation (10.4)	(58.2–71.1)	(59.3–69.4)	(44.7–56.0)	(57.1–4.2)

*The numbers 0.7 and 1.6 identify the alleles of the estrogen receptor genes that were studied (see text). Patients were either homozygous for the 1.6 kb pattern allele (had two copies of the same allele), were heterozygous (had one copy of each allele), or were homozygous for the 0.7 kb pattern allele.

age at diagnosis does not vary with genotype, we perform a one-way analysis of variance on the ages of patients in these three groups using model (10.1). In this analysis, $n = 59$, $k = 3$, and β_1, β_2 and β_3 represent the expected age of breast cancer diagnosis among patients with the 1.6/1.6, 1.6/0.7, and 0.7/0.7 genotypes, respectively. The estimates of these parameters are the average ages given in Table 10.1. The F test from this analysis equals 7.86. This statistic has $k - 1 = 2$ and $n - k = 56$ degrees of freedom. The P value associated with this test equals 0.001. Hence, we can reject the null hypothesis that these three population means are equal.

The root MSE estimate of σ from this analysis of variance is $s = \sqrt{147.25} = 12.135$. The critical value $t_{56,0.025}$ equals 2.003. Substituting these values into equation (10.3) gives that a 95% confidence interval for the age of diagnosis of women with the 1.6/0.7 genotype is $64.38 \pm 2.003 \times 12.135/\sqrt{29} = (59.9, 68.9)$. The within-group standard deviations shown in this table are quite similar, and Bartlett's test for equal standard deviations is not significant ($P = 0.58$). Hence, it is reasonable to use equation (10.3) rather than equation (10.4) to calculate the confidence intervals for the mean age at diagnosis for each genotype. In Table 10.1, these intervals are calculated for each genotype using both of these equations. Note that, in this example, these equations produce similar estimates. If the equal standard deviation assumption is true, then equation (10.3) will provide more accurate confidence intervals than equation (10.4) since it uses all of the data to calculate

Table 10.2. Comparison of mean age of breast cancer diagnosis among patients with the three estrogen receptor genotypes studied by Parl et al. (1989). The one-way analysis of variance of these data shows that there is a significant difference between the mean age of diagnosis among women with these three genotypes ($P = 0.001$).

Comparison	Difference in mean age of diagnosis	95% confidence interval	P value Eq. (10.6)	Rank-sum*
1.6/0.7 vs. 1.6/1.6	−0.264	(−8.17 to 7.65)	0.95	0.96
0.7/0.7 vs. 1.6/1.6	−14.268	(−23.2 to −5.37)	0.002	0.003
0.7/0.7 vs. 1.6/0.7	−14.004	(−21.6 to −6.43)	<0.0005	0.002

*Wilcoxon–Mann–Whitney rank-sum test

the common standard deviation estimate s. However, equation (10.4) is more robust than equation (10.3) since it does not make any assumptions about the standard deviation within each patient group.

The F test from the analysis of variance permits us to reject the null hypothesis that the mean age of diagnosis is the same for each group. Hence, it is reasonable to investigate if there are pair-wise differences in these ages (see Section 10.2). This can be done using either independent t-tests or equation (10.6). For example, the difference in average age of diagnosis between women with the 0.7/0.7 genotype and those with the 1.6/1.6 genotype is −14.268. From equation (10.6), the t statistic to test whether this difference is significantly different from zero is $t = -14.268/(12.135\sqrt{1/14 + 1/16}) = -3.21$. The P value for this statistic, which has 56 degrees of freedom, is 0.002. The 95% confidence interval for this difference using equation (10.7) is $-14.268 \pm 2.003 \times 12.135 \times \sqrt{1/14 + 1/16} = (-23.2, -5.37)$. Table 10.2 gives estimates of the difference between the mean ages of these three groups. In this table, confidence intervals are derived using equation (10.7) and P values are calculated using equation (10.6). It is clear that the age of diagnosis among women who are homozygous for the 0.7 kb pattern allele is less that that of women with the other two genotypes.

Figure 10.1 shows box plots for the age at diagnoses for the three genotypes. The vertical lines under these plots indicate the ages of diagnosis. The number of line segments equals the number of women diagnosed at each age. Although these plots are mildly asymmetric, they indicate that these age distributions are sufficiently close to normal to justify the analysis of variance given above. Of course, the Kruskal–Wallis analysis of variance is

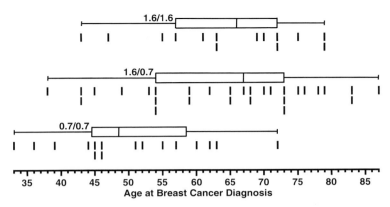

Figure 10.1

Box plots of age at breast cancer diagnosis subdivided by estrogen receptor genotype in the study by Parl et al. (1989). The vertical lines under each box plot mark the actual ages of diagnosis. The number of line segments equals the number of women diagnosed at each age. Women who were homozygous for the 0.7 pattern allele had a significantly younger age of breast cancer diagnosis than did women in the other two groups.

also valid and avoids these normality assumptions. The Kruskal–Wallis test statistic for these data is $H = 12.1$. Under the null hypothesis that the age distributions of the three patient groups are the same, H will have a chi-squared distribution with $k - 1 = 2$ degrees of freedom. The P value for this test is 0.0024, which allows us to reject this hypothesis. Note that this P value is larger (less statistically significant) than that obtained from the analogous conventional analysis of variance. This illustrates the slight loss of statistical power of the Kruskal–Wallis test, which is the cost of avoiding the normality assumptions of the conventional analysis of variance. Table 10.2 also gives the P values from pair-wise comparisons of the three groups using the Wilcoxon–Mann–Whitney rank sum test. These tests lead to the same conclusions that we obtained from the conventional analysis of variance.

10.7. One-Way Analyses of Variance using Stata

The following Stata log file and comments illustrate how to perform the one-way analysis of variance discussed in the preceding section.

```
. * 10.7.ERpolymorphism.log

. *

. * Do a one-way analysis of variance to determine whether age

. * at breast cancer diagnosis varies with estrogen receptor (ER)

. * genotype using the data of Parl et al., 1989.
```

```
. *
. use C:\WDDtext\10.7.ERpolymorphism.dta                                    {1}
. ci age                                                                    {2}

    Variable |   Obs      Mean    Std. Err.     [95% Conf. Interval]
-------------+-------------------------------------------------------
         age |    59   60.64407   1.756804      57.12744    64.16069

. by genotype: ci age                                                       {3}

_____

-> genotype = 1.6/1.6

    Variable |   Obs      Mean    Std. Err.     [95% Conf. Interval]
-------------+-------------------------------------------------------
         age |    14   64.64286   2.988269       58.1871    71.09862

_____

-> genotype = 1.6/0.7

    Variable |   Obs      Mean    Std. Err.     [95% Conf. Interval]
-------------+-------------------------------------------------------
         age |    29   64.37931   2.462234      59.33565    69.42297

_____

-> genotype = 0.7/0.7

    Variable |   Obs      Mean    Std. Err.     [95% Conf. Interval]
-------------+-------------------------------------------------------
         age |    16    50.375    2.659691       44.706      56.044

. graph age, by(genotype) box oneway                                        {4}
                                    {Graph omitted. See Figure 10.1}
. oneway age genotype                                                       {5}

                      Analysis of Variance
    Source             SS        df      MS          F      Prob > F
----------------------------------------------------------------------
Between groups      2315.73355    2   1157.86678    7.86     0.0010      {6}
Within groups       8245.79187   56   147.246283                        {7}
----------------------------------------------------------------------
    Total          10561.5254    58   182.095266

Bartlett's test for equal variances: chi2(2) = 1.0798 Prob>chi2 = 0.583    {8}
. *
. * Repeat analysis using linear regression
```

```
. *
. xi: regress age i.genotype                                          {9}
i.genotype     _Igenotype_1-3   (naturally coded; _Igenotype_1 omitted)

      Source |    SS         df       MS              Number of obs =      59
-------------+----------------------------           F( 2,    56) =    7.86
       Model | 2315.73355      2   1157.86678         Prob > F      =  0.0010
    Residual | 8245.79187     56   147.246283         R-squared     =  0.2193
-------------+----------------------------           Adj R-squared =  0.1914
       Total | 10561.5254     58   182.095266         Root MSE      =  12.135

--------------------------------------------------------------------------------
         age |    Coef.    Std. Err.    t     P>|t|     [95% Conf. Interval]
-------------+------------------------------------------------------------------
_Igenotype_2 | -.2635468   3.949057   -0.07   0.947    -8.174458    7.647365     {10}
_Igenotype_3 | -14.26786   4.440775   -3.21   0.002    -23.1638    -5.371916
       _cons |  64.64286   3.243084   19.93   0.000     58.14618    71.13953     {11}
--------------------------------------------------------------------------------

. lincom _cons + _Igenotype_2                                         {12}

 ( 1)  _Igenotype_2 + _cons = 0.0

--------------------------------------------------------------------------------
         age |    Coef.    Std. Err.    t     P>|t|     [95% Conf. Interval]
-------------+------------------------------------------------------------------
         (1) |  64.37931   2.253322   28.57   0.000     59.86536    68.89326     {13}
--------------------------------------------------------------------------------

. lincom _cons + _Igenotype_3
 ( 1)  _Igenotype_3 + _cons = 0.0

--------------------------------------------------------------------------------
         age |    Coef.    Std. Err.    t     P>|t|     [95% Conf. Interval]
-------------+------------------------------------------------------------------
         (1) |   50.375    3.033627   16.61   0.000     44.29791    56.45209
--------------------------------------------------------------------------------

. lincom _Igenotype_3 - _Igenotype_2                                  {14}

 ( 1)  _Igenotype_3 - _Igenotype_2 = 0.0

--------------------------------------------------------------------------------
         age |    Coef.    Std. Err.    t     P>|t|     [95% Conf. Interval]
-------------+------------------------------------------------------------------
         (1) | -14.00431   3.778935   -3.71   0.000     -21.57443   -6.434194
--------------------------------------------------------------------------------
```

```
. *
. * Perform a Kruskal-Wallis analysis of variance
. *
. kwallis age, by(genotype)                                          {15}

Test: Equality of populations (Kruskal-Wallis test)

genotype          _Obs     _RankSum
 1.6/1.6            14       494.00
 1.6/0.7            29       999.50
 0.7/0.7            16       276.50

chi-squared =    12.060 with 2 d.f.
probability =     0.0024

chi-squared with ties =     12.073 with 2 d.f.
probability =     0.0024

. ranksum age if genotype ~=3, by(genotype)                          {16}

Two-sample Wilcoxon rank-sum (Mann-Whitney) test

    genotype |   obs     rank sum      expected
------------+-----------------------------
    1.6/1.6 |    14         310           308
    1.6/0.7 |    29         636           638
------------+-----------------------------
    combined |    43         946           946

unadjusted variance    1488.67
adjustment for ties     -2.70
                       ------------
adjusted variance      1485.97

Ho: age(genotype==1.6/1.6) = age(genotype==1.6/0.7)
            z = 0.052
      Prob > |z|= 0.9586

. ranksum age if genotype ~=2, by(genotype)

Two-sample Wilcoxon rank-sum (Mann-Whitney) test

    genotype |   obs     rank sum      expected
-------------+-----------------------------
    1.6/1.6 |    14         289           217
    0.7/0.7 |    16         176           248
-------------+-----------------------------
    combined |    30         465           465
```

```
unadjusted variance      578.67
adjustment for ties       -1.67
                        ---------
adjusted variance        576.99

Ho: age(genotype==1.6/1.6) = age(genotype==0.7/0.7)
         z  =   2.997
   Prob > |z| =   0.0027
```

. ranksum *age* if *genotype* ~=1, by(*genotype*)

```
Two-sample Wilcoxon rank-sum (Mann-Whitney) test

   genotype |   obs    rank sum    expected
------------+-----------------------------
    1.6/0.7 |   29       798.5         667
    0.7/0.7 |   16       236.5         368
------------+-----------------------------
   combined |   45        1035        1035

unadjusted variance     1778.67
adjustment for ties       -2.23
                        --------
adjusted variance       1776.44

Ho: age(genotype==1.6/0.7) = age(genotype==0.7/0.7)
         z =  3.120
   Prob > |z|= 0.0018
```

. kwallis *age* if *genotype* ~=1, by(*genotype*)   {17}

```
Test: Equality of populations (Kruskal-Wallis test)

   genotype        _Obs      _RankSum
    1.6/0.7          29        798.50
    0.7/0.7          16        236.50

chi-squared =  9.722 with 1 d.f.
probability =  0.0018

chi-squared with ties =    9.734 with 1 d.f.
probability =     0.0018
```

Comments

1 This data set contains the age of diagnosis and estrogen receptor genotype of the 59 breast cancer patients studied by Parl et al. (1989). The
genotypes 1.6/1.6, 1.6/0.7 and 0.7/0.7 are coded 1, 2 and 3 in the variable
genotype, respectively.

2 This *ci* command calculates the mean age of diagnosis (*age*) together with the associated 95% confidence interval. This confidence interval is calculated using equation (10.4). The estimated standard error of the mean and the number of patients with non-missing ages is also given.

3 The command prefix *by genotype:* specifies that means and 95% confidence intervals are to be calculated for each of the three genotypes. The output from this and the preceding command are given in Table 10.1. The sample standard deviations are obtained by multiplying each standard error estimate by the square root of its sample size. (Alternatively, we could have used the *summarize* command.)

4 The *box* and *oneway* options of this *graph* command create a graph that is similar to Figure 10.1. In this latter figure, I used a graphics editor to add a common *x*-axis and to divide the vertical lines into line segments equal to the number of patients diagnosed at each age.

5 This *oneway* command performs a one-way analysis of variance of *age* with respect to the three distinct values of *genotype*.

6 The F statistic from this analysis equals 7.86. If the mean age of diagnosis in the target population is the same for all three genotypes, this statistic will have an F distribution with $k - 1 = 3 - 1 = 2$ and $n - k = 59 - 3 = 56$ degrees of freedom. The probability that this statistic exceeds 7.86 is 0.001.

7 The MSE estimate of σ^2 is $s^2 = 147.246$.

8 Bartlett's test for equal variances (i.e. equal standard deviations) gives a P value of 0.58.

9 This *regress* command preforms exactly the same one-way analysis of variance as the *oneway* command given above. Note that the F statistic, the P value for this statistic and the MSE estimate of σ^2 are identical to that given by the *oneway* command. The syntax of the *xi:* prefix is explained in Section 5.10. The model used by this command is equation (10.8) with $k = 3$.

10 The estimates of β_2 and β_3 in this example are $\bar{y}_2 - \bar{y}_1 = 64.379 - 64.643 = -0.264$ and $\bar{y}_3 - \bar{y}_1 = 50.375 - 64.643 = -14.268$, respectively. They are highlighted in the column labeled *Coef*. The 95% confidence intervals for β_2 and β_3 are calculated using equation (10.7). The t statistics for testing the null hypotheses that $\beta_2 = 0$ and $\beta_3 = 0$ are -0.07 and -3.21, respectively. They are calculated using equation (10.6). The highlighted values in this output are also given in Table 10.2.

11 The estimate of α is $\bar{y}_1 = 64.643$. The 95% confidence interval for α is calculated using equation (10.3). These statistics are also given in Table 10.1.

12 This *lincom* command estimates $\alpha + \beta_2$ by $\hat{\alpha} + \hat{\beta}_2 = \bar{y}_2$. A 95% confidence interval for this estimate is also given. Note that $\alpha + \beta_2$ equals the population mean age of diagnosis among women with the 1.6/0.7 genotype. Output from this and the next *lincom* command are also given in Table 10.1.

13 This confidence interval is calculated using equation (10.3).

14 This command estimates $\beta_3 - \beta_2$ by $\hat{\beta}_3 - \hat{\beta}_2 = \bar{y}_3 - \bar{y}_2 = 50.375 - 64.379 = -14.004$. The null hypothesis that $\beta_3 = \beta_2$ is the same as the hypothesis that the mean age of diagnosis in Groups 2 and 3 are equal. The confidence interval for $\beta_3 - \beta_2$ is calculated using equation (10.7). The highlighted values are also given in Table 10.2.

15 This *kwallis* command performs a Kruskal–Wallis test of *age* by *genotype*. The test statistic, adjusted for ties, equals 12.073. The associated P value equal 0.0024.

16 This command performs a Wilcoxon–Mann–Whitney rank-sum test on the age of diagnosis of women with the 1.6/1.6 genotype versus the 1.6/0.7 genotype. The P value for this test is 0.96. The next two commands perform the other two pair-wise comparisons of age by genotype using this rank-sum test. The highlighted P values are included in Table 10.2.

17 This command repeats the preceding command using the Kruskal–Wallis test. This test is equivalent to the rank-sum test when only two groups are being compared. Note that the P values from these tests both equal 0.0018

10.8. Two-Way Analysis of Variance, Analysis of Covariance, and Other Models

Fixed-effects analyses of variance generalize to a wide variety of complex models. For example, suppose that hypertensive patients were treated with either a placebo, a diuretic alone, a beta-blocker alone, or with both a diuretic and a beta-blocker. Then a model of the effect of treatment on diastolic blood pressure (DBP) might be

$$y_i = \alpha + \beta_1 x_{i1} + \beta_2 x_{i2} + \varepsilon_i, \tag{10.10}$$

where

α, β_1 and β_2 are unknown parameters,

$$x_{i1} = \begin{cases} 1: & i^{\text{th}} \text{ patient is on a diuretic} \\ 0: & \text{otherwise,} \end{cases}$$

$$x_{i2} = \begin{cases} 1: i^{\text{th}} \text{ patient is on a beta-blocker} \\ 0: \text{otherwise,} \end{cases}$$

y_i is the DBP of the ith patient after some standard interval of therapy, and ε_i are error terms that are independently and normally distributed with mean zero and standard deviation σ.

Model (10.10) is an example of a fixed-effects, **two-way analysis of variance**. It is called two-way because each patient is simultaneously influenced by two covariates – in this case whether she did, or did not, receive a diuretic or a beta-blocker. A critical feature of this model is that each patient's blood pressure is only observed once. It is this feature that makes the independence assumption for the error term reasonable and makes this a fixed-effects model. In this model, α is the mean DBP of patients on placebo, $\alpha + \beta_1$ is the mean DBP of patients on the diuretic alone, and $\alpha + \beta_2$ is the mean DBP of patients on the beta-blocker alone. The model is additive since it assumes that the mean DBP of patients on both drugs is $\alpha + \beta_1 + \beta_2$. If this assumption is unreasonable we can add an interaction term as in Section 3.12.

Another possibility is to mix continuous and indicator variables in the same model. Inference from these models is called **analysis of covariance**. For example, we could add the patient's age to model (10.10). This gives

$$y_i = \alpha + \beta_1 x_{i1} + \beta_2 x_{i2} + \beta_3 \times age_i + \varepsilon_i, \tag{10.11}$$

where age_i is the ith patient's age, β_3 is the parameter associated with age, and the other terms are as defined in model (10.10). The analysis of model (10.11) would be an example of analysis of covariance. There is a vast statistical literature on the analysis of variance and covariance. The interested reader will find references to some good texts on this topic in Section 10.9. Note, however, that models (10.10) and (10.11) are both special cases of model (3.1). Thus, we can usually reformulate any fixed-effects analysis of variance or covariance problem into a multiple linear regression problem by choosing suitably defined indicator and continuous covariates.

10.9. Additional Reading

Armitage and Berry (1994) and
Steel and Torrie (1980) provide additional discussion of fixed-effects analysis of variance and covariance.
Cochran and Cox (1957) is a classic text that documents the extraordinary ingenuity and effort that was devoted in the last century to devise methods

of experimental design and analysis of variance that could be implemented with electric calculators.

Searle (1987) is a more mathematically advanced text on linear models, including analysis of variance.

Parl et al. (1989) studied the relationship between age of breast cancer diagnosis and a polymorphism in the estrogen receptor gene. We use their data to illustrate fixed-effects one-way analysis of variance.

Royall (1997) provides an excellent introduction to the foundations of statistical inference. This introduction is written from a likelihood perspective, of which Royall is a leading advocate.

Cox and Hinkley (1974) provide a concise summary of the different fundamental approaches to statistical inference.

Dupont (1983) and

Dupont (1986) provide two examples of how classical inference can lead to unsatisfactory conclusions.

Bartlett (1937) is the original reference for Bartlett's test of equal standard deviations.

Kruskal and Wallis (1952) is the original reference for the Kruskal–Wallis test.

Wilcoxon (1945) and

Mann and Whitney (1947) are the original references on the Wilcoxon–Mann–Whitney rank-sum test.

10.10. Exercises

1 Perform a one-way analysis of variance on the age of entry biopsy in the three different diagnostic groups of women from the Nashville Breast Cohort (see Section 6.19). In question 5 of Chapter 6 you were also asked to compare these ages. If you answered this previous question by performing t tests, what additional information does the analysis of variance provide you that the individual t tests did not?

2 Draw box plots of the age of entry biopsy in the Nashville Breast Cohort subdivided by diagnosis. In view of these plots, is a one-way analysis of variance a reasonable approach to analyzing these data?

3 Perform a Kruskal–Wallis analysis of variance for the age of entry biopsy in these three groups. Contrast your answer to that for question 1.

4 Perform Wilcoxon–Mann–Whitney rank-sum tests of the age of biopsy for each pair of diagnostic groups in the Nashville Breast Cohort. Contrast your answer with that for question 5 of Chapter 6.

11

Repeated-Measures Analysis of Variance

Repeated-measures analysis of variance is concerned with study designs in which the same patient is observed repeatedly over time. In analyzing these data, we must take into consideration the fact that the error components of repeated observations on the same patient are usually correlated. This is a critical difference between repeated-measures and fixed-effects designs. In a repeated-measures experiment, the fundamental unit of observation is the patient. We seek to make inferences about members of a target population who are treated in the same way as our study subjects. Using a fixed-effects method of analysis on repeated-measures data can lead to wildly exaggerated levels of statistical significance since we have many more observations than patients. For this reason, it is essential that studies with repeated-measures designs be always analyzed with methods that account for the repeated measurements on study subjects.

11.1. Example: Effect of Race and Dose of Isoproterenol on Blood Flow

Lang et al. (1995) studied the effect of isoproterenol, a β-adrenergic agonist, on forearm blood flow in a group of 22 normotensive men. Nine of the study subjects were black and 13 were white. Each subject's blood flow was measured at baseline and then at escalating doses of isoproterenol. Figure 11.1 shows the mean blood flow at each dose subdivided by race. The standard deviations of these flows are also shown.

At first glance, the data in Figure 11.1 look very much like that from a fixed-effects two-way analysis of variance in that each blood flow measurement is simultaneously affected by the patient's race and isoproterenol dose. The fixed-effects model, however, provides a poor fit because each patient is observed at each dose. Observations on the same patient are likely to be correlated, and the closer the dose, the higher the correlation is likely to be. In a fixed-effects model, all of the error terms are assumed to be independent. This implies that the probability that a patient's response is greater than the mean value for his race at the specified dose is in no way affected by his

11.1. Example: Effect of race and dose of isoproterenol on blood flow

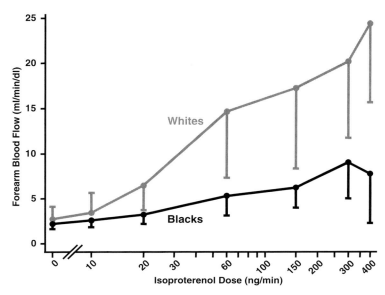

Figure 11.1

Mean rates of forearm blood flow in normotensive white and black men in response to different doses of isoproterenol. The vertical bars indicate the estimated standard deviations within each racial group at each dose (Lang et al., 1995).

response at an earlier dose. In fact, if a patient's response at one dose is well above average, his response at the next is more likely to be above average than below. This invalidates the independence assumption of the fixed-effects model. It is important to obtain an intuitive feel for the correlation structure of data from individual patients. One way to do this is shown in Figure 11.2. In this figure, straight lines connect observations from the same patient. Note, that these lines usually do not cross, indicating a high degree of correlation between observations from the same patient. Both Figures 11.1 and 11.2 suggest that the response of men to escalating doses of isoproterenol tends to be greater in whites than in blacks.

Graphs like Figure 11.2 can become unintelligible when the number of subjects is large. In this situation, it is best to connect the observations from a representative sub-sample of patients. For example, we might calculate the mean response for each patient. We could then identify those patients with the lowest and highest mean response as well as those patients whose mean response corresponds to the 5th, 10th, 20th, 30th, 40th, 50th, 60th, 70th, 80th, 90th and 95th percentile of the entire sample. Connecting the observations for these 13 patients gives a feel for the degree of correlation of observations from the same subject without overwhelming the graph with interconnecting

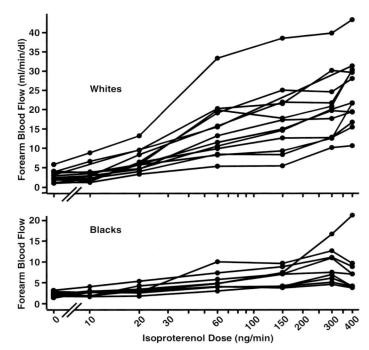

Figure 11.2   Plots of forearm blood flow against isoproterenol dose for white and black men. Straight lines connect observations from the same study subjects. Note that patients who have high, medium or low flows at one dose tend to have high, medium or low flows at other doses, respectively. This indicates that blood flows from the same patient are strongly correlated (Lang et al., 1995).

lines. Diggle et al. (1994) provide an excellent discussion of exploratory methods of graphing repeated measures data.

11.2. Exploratory Analysis of Repeated Measures Data using Stata

The following log file and comments illustrates how to produce graphs similar to Figures 11.1 and 11.2. It also reformats the data from one record per patient to one record per observation. This latter format will facilitate the analysis of these data.

```
. * 11.2.Isoproterenol.log
. *
. * Plot mean forearm blood flow by race and log dose of isoproterenol
. * using the data of Lang et al. (1995). Show standard deviation for
. * each race at each drug level.
```

```
. *
. use C:\WDDtext\11.2.Isoproterenol.dta, clear
. table race, row                                                    {1}

--------------------
    Race |     Freq.
---------+----------
   White |        13
   Black |         9
         |
   Total |        22
--------------------

. list if id == 1 id == 22                                           {2}

        id     race    fbf0    fbf10    fbf20    fbf60    fbf150    fbf300    fbf400
 1.      1    White       1      1.4      6.4     19.1        25      24.6        28
22.     22    Black     2.1      1.9        3      4.8       7.4      16.7      21.2

. generate baseline = fbf0                                           {3}

. *
. * Convert data from one record per patient to one record per observation.
. *
. reshape long fbf,  i(id) j(dose)                                   {4}
(note: j = 0 10 20 60 150 300 400)

Data                               wide    ->     long
-------------------------------------------------------------
Number of obs.                       22    ->      154
Number of variables                  10    ->        5
j variable (7 values)                       ->     dose
xij variables:
                      fbf0 fbf10 ... fbf400    ->     fbf
-------------------------------------------------------------

. list if id == 1 | id == 22                                         {5}

        id    dose     race     fbf    baseline
 1.      1       0    White       1           1
 2.      1      10    White     1.4           1
 3.      1      20    White     6.4           1
 4.      1      60    White    19.1           1
 5.      1     150    White      25           1
 6.      1     300    White    24.6           1
```

```
  7.     1     400     White      28              1
148.    22       0     Black     2.1            2.1
149.    22      10     Black     1.9            2.1
150.    22      20     Black       3            2.1
151.    22      60     Black     4.8            2.1
152.    22     150     Black     7.4            2.1
153.    22     300     Black    16.7            2.1
154.    22     400     Black    21.2            2.1
```

```
. generate delta_fbf = fbf - baseline
(4 missing values generated)

. label variable delta_fbf "Change in Forearm Blood Flow"

. label variable dose "Isoproterenol Dose (ng/min)"

. generate plotdose = dose

. replace plotdose = 6 if dose == 0                                          {6}
(22 real changes made)

. label variable plotdose "Isoproterenol Dose (ng/min)"

. generate logdose = log(dose)
(22 missing values generated)

. label variable logdose "Log Isoproterenol Dose"

. *
. * Save long format of data for subsequent analyses
. *
. save C:\WDDtext\11.2.Long.Isoproterenol.dta, replace
file C:\WDDtext\11.2.Long.Isoproterenol.dta saved
. *
. * Generate Figure 11.1
. *
. collapse (mean) fbfbar = fbf (sd) sd = fbf, by(race plotdose)             {7}

. generate blackfbf = .
(14 missing values generated)

. generate whitefbf = .
(14 missing values generated)

. generate whitesd = .
(14 missing values generated)

. generate blacksd = .
(14 missing values generated)
```

```
. replace whitefbf = fbfbar if race == 1                                    {8}
(7 real changes made)

. replace blackfbf = fbfbar if race == 2
(7 real changes made)

. replace blacksd = sd if race == 2
(7 real changes made)

. replace whitesd = sd if race == 1
(7 real changes made)

. label variable whitefbf "Forearm Blood Flow (ml/min/dl)"

. label variable blackfbf "Forearm Blood Flow (ml/min/dl)"

. generate wsdbar = whitefbf - whitesd                                      {9}
(7 missing values generated)

. generate bsdbar = blackfbf - blacksd
(7 missing values generated)

. replace wsdbar = whitefbf + whitesd if plotdose < 20                      {10}
(2 real changes made)

. graph whitefbf blackfbf wsdbar whitefbf bsdbar blackfbf plotdose, xlog    {11}
> xlabel(10,20,60,100,150,200,300,400) xtick(6,30,40,50,70,80,90,250,300,350)
> ylabel(0 5 10 15 20 25) c(llIIII) s(OOiiii) lltitle(Forearm Blood Flow)
> (ml/min/dl)) gap(3)
```
                                            {Graph omitted. See Figure 11.1}

```
. *
. * Plot individual responses for white and black patients
. *
. use C:\WDDtext\11.2.Long.Isoproterenol.dta, clear                         {12}
. sort id plotdose

. *
. * Plot responses for white patients.
. *
. graph fbf plotdose if race==1, xlog xlabel(10,20,30,60,100,150,200,300,400)
> xtick(6,30,40,50,70,80,90,250,300,350) ylabel(0 5 to 40) connect(L)       {13}
> symbol(O) lltitle(Forearm Blood Flow (ml/min/dl)) gap (3)
```
                                    {Graph ommitted. See upper panel of Figure 11.2}

```
. *
. * Plot responses for black patients.
. *
. graph fbf plotdose if race==2, xlog xlabel(10,20,30,60,100,150,200,300,400)
```

```
> xtick(6,30,40,50,70,80,90,250,300,350) ylabel(0 5 to 40) connect(L)
> symbol(O) l1title(Forearm Blood Flow (ml/min/dl)) gap(3)
```
                        {Graph ommitted. See lower panel of Figure 11.2}

Comments

1 *11.2.Isoproterenol.dta* contains one record per patient. Lang et al. (1995) studied 13 white subjects and nine black subjects.

2 We list the variables in the first and last record of this file. In addition to race and patient identification number there are seven variables recording the patient's forearm blood flow at different doses: *fbf0* records the baseline blood-flow, *fbf10* the blood flow at 10 ng/min, *fbf20* the blood flow at 20 ng/min, et cetera.

3 We set baseline equal to *fbf0* for use in subsequent calculations.

4 The *reshape long* command converts data from one record per patient to one record per observation. In this command, *i(id)* specifies that the *id* variable identifies observations from the same subject. The variable *fbf* is the first three letters of variables *fbf0, fbf10, ... , fbf400*; *j(dose)* defines *dose* to be a new variable whose values are the trailing digits in the names of the variables *fbf0, fbf10, ... , fbf400*. That is, *dose* will take the values 0, 10, 20, ... , 300, 400. One record will be created for each value of *fbf0, fbf10, ... , fbf400*. Other variables in the file that are not included in this command (like *race* or *baseline*) are assumed not to vary with *dose* and are replicated in each record for each specific patient.

5 This *list* command shows the effect of the preceding *reshape long* command. There are now seven records that record the data for the patient with *id* = 1; *fbf* records the forearm blood pressure for this patient at the different doses of isoproterenol. Note that the values of *race* and *baseline* remain constant in all records with the same value of *id*.

6 We want to create Figures 11.1 and 11.2 that plot dose on a logarithmic scale. We also want to include the baseline dose of zero on these figures. Since the logarithm of zero is undefined, we create a new variable called *plotdose* that equals *dose* for all values greater than zero and equals 6 when *dose* = 0. We will use a graphics editor to relabel this value zero with a break in the *x*-axis when we create these figures.

7 This *collapse* command compresses the data to a single record for each unique combination of *race* and *dose*. Two new variables called *fbfbar* and *sd* are created. The variable *fbfbar* equals the mean of all values of *fbf* that have identical values of *race* and *plotdose*; *sd* is the standard deviation of these values. Hence, *fbfbar* and *sd* record the mean and standard deviation of the forearm blood flow at each dose within each race.

8 The variable *whitefbf* equals the mean forearm blood flow for white subjects and is missing for black subjects; *blackfbf* is similarly defined for black subjects. The variables *blacksd* and *whitesd* give the standard deviations for black and white subjects, respectively.

9 The distance between *whitefbf* and *wsdbar* equals the standard deviation of the forearm blood flow for white subjects at each dose; *bsdbar* is similarly defined for black patients.

10 In Figure 11.1 we will draw bars indicating standard deviations, which will hang from the associated mean forearm blood flows. This works well except for the baseline and 10 ng doses, where the mean values for blacks and whites are very close. To avoid collisions between the standard deviation bars for the two races, we will draw the white standard deviations extending above the means for these two doses. This *replace* command accomplishes this task.

11 The *xlog* option of the *graph* command causes the *x*-axis to be drawn on a logarithmic scale. This *graph* command creates a graph that is similar to Figure 11.1. In this figure I used a graphic editor to relabel the baseline dose 0, break the *x*-axis between 0 and 10, write the *x*-axis labels at a slant for increased legibility, and label the two curves *White* and *Black*.

12 We restore the long form of the data set. Note that this data set was destroyed in memory by the preceding *collapse* command.

13 The *connect(L)* option specifies that straight lines are to connect consecutive points as long as the values of the *x*-variable, *plotdose*, are increasing. Otherwise the points are not connected. Note that in the preceding command we sorted the data set by *id* and *plotdose*. This has the effect of grouping all observations on the same patient together and of ordering the values on each patient by increasing values of *plotdose*. Hence, *connect(L)* will connect the values for each patient but will not connected the last value of one patient with the first value of the next. The result is the upper panel of Figure 11.2.

11.3. Response Feature Analysis

The simplest approach to analyzing repeated measures data is a **response feature analysis**. The basic idea is to reduce the multiple responses on each patient to a single biologically meaningful response that captures the patient attribute of greatest interest. This response measure is then analyzed in a fixed-effects one-way analysis of variance. Examples of a response feature that may be useful are an area under the curve or a regression slope derived from the observations on an individual patient. The great advantage of this approach is that since we analyze a single value per patient we do not need to worry about the correlation structure on the multiple observations on each patient. We do need to assume that the observations on separate patients are independent, but this is usually reasonable. Another advantage is its simplicity. It is easy for non-statisticians to understand a response feature analysis. More complex analyses may appear to your colleagues as a black box from which P values and confidence intervals magically arise. Also, more complex methods can be misleading if they are based on models that fit the data poorly. Another advantage of this method is that it can handle situations where some patients have missing values on some observations. The disadvantage of the response feature analysis is that we may lose some power by ignoring information that is available in the correlation structure of observations from individual patients.

11.4. Example: The Isoproterenol Data Set

Figure 11.2 suggests that there is a linear relationship between forearm blood flow and the log dose of isoproterenol in both blacks and whites. The hypothesis of greatest interest in this data set is whether whites are, in general, more responsive to increasing doses of isoproterenol than blacks. There is a small degree of variation in the baseline blood flow levels and the average baseline blood flow is slightly larger in whites than blacks (see Figure 11.1). In order to keep these facts from complicating the interpretation of our analysis, we will use as our dependent variable the change in blood flow from baseline for each patient. Figure 11.3 shows a scatter plot of the responses for the first patient ($id = 1$) together with the linear regression line for change in blood flow against log dose of isoproterenol. As can be seen from this figure, this model provides an excellent fit for this patient. The quality of the model fit for the other patients is similar. The estimate of the regression slope parameter for this patient is 7.18. We calculate the corresponding slope estimates for all the other patients in this experiment. These slopes are shown as vertical lines for black and white subjects in Figure 11.4. Box plots for black and white patients are also shown. The difference in response of blacks and whites is quite marked. There are only two black subjects whose slopes are greater than the lowest slope for a white patient. There are outliers in both the black and white subject groups. For this reason we will analyze these slopes using the Wilcoxon–Mann–Whitney rank-sum test. (Had there been three or more racial groups we would have used a one-way analysis of variance or a Kruskal–Wallis test.) The Wilcoxon–Mann–Whitney test gives a P value of 0.0006. Hence, it is clear that the markedly stronger response of whites to increasing doses of isoproterenol can not be explained by chance.

11.4. Example: The isoproterenol data set

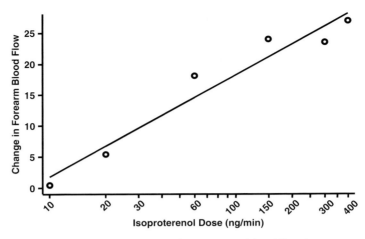

Figure 11.3   Scatter plot of change from baseline forearm blood flow in response to escalating isoproterenol dose for a single patient (*id* = 1). Note that dose is plotted on a logarithmic scale. The linear regression line of change in blood flow against log dose is also plotted and fits these data well. The slope of this regression line for this patient is 7.18. We calculate a similar slope for every patient in the study. These slopes are plotted in Figure 11.4.

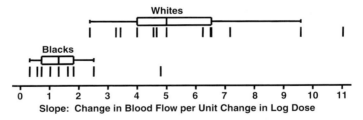

Figure 11.4   Box plots of the individual regresson slopes in white and black patients treated with escalating doses of isoproterenol by Lang et al. (1995). Each vertical bar represents the regression slope of change in forearm blood flow against log dose of isoproterenol for an individual subject. These slopes were analyzed using the Wilcoxon–Mann–Whitney rank-sum test, which showed that slopes for white study subjects were significantly higher than those for black study subjects ($P = 0.0006$).

Of course, one needs to be very cautious about inferring that this difference in response between blacks and whites is of genetic origin. This is because genetic and environmental factors are highly confounded in our society. Hence, it is possible that race may be a marker of some environmental difference that explains these results. Interested readers can find additional research on this topic in papers by Xie et al. (1999 and 2000).

Our response feature analysis establishes that there is a significant difference in the response of blacks and whites to increasing doses of isoproterenol.

Table 11.1. Effect of race and dose of isoproterenol on change from baseline in forearm blood flow (Lang et al., 1995). Comparisons between black and white men at each dose were made using *t* tests with unequal variances. A response feature analysis was used to demonstrate a significant difference in the response of blacks and whites to escalating doses of isoproterenol (see Section 11.4).

	Dose of isoproterenol (ng/min)					
	10	20	60	150	300	400
White subjects						
Mean change from baseline	0.734	3.78	11.9	14.6	17.5	21.7
Standard error	0.309	0.601	1.77	2.32	2.13	2.16
95% confidence interval	0.054 to 1.4	2.5 to 5.1	8.1 to 16	9.5 to 20	13 to 22	17 to 26
Black subjects						
Mean change from baseline	0.397	1.03	3.12	4.05	6.88	5.59
Standard error	0.207	0.313	0.607	0.651	1.30	1.80
95% confidence interval	−0.081 to 0.87	0.31 to 1.8	1.7 to 4.5	2.6 to 5.6	3.9 to 9.9	1.4 to 9.7
Mean difference						
White − black	0.338	2.75	8.82	10.5	10.6	16.1
95% confidence interval	−0.44 to 1.1	1.3 to 4.2	4.8 to 13	5.3 to 16	5.4 to 16	10 to 22
P value	0.38	0.0009	0.0003	0.0008	0.0005	<0.0001

This justifies determining which doses induce a significant effect using the same logic as in Fisher's protected LSD procedure (see Section 10.2). Table 11.1 shows the results of these sub-analyses. The differences in change from baseline between blacks and whites at each dose in this table are assessed using independent *t* tests. The standard errors for blacks tend to be lower than for whites and Bartlett's test for equal variances is significant at doses 20, 60, and 150. For this reason, we use Satterthwaite's *t* test, which assumes unequal variances (see Section 1.4.13). Equations (1.9) and (1.11) are used to derive the *P* values and confidence intervals, respectively, for the differences in change from baseline given in Table 11.1. This table provides convincing evidence that the response to treatment is greater for whites than blacks at all doses greater than or equal to 20 ng/min.

11.5. Response Feature Analysis using Stata

The following log file and comments illustrate how to perform the response feature analysis described in the preceding section.

```
. * 11.5.Isoproterenol.log
. *
```

```
. * Perform a response feature analysis of the effect of race and dose of
. * isoproterenol on blood flow using the data of Lang et al. (1995). For
. * each patient, we will perform separate linear regressions of change in
. * blood flow against log dose of isoproterenol. The response feature that
. * we will use is the slope of each individual regression curve.
. *
. use C:\WDDtext\11.2.Long.Isoproterenol.dta, clear

. *
. * Calculate the regression slope for the first patient
. *
. regress delta_fbf logdose if id == 1                                    {1}

      Source |       SS       df       MS              Number of obs =       6
-------------+------------------------------           F(  1,     4) =   71.86
       Model |  570.114431     1   570.114431          Prob > F      =  0.0011
    Residual |  31.7339077     4   7.93347694          R-squared     =  0.9473
-------------+------------------------------           Adj R-squared =  0.9341
       Total |  601.848339     5   120.369668          Root MSE      =  2.8166

------------------------------------------------------------------------------
    delta_fbf |     Coef.   Std. Err.      t    P>|t|    [95% Conf. Interval]
-------------+----------------------------------------------------------------
     logdose |   7.181315   .8471392     8.48   0.001     4.82928    9.533351
       _cons |  -14.82031   3.860099    -3.84   0.018    -25.53767   -4.10296
------------------------------------------------------------------------------

. predict yhat
(option xb assumed; fitted values)
(22 missing values generated)

. graph delta_fbf yhat dose if dose ~= 0 & id == 1,s(Oi) c(.l) xlog         {2}
> xlabel(10,20,30,60,100,150,200,300,400) xtick(30,40,50,70,80,90,250,300,350)
> ylabel(0 5 to 25) gap(3)
```

{Graph omitted. See Figure 11.3}

```
. *
. * Calculate some intra-patient statistics
. *
. sort id

. by id: egen ldmean = mean(logdose)                                       {3}

. by id: egen delta_fbfmean = mean(delta_fbf)                              {4}

. by id: egen ldsd = sd(logdose)                                           {5}

. by id: egen delta_fbfsd = sd(delta_fbf)                                  {6}
```

```
. by id: egen n = count(delta_fbf*logdose)                              {7}

. generate cross = (delta_fbf - delta_fbfmean)*(logdose - ldmean)/(n - 1)   {8}
(26 missing values generated)

. *
. * cov is the within-patient covariance
. *
. by id: egen cov = sum(cross)                                          {9}

. *
. * r is the within patient correlation coefficient
. *
. generate r = cov/(ldsd*delta_fbfsd)                                   {10}

. *
. * Calculate slope coefficient for each patient
. *
. generate slope = r*delta_fbfsd/ldsd                                   {11}

. *
. * Reduce the data set to the last record for each patient.
. *
. by id: keep if _n == _N                                               {12}
(132 observations deleted)

. list id slope race                                                    {13}

          id      slope    race
  1.       1    7.181315   White
  2.       2    6.539237   White
  3.       3    3.999704   White
  4.       4    4.665485   White
  5.       5    4.557809   White
  6.       6    6.252436   White
  7.       7    2.385183   White
  8.       8   11.03753    White
  9.       9    9.590916   White
 10.      10    6.515281   White
 11.      11    3.280572   White
 12.      12    3.434072   White
 13.      13    5.004545   White
 14.      14    .5887727   Black
 15.      15    1.828892   Black
```

```
16.      16    .3241574    Black
17.      17    1.31807     Black
18.      18    1.630882    Black
19.      19    .7392464    Black
20.      20    2.513615    Black
21.      21    1.031773    Black
22.      22    4.805953    Black
```

```
. set textsize 120
```

```
. graph slope, by(race) oneway box                                        {14}
```
                                              {Graph omitted. See Figure 11.4}

```
. *
. * Do ranksum test on slopes.
. *
. ranksum slope, by(race)                                                  {15}
```

```
Two-sample Wilcoxon rank-sum (Mann-Whitney) test
         race |    obs    rank sum    expected
--------------+---------------------------------
        White |     13         201       149.5
        Black |      9          52       103.5
--------------+---------------------------------
     combined |     22         253         253

unadjusted variance         224.25
adjustment for ties          -0.00
                         ----------
adjusted variance           224.25
```

Ho: slope(race==White) = slope(race==Black)
          z = 3.439
   Prob > |z| = 0.0006

```
. *
. * Do t tests comparing change in blood flow in blacks and whites at
. * different doses
. *
. use C:\WDDtext\11.2.Long.Isoproterenol.dta, clear                        {16}
```

```
. sort dose
```

```
. drop if dose == 0
(22 observations deleted)
```

```
. by dose: ttest delta_fbf, by(race) unequal                              {17}
```

```
-> dose = 10
Two-sample t test with unequal variances
------------------------------------------------------------------------------
    Group |    Obs      Mean    Std. Err.   Std. Dev.   [95% Conf. Interval]
----------+-------------------------------------------------------------------
    White |     12   .7341667   .3088259   1.069804    .0544455    1.413888
    Black |      9   .3966667   .2071634   .6214902   -.081053     .8743863
----------+-------------------------------------------------------------------
 combined |     21   .5895238   .1967903   .9018064    .1790265    1.000021
----------+-------------------------------------------------------------------
     diff |             .3375   .3718737              -.4434982    1.118498
------------------------------------------------------------------------------
Satterthwaite's degrees of freedom:  18.0903
               Ho: mean(White) - mean(Black) = diff = 0

   Ha: diff < 0              Ha: diff ~= 0              Ha: diff > 0
      t =    0.9076              t =    0.9076              t =    0.9076
    P < t =  0.8120        P > |t|  =    0.3760        P > t =    0.1880
```

```
-> dose = 20

Two-sample t test with unequal variances
------------------------------------------------------------------------------
    Group |    Obs      Mean    Std. Err.   Std. Dev.   [95% Conf. Interval]
----------+-------------------------------------------------------------------
    White |     12   3.775833   .6011875   2.082575    2.452628    5.099038
    Black |      9       1.03   .3130229   .9390686    .308168     1.751832
----------+-------------------------------------------------------------------
 combined |     21   2.599048   .4719216   2.162616    1.614636    3.583459
----------+-------------------------------------------------------------------
     diff |          2.745833   .6777977               1.309989    4.181677

------------------------------------------------------------------------------
Satterthwaite's degrees of freedom: 16.1415
               Ho: mean(White) - mean(Black) = diff = 0

   Ha: diff < 0              Ha: diff ~= 0              Ha: diff > 0
      t =    4.0511              t =    4.0511              t =    4.0511
    P < t =  0.9995        P > |t|  =    0.0009        P > t =    0.0005
```
{Output omitted. See Table 11.1}

```
-> dose = 400
Two-sample t test with unequal variances
```

Group	Obs	Mean	Std. Err.	Std. Dev.	[95% Conf. Interval]	
White	13	21.69308	2.163637	7.801104	16.97892	26.40724
Black	9	5.586667	1.80355	5.410649	1.427673	9.74566
combined	22	15.10409	2.252517	10.56524	10.41972	19.78846
diff		16.10641	2.816756		10.2306	21.98222

```
Satterthwaite's degrees of freedom: 19.9917
                    Ho: mean(White) - mean(Black) = diff = 0
       Ha: diff < 0                Ha: diff ~= 0                Ha: diff > 0
       t =    5.7181              t =     5.7181              t =    5.7181
     P < t =    1.0000          P > |t| =    0.0000          P > t =    0.0000
```

Comments

1 We regress change in blood flow against log dose of isoproterenol for the observations from the first patient. Note that *logdose* is missing when *dose* = 0. Hence, only the six positive doses are included in this analysis. The regression slope for this patient is 7.18. We could obtain the slopes for all 22 patients with the command

```
by id: regress delta_fbf logdose
```

However, this would require extracting the slope estimates by hand and re-entering them into Stata. This is somewhat tedious to do and is prone to transcription error. Alternatively, we can calculate these slopes explicitly for each patient using equation (2.6), which we will do below.

2 This graph shows the regression line and individual data points for the first patient. It is similar to Figure 11.3.

3 The command *egen xbar = mean(x)* creates a new variable *xbar* that equals the mean of *x* over the entire data set. When preceded with the *by z:* prefix, this command calculates separate means of *x* from subsamples of the data that have identical values of *z*. Hence, this command calculates *ldmean* to equal the mean log dose of isoproterenol for the ith subject. Missing values are excluded from this mean. In the calculations given below we will denote this mean $\bar{x}$. The individual values of *logdose* for the ith patient will be denoted x_j.

In this example, *ldmean* is constant for all patients except patient 8 who has missing blood flow values at several doses.

4 This command calculates *delta_fbfmean* to equal the mean change in forearm blood flow for the ith subject. We will denote this value $\bar{y}$. The individual values of *delta_fbf* for the ith patient will be denoted y_j.

5 This command calculates *ldsd* to equal the estimated standard deviation of *logdose* for the ith patient, which we denote s_x.

6 The variable *delta_fbfsd* equals the standard deviation of *delta_fbf* for the ith patient, which we denote s_y.

7 This command defines n to be the number of non-missing values of *delta_fbf*logdose* for the ith patient; *delta_fbf*logdose* is missing if either *delta_fbf* or *logdose* is missing.

8 This generate command calculates *cross* to equal $(y_j - \bar{y})(x_j - \bar{x})/(n-1)$.

9 This *egen* command calculates *cov* to equal the sum of *cross* over all records with identical values of *id*. In other words, *cov* is the sample covariance of *delta_fbf* with *logdose* for the ith patient, which was defined in equation (2.1) to be $s_{xy} = \sum (y_j - \bar{y})(x_j - \bar{x})/(n-1)$.

10 The variable $r = s_{xy}/(s_x s_y)$ is the sample correlation coefficient for the ith patient (see equation (2.2)).

11 The variable $slope = b = rs_y/s_x$ is the slope estimate of the regression line for the ith patient (see equation (2.6)).

12 We still have one record per observation sorted by *id*. When used with the *by id:* prefix, the system constant _*N* equals the number of records with the current value of *id*; _*n* is set to 1 for the first record with a new value of *id* and is incremented by 1 for each succeeding record with the same *id* value. Hence, this *keep* command deletes all but the last record corresponding to each patient. (Note that *slope* is constant for all records corresponding to the same patient. Thus, it does not matter which of the available records we keep for each patient.)

13 We list the individual slope estimates for each patient. Note that the highlighted slope estimate for the first patient is identical to the estimate obtained earlier with the *regress* command.

14 This graph, which is similar to Figure 11.4, highlights the difference in the distribution of slope estimates between blacks and whites.

15 This *ranksum* command performs a Wilcoxon–Mann–Whitney rank sum test of the null hypothesis that the distribution of slopes is the same for both races. The test is highly significant, giving a P value of 0.0006.

16 The preceding *keep* command deleted most of the data. We must read in the data set before performing *t* tests at the different doses.

17 This *ttest* command performs independent *t* tests of *delta_fbf* in blacks and whites at each dose of isoproterenol. The output for doses 60, 150 and 300 have been omitted. The highlighted output from this command is also given in Table 11.1.

11.6. The Area-Under-the-Curve Response Feature

A response feature that is often useful in response feature analysis is the **area under the curve**. Suppose that $y_i(t)$ is the response from the ith patient at time t. Suppose further that we measure this response at times $t_1, t_2, \ldots, t_n$, and that $y_{ij} = y_i(t_j)$, for $j = 1, 2, \ldots, n$. We can estimate the area under the curve $y_i(t)$ between t_1 and t_n as follows. Draw a scatterplot of y_{ij} against t_j for $j = 1, 2, \ldots, n$. Then, draw straight lines connecting the points (t_1, y_{i1}), $(t_2, y_{i2}), \ldots, (t_n, y_{in})$. We estimate the area under the curve to be the area under these lines. Specifically, the area under the line from (t_j, y_{ij}) to $(t_{j+1}, y_{i, j+1})$ is

$$\left(\frac{y_{ij} + y_{i, j+1}}{2} \right) (t_{j+1} - t_j).$$

Hence, the area under the entire curve is estimated by

$$\sum_{j=1}^{n-1} \left(\frac{y_{ij} + y_{i, j+1}}{2} \right) (t_{j+1} - t_j). \tag{11.1}$$

For example, if $n = 3$, $t_1 = 0$, $t_2 = 1$, $t_3 = 3$, $y_{i1} = 4$, $y_{i2} = 8$ and $y_{i3} = 6$ then equation (11.1) reduces to

$$\left(\frac{4 + 8}{2} \right) (1 - 0) + \left(\frac{8 + 6}{2} \right) (3 - 1) = 20.$$

In a response feature analysis based on area under the curve, we use equation (11.1) to calculate this area for each patient and then perform a one-way analysis of variance on these areas.

Equation (11.1) can be implemented in Stata as follows. Suppose that a Stata data set with repeated-measures data has one record per observation. Let the variables *id*, *time*, and *response* indicate the patient's identification number, time of observation, and response, respectively. Then the area under the response curve for study subjects can be calculated by using the following Stata code:

```
sort id time
*
* Delete records with missing values for time or response
*
drop if time == .| response  == .
generate area=(response+response[_n+1])*(time[_n+1]-time)/2 if id==id[_n+1]
collapse (sum) area = area, by(id)
*
* The variable 'area' is now the area under the curve for each patient
* defined by equation (11.1). The data file contains one record per
* patient.
*
```

11.7. Generalized Estimating Equations

There are a number of excellent methods for analyzing repeated measures data. One of these is **generalized estimating equations (GEE)** analysis. This approach extends the generalized linear model so that it can handle repeated measures data (Zeger and Liang, 1986). Suppose that we observe an unbiased sample of n patients from some target population and that the ith patient is observed on n_i separate occasions. Let y_{ij} be the response of the ith patient at her j^{th} observation and let $x_{ij1}, x_{ij2}, \ldots, x_{ijq}$ be q covariates that are measured on her at this time. Let $\mathbf{x}_{ij} = (x_{ij1}, x_{ij2}, \ldots, x_{ijq})$ denote the values of all of the covariates for the ith patient at her j^{th} observation. Then the model used by GEE analysis assumes that:

(i) The distribution of y_{ij} belongs to the exponential family of distributions. This is a large family that includes the normal, binomial, and Poisson distributions; y_{ij} is called the random component of the model.

(ii) The expected value of y_{ij} given the patient's covariates $x_{ij1}, x_{ij2}, \ldots,$ x_{ijq} is related to the model parameters through an equation of the form

$$g[E[y_{ij} \mid \mathbf{x}_{ij}]] = \alpha + \beta_1 x_{ij1} + \beta_2 x_{ij2} + \cdots + \beta_q x_{ijq}. \qquad (11.2)$$

In equation (11.2), $\alpha, \beta_1, \beta_2, \ldots,$ and β_q are unknown parameters and g is a smooth function that is either always increasing or always decreasing over the range of y_{ij}. The function g is the link function for the model; $\alpha + \beta_1 x_{ij1} + \beta_2 x_{ij2} + \cdots + \beta_q x_{ijq}$ is the linear predictor.

(iii) Responses from different patients are mutually independent.

When there is only one observation per patient ($n_i = 1$ for all i), model (11.2) is, in fact, the generalized linear model. In this case, when g is the identity function ($g[y] = y$), and y_{ij} is normally distributed, (11.2) reduces to multiple linear regression; when g is the logit function and y_{ij} has a binomial distribution, (11.2) describes logistic regression; when g is the logarithmic function and y_{ij} has a Poisson distribution, this model becomes Poisson regression. Model (11.2) differs from the generalized linear model in that it does not make any assumptions about how observations on the same patient are correlated.

11.8. Common Correlation Structures

Let ρ_{jk} denote the population correlation coefficient between the jth and k^{th} observations on the same patient. If all patients have n observations, we express the correlation structure for each patient's observations as the following square array of correlation coefficients:

$$
\mathbf{R} = \begin{bmatrix}
1 & \rho_{12} & \rho_{13} & \cdots & \rho_{1n} \\
\rho_{21} & 1 & \rho_{23} & \cdots & \rho_{2n} \\
\rho_{31} & \rho_{32} & 1 & \cdots & \rho_{3n} \\
\vdots & \vdots & \vdots & \ddots & \vdots \\
\rho_{n1} & \rho_{n2} & \rho_{n3} & \cdots & 1
\end{bmatrix}.
\tag{11.3}
$$

$\mathbf{R}$ is called the **correlation matrix** for repeated observations on study subjects. In this matrix, the coefficient in the jth row and k^{th} column is the correlation coefficient between the jth and k^{th} observations. The diagonal elements are always 1 since any observation will be perfectly correlated with itself. Any correlation matrix will be symmetric about the diagonal that runs from upper left to lower right. This is because the correlation between the jth and k^{th} observation equals the correlation between the kth and j^{th} observation.

There are a number of special correlation structures that come up in various models. However, we will only need to mention two of these here. The first is the **unstructured correlation** matrix given by equation (11.3). Although this matrix makes no assumptions about the correlation structure it requires $n(n-1)/2$ correlation parameters. Estimating this large number of parameters may be difficult if the number of observations per patient is large. The second is the **exchangeable correlation** structure, which assumes that

$$
\mathbf{R} = \begin{bmatrix}
1 & \rho & \rho & \cdots & \rho \\
\rho & 1 & \rho & \cdots & \rho \\
\rho & \rho & 1 & \cdots & \rho \\
\vdots & \vdots & \vdots & \ddots & \vdots \\
\rho & \rho & \rho & \cdots & 1
\end{bmatrix}.
\tag{11.4}
$$

In other words, the exchangeable structure assumes that any two distinct observations from the same patient have the same correlation coefficient ρ. Many data sets have much more complicated correlation structures. In particular, observations on a patient taken closer in time are often more correlated than observations taken far apart. Also, the correlation structure is not necessarily the same for all patients. Nevertheless, the exchangeable correlation structure will meet our needs for GEE analysis. This is because a GEE analysis requires only a rough estimate of this structure to get started. Its final parameter estimates are not usually dependent on the accuracy of our initial assumptions about the correlation matrix.

11.9. GEE Analysis and the Huber–White Sandwich Estimator

GEE analysis is computationally and methodologically complex (Diggle et al., 1994). However, the basic idea of the analysis can be summarized as follows:

1 We select a working correlation matrix $\mathbf{R}_i$ for each patient. $\mathbf{R}_i$, the matrix for the ith patient, can be quite complicated, but need not be. An exchangeable correlation structure usually works just fine. From this, we estimate the working variance–covariance matrix for the ith patient. This is a function of both the working correlation matrix and the link function g. For example, if we use an exchangeable correlation structure, the identity link function, and a normal random component then the working variance–covariance matrix specifies that y_{ij} will have variance σ^2 and that the covariance between any two distinct observations on the ith patient will equal $\rho\sigma^2$.

2 Using the working variance–covariance structure we obtain estimates of the model parameters. This is done using a technique called **quasi-likelihood**, which is related to maximum likelihood estimation but does not require the likelihood function to be fully specified.

3 We estimate the variance–covariance matrix of our model parameters using a technique called the **Huber–White sandwich estimator**.

4 We use our parameter estimates and the Huber–White variance–covariance matrix to test hypotheses or construct confidence intervals from relevant weighted sums of the parameter estimates (see Sections 5.14 through 5.16).

What is truly amazing about this technique is that, under mild regularity conditions, the Huber–White variance–covariance estimate converges to the true variance–covariance matrix of the parameter estimates as n gets large.

This is so even when the working correlation matrix is incorrectly specified. Thus, we can specify a very simple working matrix such as the exchangeable correlation matrix for models in which none of the observations obey this structure and the correlation structure may vary for different study subjects. This result holds, however, "... only when there is a diminishing fraction of missing data or when the data are missing completely at random" (Zeger and Liang, 1986). For this reason, it is sometimes prudent to drop patients with missing response values from the analysis.

When there is a large proportion of patients who have at least one missing response value, it may not be reasonable to delete all of these patients from the analysis. In this case, if you include all of the patients in your analysis, then the validity of your choice of working correlation matrix can become important; if the true correlation structure cannot be reasonably modeled by any of the working correlation matrices provided by your statistical software, then GEE may not be the best approach to analyzing your data.

11.10. Example: Analyzing the Isoproterenol Data with GEE

Suppose that in model (11.2), y_{ij} is a normally distributed random component and $g[y] = y$ is the identity link function. Then model (11.2) reduces to

$$E[y_{ij}|\mathbf{x}_{ij}] = \alpha + \beta_1 x_{ij1} + \beta_2 x_{ij2} + \cdots + \beta_q x_{ijq}. \tag{11.5}$$

Model (11.5) is a special case of the GEE model (11.2). We now analyze the blood flow, race and isoproterenol data set of Lang et al. (1995) using this model. Let

y_{ij} be the change from baseline in forearm blood flow for the ith patient at the jth dose of isoproterenol,

$$white_i = \begin{cases} 1: & \text{if the } i^{\text{th}} \text{ patient is white} \\ 0: & \text{if he is black, and} \end{cases}$$

$$dose_{jk} = \begin{cases} 1: & \text{if } j = k \\ 0: & \text{otherwise.} \end{cases}$$

We will assume that y_{ij} is normally distributed and

$$E[y_{ij} \mid white_i, j] = \alpha + \beta \times white_i$$

$$+ \sum_{k=2}^{6} (\gamma_k dose_{jk} + \delta_k \times white_i \times dose_{jk}), \tag{11.6}$$

where $\alpha, \beta, \{\gamma_k, \delta_k : k = 2, \ldots, 6\}$ are the model parameters. Model (11.6) is a special case of model (11.5). Note that this model implies that the expected change in blood flow is

α for a black man on the first dose, $\qquad\qquad\qquad\qquad\qquad$ (11.7)

$\alpha + \beta$ for a white man on the first dose, $\qquad\qquad\qquad\qquad$ (11.8)

$\alpha + \gamma_j$ for a black man on the jth dose with $j > 1$, and $\qquad$ (11.9)

$\alpha + \beta + \gamma_j + \delta_j$ for a white man on the jth dose with $j > 1$. $\quad$ (11.10)

It must be noted that patient 8 in this study has four missing blood flow measurements. This concentration of missing values in one patient causes the choice of the working correlation matrix to have an appreciable effect on our model estimates. Regardless of the working correlation matrix, the working variance for y_{ij} in model (11.5) is constant. Figure 11.2 suggests that this variance is greater for whites than blacks and increases with increasing dose. Hence, it is troubling to have our parameter estimates affected by a working correlation matrix that we know is wrong. Also, the Huber–White variance–covariance estimate is only valid when the missing values are few and randomly distributed. For these reasons, we delete patient 8 from our analysis. This results in parameter estimates and a Huber–White variance–covariance estimate that are unaffected by our choice of the working correlation matrix.

Let $\hat{\alpha}, \hat{\beta}, \{\hat{\gamma}_k, \hat{\delta}_k : k = 2, \ldots, 6\}$ denote the GEE parameter estimates from the model. Then our estimates of the mean change in blood flow in blacks and whites at the different doses are given by equations (11.7) through (11.10) with the parameter estimates substituting for the true parameter values. Subtracting the estimate of equation (11.7) from that for equation (11.8) gives the estimated mean difference in change in flow between whites and blacks at dose 1, which is

$$(\hat{\alpha} + \hat{\beta}) - \hat{\alpha} = \hat{\beta}. \qquad\qquad\qquad\qquad\qquad (11.11)$$

Subtracting the estimate of equation (11.9) from that for equation (11.10) gives the estimated mean difference in change in flow between whites and blacks at dose $j > 1$, which is

$$(\hat{\alpha} + \hat{\beta} + \hat{\gamma}_j + \hat{\delta}_j) - (\hat{\alpha} + \hat{\gamma}_j) = (\hat{\beta} + \hat{\delta}_j). \qquad\qquad (11.12)$$

Tests of significance and 95% confidence intervals can be calculated for these estimates using the Huber–White variance–covariance matrix. This is done in the same way as was illustrated in Sections 5.14 through 5.16. These estimates, standard errors, confidence intervals and P values are given in Table 11.2.

Table 11.2. Effect of race and dose of isoproterenol on change from baseline in forearm blood flow (Lang et al., 1995). This table was produced using a generalized estimating equation (GEE) analysis. Note that the confidence intervals in this table are slightly narrower than the corresponding intervals in Table 11.1. This GEE analysis is slightly more powerful than the response feature analysis that produced Table 11.1.

	Dose of isoproterenol (ng/min)					
	10	20	60	150	300	400
White subjects						
Mean change from baseline	0.734	3.78	11.9	14.6	17.5	21.2
Standard error	0.303	0.590	1.88	2.27	2.09	2.23
95% confidence interval	0.14 to 1.3	2.6 to 4.9	8.2 to 16	10 to 19	13 to 22	17 to 26
Black subjects						
Mean change from baseline	0.397	1.03	3.12	4.05	6.88	5.59
Standard error	0.200	0.302	0.586	0.629	1.26	1.74
95% confidence interval	0.0044 to 0.79	0.44 to 1.6	2.0 to 4.3	2.8 to 5.3	4.4 to 9.3	2.2 to 9.0
Mean difference						
White – black	0.338	2.75	8.79	10.5	10.6	15.6
95% confidence interval	−0.37 to 1.0	1.4 to 4.0	4.9 to 13	5.9 to 15	5.9 to 15	10 to 21
P value	0.35	<0.0005	<0.0005	<0.0005	<0.0005	<0.0001

Testing the null hypothesis that there is no interaction between race and dose on blood flow is equivalent to testing the null hypothesis that the effects of race and dose on blood flow are additive. In other words, we test the null hypothesis that $\delta_2 = \delta_3 = \delta_4 = \delta_5 = \delta_6 = 0$. Under this null hypothesis a chi-squared statistic can be calculated that has as many degrees of freedom as there are interaction parameters (in this case five). This statistic equals 40.41, which is highly significant ($P < 0.00005$). Hence, we can conclude that the observed interaction is certainly not due to chance.

The GEE and response feature analysis (RFA) in Tables 11.2 and 11.1 should be compared. Note that the mean changes in blood flow in the two races and six dose levels are very similar. They would be identical were if not for the fact that patient 8 is excluded from the GEE analysis but is included in the RFA. This is a challenging data set to analyze in view of the fact that the standard deviation of the response variable increases with dose and differs between the races. The GEE analysis does an excellent job at modeling this variation. Note how the standard errors in Table 11.2 increase from black subjects to white subjects at any dose or from low dose to high dose within either race. Figure 11.5 compares the mean difference between blacks and whites at the six different doses. The white and gray

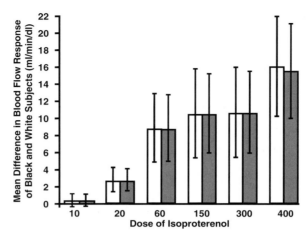

Figure 11.5   This graph shows the mean differences between black and white study subjects given at the botton of Tables 11.1 and 11.2. The white and gray bars are from the response feature analysis (RFA) and generalized estimating equation (GEE) analysis, respectively. The vertical lines give the 95% confidence intervals for these differences. These analyses give very similar results. The GEE analysis is slighly more powerful than the RFA as is indicated by the slightly narrower confidence intervals of the GEE results.

bars are from the RFA and GEE analyses, respectively. Note that these two analyses provide very similar results for these data. The GEE analysis is slightly more powerful than the RFA as is indicated by the slightly narrower confidence intervals for its estimates. This increase in power is achieved at a cost of considerable methodological complexity in the GEE model. The GEE approach constitutes an impressive intellectual achievement and is a valuable tool for advanced statistical analysis. Nevertheless, RFA is a simple and easily understood approach to repeated measures analysis that can, as in this example, approach the power of a GEE analysis. At the very least, it is worth considering as a crosscheck against more sophisticated multiple regression models for repeated measures data.

11.11. Using Stata to Analyze the Isoproterenol Data Set Using GEE

The following log file and comments illustrate how to perform the GEE analysis from Section 11.10 using Stata.

```
. * 11.11.Isoproterenol.log
. *
. * Perform a GEE analyses of the effect of race and dose of isoproterenol
. * on blood flow using the data of Lang et al. (1995).
. *
. use C:\WDDtext\11.2.Long.Isoproterenol.dta, clear
. drop if dose == 0 | id == 8                                         {1}
(28 observations deleted)
. generate white = race == 1
. *
. * Analyze data using classification variables with interaction
. *
. xi: xtgee delta_fbf i.dose*white, i(id) robust                      {2}
i.dose             _Idose_1-6              (_Idose_1 for dose==10 omitted)
i.dose*white       _IdosXwhite_#           (coded as above)

Iteration 1: tolerance = 2.061e-13

GEE population-averaged model          Number of obs     =      126
Group variable:                    id  Number of groups  =       21
Link:                        identity  Obs per group: min =        6
Family:                      Gaussian                 avg =      6.0
Correlation:             exchangeable                 max =        6
                                       Wald chi2(11)     =   506.86
Scale parameter:          23.50629     Prob > chi2       =   0.0000
                     (standard errors adjusted for clustering on id)
-----------------------------------------------------------------------------
              |              Semi-robust
    delta_fbf |    Coef.    Std. Err.     z    P>|z|    [95% Conf. Interval]
--------------+--------------------------------------------------------------
     _Idose_2 |  .6333333   .2706638    2.34   0.019   .1028421   1.163825
     _Idose_3 |  2.724445   .6585882    4.14   0.000   1.433635   4.015254
     _Idose_4 |  3.656667   .7054437    5.18   0.000   2.274022   5.039311
     _Idose_5 |  6.478889   1.360126    4.76   0.000   3.813091   9.144687
     _Idose_6 |      5.19   1.830717    2.83   0.005   1.601861    8.77814
        white |     .3375    .363115    0.93   0.353  -.3741922   1.049192 {3}
 _IdosXwhit~2 |  2.408333   .5090358    4.73   0.000   1.410642   3.406025
 _IdosXwhit~3 |  8.450556   1.823352    4.63   0.000   4.876852   12.02426
 _IdosXwhit~4 |  10.17667    2.20775    4.61   0.000   5.849557   14.50378
 _IdosXwhit~5 |  10.30444   2.305474    4.47   0.000   5.785798   14.82309
 _IdosXwhit~6 |  15.22667   2.748106    5.54   0.000   9.840479   20.61285
        _cons |  .3966667   .2001388    1.98   0.047   .0044017   .7889316 {4}
-----------------------------------------------------------------------------
```

```
. lincom _cons + white                                                    {5}
( 1) white + _cons = 0.0
------------------------------------------------------------------------------
delta_fbf |     Coef.    Std. Err.      z    P>|z|    [95% Conf. Interval]
----------+-------------------------------------------------------------------
      (1) |   .7341667     .30298     2.42   0.015    .1403367    1.327997
------------------------------------------------------------------------------

. lincom _cons + _Idose_2                                                  {6}
( 1) _Idose_2 + _cons = 0.0
------------------------------------------------------------------------------
delta_fbf |     Coef.    Std. Err.      z    P>|z|    [95% Conf. Interval]
----------+-------------------------------------------------------------------
      (1) |     1.03     .3024088    3.41   0.001    .4372896    1.62271
------------------------------------------------------------------------------

. lincom _cons + _Idose_2 + white + _IdosXwhite_2                          {7}
( 1) _Idose_2 + white + _IdosXwhite_2 + _cons = 0.0
------------------------------------------------------------------------------
delta_fbf |     Coef.    Std. Err.      z    P>|z|    [95% Conf. Interval]
----------+-------------------------------------------------------------------
      (1) |   3.775833    .5898076   6.40   0.000    2.619832    4.931835
------------------------------------------------------------------------------

. lincom                  white + _IdosXwhite_2                            {8}
( 1)  white + _IdosXwhite_2 = 0.0
------------------------------------------------------------------------------
delta_fbf |     Coef.    Std. Err.      z    P>|z|    [95% Conf. Interval]
----------+-------------------------------------------------------------------
      (1) |   2.745833    .6628153   4.14   0.000    1.446739    4.044927
------------------------------------------------------------------------------

. lincom _cons + _Idose_3
                                            {output omitted. See Table 11.2}

. lincom _cons + _Idose_3 + white + _IdosXwhite_3
                                            {output omitted. See Table 11.2}

. lincom                  white + _IdosXwhite_3
                                            {output omitted. See Table 11.2}

. lincom _cons + _Idose_4
                                            {output omitted. See Table 11.2}

. lincom _cons + _Idose_4 + white + _IdosXwhite_4
                                            {output omitted. See Table 11.2}
```

```
. lincom                         white + _IdosXwhite_4
```
{output omitted. See Table 11.2}
```
. lincom _cons + _Idose_5
```
{output omitted. See Table 11.2}
```
. lincom _cons + _Idose_5 + white + _IdosXwhite_5
```
{output omitted. See Table 11.2}
```
. lincom                         white + _IdosXwhite_5
```
{output omitted. See Table 11.2}
```
. lincom _cons + _Idose_6
( 1) _Idose_6 + _cons = 0.0
-----------------------------------------------------------------------
delta_fbf |    Coef.    Std. Err.      z     P>|z|    [95% Conf. Interval]
----------+------------------------------------------------------------
      (1) |  5.586667   1.742395    3.21   0.001    2.171636    9.001698
-----------------------------------------------------------------------
```
```
. lincom _cons + _Idose_6 + white + _IdosXwhite_6
(1) _Idose_6 + white + _IdosXwhite_6 + _cons = 0.0
-----------------------------------------------------------------------
delta_fbf |    Coef.    Std. Err.      z     P>|z|    [95% Conf. Interval]
----------+------------------------------------------------------------
      (1) |  21.15083   2.233954    9.47   0.000    16.77236    25.5293
-----------------------------------------------------------------------
```
```
. lincom                         white + _IdosXwhite_6
(1) white + _IdosXwhite_6 = 0.0
-----------------------------------------------------------------------
delta_fbf |    Coef.    Std. Err.      z     P>|z|    [95% Conf. Interval]
----------+------------------------------------------------------------
      (1) |  15.56417   2.833106    5.49   0.000    10.01138    21.11695
-----------------------------------------------------------------------
```
```
. test _IdosXwhite_2 _IdosXwhite_3 _IdosXwhite_4 _IdosXwhite_5 _IdosXwhite_6
```
{9}
```
(1)   _IdosXwhite_2 = 0.0
(2)   _IdosXwhite_3 = 0.0
(3)   _IdosXwhite_4 = 0.0
(4)   _IdosXwhite_5 = 0.0
(5)   _IdosXwhite_6 = 0.0


       chi2( 5) = 40.41
     Prob > chi2 =   0.0000
```

Comments

1 We drop all records with *dose* = 0 or *id* = 8. When *dose* = 0, the change from baseline, *delta_fbf*, is, by definition, zero. We eliminate these records as they provide no useful information to our analyses. Patient 8 has four missing values. These missing values have an adverse effect on our analysis. For this reason we eliminate all observations on this patient (see Sections 11.9 and 11.10).

2 This *xtgee* command analyzes model (11.6). The syntax of *i.dose*white* is analogous to that used for the logistic command in Section 5.23 (see also comment 8 of Section 9.3). The default link function is the identity function. For the identity link function the default random component is the normal distribution. Hence, we do not need to specify either of these aspects of our model explicitly in this command. The *i(id)* option specifies *id* to be the variable that identifies all observations made on the same patient. The exchangeable correlation structure is the default working correlation structure, which we use here. The *robust* option specifies that the Huber–White sandwich estimator is to be used. The table of coefficients generated by this command is similar to that produced by other Stata regression commands.

   Note that if we had not used the *robust* option the model would have assumed that the exchangeable correlation structure was true. This would have led to inaccurate confidence intervals for our estimates. I strongly recommend that this option always be used in any GEE analysis.

3 The highlighted terms are the estimated mean, *P* value and 95% confidence interval for the difference in response between white and black men on the first dose of isoproterenol (10 ng/min). The parameter estimate associated with the *white* covariate is $\hat{\beta} = 0.3375$ in model (11.6). The highlighted values in this and in subsequent lines of output are entered into Table 11.2.

4 The highlighted terms are the estimated mean, standard error and 95% confidence interval for black men on the first dose of isoproterenol. The parameter estimate associated with *_cons* is $\hat{\alpha} = 0.3967$.

5 This command calculates $\hat{\alpha} + \hat{\beta}$, the mean response for white men at the first dose of isoproterenol, together with related statistics.

6 This command calculates $\hat{\alpha} + \hat{\gamma}_2$, the mean response for black men at the second dose of isoproterenol, together with related statistics.

7 This command calculates $\hat{\alpha} + \hat{\beta} + \hat{\gamma}_2 + \hat{\delta}_2$, the mean response for white men at the second dose of isoproterenol, together with related statistics.

8 This command calculates $\hat{\beta} + \hat{\delta}_2$, the mean difference in response between white and black men at the second dose of isoproterenol, together with

related statistics. Analogous *lincom* commands are also given for dose 3, 4, 5, and 6.

9 This command tests the null hypothesis that the interaction parameters $\delta_2, \delta_3, \delta_4, \delta_5,$ and δ_6 are simultaneously equal to zero. That is, it tests the null hypothesis that the effects of race and dose on change in blood flow are additive. This test, which has five degrees of freedom, gives $P < 0.00005$, which allows us to reject the null hypothesis with overwhelming statistical significance.

11.12. GEE Analyses with Logistic or Poisson Models

GEE analyses can be applied to any generalized linear model with repeated measures data. For logistic regression we use the logit link function and a binomial random component. For Poisson regression we use the logarithmic link function and a Poisson random component. In Stata, the syntax for specifying these terms is the same as in the *glm* command. For logistic regression, we use the *link(logit)* and *family(binomial)* options to specify the link function and random component, respectively. For Poisson regression, these options are *link(log)* and *family(poisson)*. Additional discussion on these techniques is given by Diggle et al. (1994).

11.13. Additional Reading

Crowder and Hand (1990) and

Diggle et al. (1994) are excellent texts on repeated measures data analysis. Diggle et al. (1994) is the definitive text on GEE analysis at this time.

Lang et al. (1995) studied the effects of race and dose of isoproterenol on forearm blood flow. We used data from their study to illustrate repeated measures analyses of variance.

Xie et al. (1999) and

Xie et al. (2000) have done additional research on the relationship between blood flow and isoproterenol dose in different races.

Liang and Zeger (1986) and

Zeger and Liang (1986) are the original references on generalized estimating equation analysis.

Huber (1967),

White (1980) and

White (1982) are the original references for the Huber–White sandwich estimator.

11.14. Exercises

1 Create a repeated measures data set in Stata with one record per patient. Calculate the area under the curve for these patients using code similar to that given in Section 11.6. Confirm by hand calculations that your program calculates this area properly. Explain why this code correctly calculates equation (11.1)

2 In the Ibuprofen in Sepsis clinical trial each patient's temperature was measured at baseline, after two and four hours, and then every four hours until 44 hours after entry into the study. Ibuprofen treatment in the intervention group was stopped at 44 hours. Three additional temperatures were recorded at 72, 96 and 120 hours after baseline (see the *11.ex.-Sepsis.dat* data set). Draw exploratory graphs to investigate the relationship between treatment and body temperature in this study.

3 Perform a response feature analysis of body temperature and treatment in the Ibuprofen in Sepsis study. What response feature do you think is most appropriate to use in this analysis?

4 For the response feature chosen in question 3, draw box plots of this statistic for patients in the intervention and control groups. Calculate a 95% confidence interval for the difference in this response feature between patients in the ibuprofen and control groups. Can we conclude that ibuprofen changes the body temperature profile in septic patients?

5 At what times can we conclude that body temperature was reduced in the ibuprofen group compared to controls?

6 Repeat question 7 using a GEE analysis. Do you get similar answers? Note that a sizable fraction of patients had at least one missing temperature reading. How have you dealt with these missing values in your analysis? What are the strengths and weaknesses of these two approaches?

7 Experiment with different working correlation structures in your answer to question 6. Does your choice of working correlation structure affect your answers?

8 Lang et al. (1995) reported impressive physiologic differences in the response of a group of white and black men to escalating doses of isoproterenol. Suppose that you wanted to determine whether these differences were due to genetic or environmental factors. What additional experiments might you wish to perform to try to settle this question? What sort of evidence would you consider to be conclusive that this difference has a genetic etiology?

Appendix: Summary of Stata Commands Used in this Text

The following tables list the Stata commands and command components that are used in this text. A terse indication of the function of each command is also given. See the Stata reference manuals for a complete explanation of these commands. Section numbers show where the command is explained or first illustrated in this text.

Data Manipulation

Command	Function	Section
* comment	Any command that starts with an asteric is ignored.	1.3.2
by varlist: egen newvar = function(expression)	Define newvar to equal some function of expression within groups defined by varlist. Acceptable functions include count, mean, sd, and sum.	11.5
codebook varlist	Describe variables in the spreadsheet editor (memory).	1.4.11
collapse (mean) newvar = varname, by(varlist)	Make dataset with one record for each distinct combination of values in varlist; newvar equals the mean of all values of varname in records with identical values of the variables in varlist.	11.2
collapse (sd) newvar = varname, by(varlist)	This command is similar to the preceding one except that now newvar equals the standard deviation of varname in records with identical values of the variables in varlist.	11.2
collapse (sum) newvar = varname, by(varlist)	This command is similar to the preceding one except that now newvar equals the sum of values of varname.	5.29
describe varlist	Summarize variables in memory (see also codebook).	1.3.2
drop varlist	Drop variables in varlist from memory.	3.21
drop if expression	Drop observations from memory where expression is true.	3.17.1

Data Manipulation (*cont.*)

Command	Function	Section
edit	Edit data in memory.	1.3.2
egen *newvar* = count(*expression*)	Define *newvar* to equal the number of records with non-missing values of *expression*.	11.5
egen *newvar* = mean(*expression*)	Define *newvar* to equal the mean value of *expression*.	11.5
egen *newvar* = sd(*expression*)	Define *newvar* to equal the standard deviation of *expression*.	11.5
egen *newvar* = sum(*expression*)	Define *newvar* to equal the sum of *expression*.	11.5
expand *expression*	Add max[*expression* − 1, 0] duplicate observations for each current observation.	7.11
format *varlist* %*fmt*	Assign the %*fmt* display format to the variables in *varlist*.	2.12
generate *newvar* = *expression*	Define a new variable equal to *expression*.	1.4.14
keep *varlist*	Keep *varlist* variables in memory. Drop all others.	1.4.11
keep if *expression*	Keep only observations where *expression* is true.	1.3.11
label define *lblname* # "*label*" # "*label*" … # "*label*"	Define the label *lblname*.	4.21
label values *varname* *lblname*	Assign a value label *lblname* to a variable *varname*.	4.21
label variable *varname* "*label*"	Assign a label to the variable *varname*.	2.18
log close	Close log file.	1.3.6
log using \ *foldername*\ *filename*	Open a log file called *filename* in the *foldername* folder.	1.3.6
recode *varname* 1 3 = 10 5/7 = 11 * = 12	Recode *varname* values 1 and 3 as 10, 5 through 7 as 11 and all other values as 12.	5.20
rename *oldvar* *newvar*	Change the name of the variable *oldvar* to *newvar*.	4.21
replace *oldvar* = *expression1* if *expression2*	Redefine an old variable if *expression2* is true.	3.16
reshape long *varlist*, i(*idvar*) j(*subvar*)	Convert data from wide to long format; *idvar* identifies observations on the same patient; *subvar* identifies sub-observations on each patient.	11.2
save *filename*, replace	Store memory data set in a file called *filename*. Overwrite any existing file with the same name.	4.21
set memory #	Set memory size to # kilobytes.	7.7
set textsize #	Set text to #% of normal on graphs.	3.11.1
sort *varlist*	Sort data records in ascending order by values in *varlist*.	1.3.6
use "*stata_data_file*", clear	Load new data file, purge old data from memory.	1.3.2

Command Qualifiers (insert before comma)

Qualifier	Function	Section
if *expression*	Apply command to observations where *expression* is true.	1.4.11
in *range*	Apply command to observations in *range*.	1.3.2
in 5/25	Apply command to observations 5 through 25.	1.3.2
in −5/−1	Apply command to 5th from last through last observation.	3.21
[freq = *varname*]	Weight each observation by the value of *varname* by replacing each record with *varname* identical records and doing an unweighted analysis.	4.18, 4.22

Analysis Commands

Command	Function	Section
centile *varlist*, centile(*numlist*)	Produce a table of percentiles specified by *numlist* for the variables in *varlist*.	8.9
cc *var_case var_control*	Calculate simple odds-ratio for a case-control study.	4.22
cc *var_case var_control*, by(*varcon*)	Calculate Mantel–Haenszel odds-ratio adjusted for *varcon*.	5.5
cc *var_case var_control*, woolf	Calculate odds-ratio for case-control study using Woolf's method to derive a confidence interval.	4.22
ci *varlist*	Calculate standard errors and confidence intervals for variables in *varlist*.	10.7
display *expression*	Calculate *expression* and show result.	2.12
dotplot *varname*, by(*groupvar*) center	Draw centered dotplots of *varname* by *groupvar*.	1.3.2
glm *depvar varlist*, family(*familyname*) link(*linkname*)	Generalized linear models.	4.11
glm *depvar varlist*, family(binomial) link(logit)	Logistic regression: Bernoulli dependent variable.	4.11
glm *depvar varlist*, family(binomial *denom*) link(logit)	Logistic regression with *depvar* events in *denom* trials.	4.18
glm *depvar varlist*, family(poisson) link(log) lnoffset(*patientyears*)	Poisson regression with *depvar* events in *patientyears* patient-years of observation.	8.7
glm *depvar varlist*, family(poisson) link(log) lnoffset(*patientyears*) eform	Poisson regression. Exponentiate the regression coefficients in the output table.	8.12

Analysis Commands (*cont.*)

Command	Function	Section
graph *var*, bin(#)	Draw a histogram of *var* with # bars. *y*-axis is proportion of subjects.	1.3.6
graph *var*, bin(#) freq	Draw a histogram of *var* with # bars. *y*-axis is number of subjects.	4.18
graph *var*, box by(*groupvar*)	Draw boxplots of *var* for each distinct value of *groupvar*.	1.3.6
graph *var*, box oneway by(*groupvar*)	Draw horizontal boxplots and one-dimensional scatterplots of *var* for each distinct value of *groupvar*.	10.7
graph *var1 var2*, bar by(*varstrat*)	Grouped bar graph of *var1* and *var2* stratified by *varstrat*.	9.3
graph *y1 y2 x*, connect(.l) symbol(oi)	Draw scatter plot of *y1* vs. *x*. Graph *y2* vs. *x*, connect points, no symbol.	2.12
graph *y x*, connect(l[−#])	Graph *y* vs. *x*. Connect points with a dashed line.	2.20
graph *y x*, connect(L)	Graph *y* vs. *x*. Connect consecutive points with a straight line if the values of *x* are increasing.	11.2
graph *y1 y2 x*, connect(II) symbol(ii)	Draw error bars connecting *y1* to *y2* as a function of *x*.	4.18
graph *y x*, connect(J) symbol(i)	Plot a step function of *y* against *x*.	6.9
graph *y x*, symbol(O)	Scatter plot of *y* vs. *x* using large circles.	2.12
graph *varlist*, matrix label symbol(o) connect(s) band(#)	Plot matrix scatterplot of variables in *varlist*. Estimate regression lines with # median bands and cubic splines.	3.11.1
iri *#a #b #Na #Nb*	Calculate relative risk from incidence data; *#a* and *#b* are the number of exposed and unexposed cases observed during *#Na* and *#Nb* person-years of follow-up.	8.2
ksm *yvar xvar*, lowess bwidth(#) gen(*newvar*)	Plot lowess curve of *yvar* vs. *xvar* with bandwidth #. Save lowess regression line as *newvar*.	2.14
kwallis *var*, by(*groupvar*)	Perform a Kruskal–Wallis test of *var* by *groupvar*.	10.7
list *varlist*	List values of variables in *varlist*.	1.3.2
list *varlist*, nodisplay	List values of variables in *varlist* with tabular format.	5.29
logistic *depvar varlist*	Logistic regression: regress *depvar* against variables in *varlist*.	4.13.1, 5.9
oneway *responsevar factorvar*	One-way analysis of variance of *responsevar* in groups defined by *factorvar*.	10.7

Analysis Commands (*cont.*)

Command	Function	Section
ranksum *var*, by(*groupvar*)	Perform a Wilcoxon–Mann–Whitney rank sum test of *var* by *groupvar*.	10.7
regress *depvar varlist*, level(#)	Regress *depvar* against variables in *varlist*.	2.12, 3.16
stcox *varlist*	Proportional hazard regression analysis with independent variables given by *varlist*. A *stset* statement defines failure. Exponentiated model coefficients are given.	6.16
stcox *varlist1*, strata(*varlist2*)	Stratified proportional hazard regression analysis with strata defined by the values of variables in *varlist2*.	7.8
stcox *varlist*, mgale(*newvar*)	Cox hazard regression analysis. Define *newvar* to be the martingale-residual for each patient.	7.7
stset *timevar*, failure(*failvar*)	Declare *timevar* and *failvar* to be time and failure variables, respectively. *failvar* $\neq 0$ denotes failure.	6.9
stset *exittime*, id(*idvar*) enter(time *entrytime*) failure(*failvar*)	Declare *entrytime*, *exittime* and *failvar* to be the entry time, exit time and failure variables, respectively. id(*idvar*) is a patient identification variable needed for time-dependent hazard regression analysis.	7.9.4 7.11
sts generate *var* = survfcn	Define *var* to equal one of several functions related to survival analyses.	6.9
sts graph, by(*varlist*)	Kaplan–Meier survival plots. Plot a separate curve for each combination of distinct values of the variables in *varlist*. Must be preceded by a *stset* statement.	6.9
sts graph, gwood lost	Kaplan–Meier survival plots showing number of patients censored with 95% confidence bands.	6.9
sts graph, by(*varlist*) failure	Kaplan–Meier cumulative mortality plot.	7.7
sts list, by(*varlist*)	List estimated survival function by patient groups defined by unique combinations of values of *varlist*.	6.9
sts test *varlist*	Perform logrank test on groups defined by the values of *varlist*.	6.9
summarize *varlist*, detail	Summarize variables in *varlist*.	1.3.6
sw regress *depvar varlist*, forward pe(#)	Automatic linear regression: forward covariate selection.	3.17.1
sw regress *depvar varlist*, pr(#)	Automatic linear regression: backward covariate selection.	3.17.2
sw regress *depvar varlist*, forward pe(#) pr(#)	Automatic linear regression: stepwise forward covariate selection.	3.17.3
sw regress *depvar varlist*, pe(#) pr(#)	Automatic linear regression: stepwise backward covariate selection.	3.17.4

Analysis Commands (*cont.*)

Command	Function	Section
table *rowvar colvar*	Two-way frequency tables of values of *rowvar* by *colvar*.	5.5
table *rowvar colvar*, row col	Two-way frequency tables with row and column totals.	5.20
table *rowvar colvar*, by(*varlist*)	Two-way frequency tables of values of *rowvar* by *colvar* for each unique combination of values of *varlist*.	5.5
table *rowvar colvar*, contents(sum *varname*)	Create a table of sums of *varname* cross-tabulated by *rowvar* and *colvar*.	8.9
tabulate *varname*	Frequency table of *varname* with percentages and cumulative percentages.	3.21
tabulate *varname1 varname2*, column row	Two-way frequency tables with row and column percentages.	5.11.1
ttest *var1* = *var2*	Paired *t*-test of *var1* vs. *var2*.	1.4.11
ttest *var*, by(*groupvar*)	Independent *t*-test of *var* in groups defined by *groupvar*.	1.4.14
ttest *var*, by(*groupvar*) unequal	Independent *t*-test of *var* in groups defined by *groupvar*. Variances assumed unequal.	1.4.14
xi: glm *depvar varlist* i.*catvar*, family(*dist*) link(*linkfcn*)	Glm with dichotomous indicator variables replacing a categorical variable *catvar*.	8.12
xi: glm *depvar varlist* i.*var1**i .*var2*, family(*dist*) link(*linkfcn*)	Glm with dichotomous indicator variables replacing categorical variables *var1*, *var2*. All two-way interaction terms are also generated.	9.3
xi: logistic *depvar varlist* i.*catvar*	Logistic regression with dichotomous indicator variables replacing a categorical variable *catvar*.	5.10
xi: logistic *depvar varlist* i.*var1**i .*var2*	Logistic regression with dichotomous indicator variables replacing categorical variables *var1* and *var2*. All two-way interaction terms are also generated.	5.23
xi: stcox *varlist* i.*varname*	Proportional hazards regression with dichotomous indicator variables replacing categorical variable *varname*.	7.7
xi: stcox *varlist* i.*var1**i.*var2*	Proportional hazards regression with dichotomous indicator variables replacing categorical variables *var1* and *var2*. All two-way interaction terms are also generated.	7.7
xtgee *depvar varlist*, family(family) link(link) corr(correlation) i(*idname*) t(*tname*)	Perform a generalized estimating equation analysis in regressing *depvar* against the variables in *varlist*.	11.11

Post Estimation Commands (affected by preceding regression command)

Command	Function	Section
lincom *expression*	Calculate *expression* and a 95% CI associated with *expression*.	5.20, 10.7
lincom *expression*, or	Calculate exp[*espression*] with associated 95% CI. The *hr* and *irr* options perform the same calculations.	5.20, 7.7, 8.7
predict *newvar*, cooksd	Set *newvar* = Cook's D.	3.21
predict *newvar*, csnell	Set *newvar* = Cox–Snell residual.	7.7
predict *newvar*, ccsnell	Set *newvar* = Cox–Snell residual in the last record for each patient – used with multiple records per patient.	7.10.1
predict *newvar*, dfbeta(*varname*)	Set *newvar* = delta beta statistic for the *varname* covariate in the linear regression model.	3.21
predict *newvar*, h	Set *newvar* = leverage.	3.16
predict *newvar*, rstudent	Set *newvar* = studentized residual.	2.16, 3.21
predict *newvar*, standardized deviance	Set *newvar* = standardized deviance residual.	9.5
predict *newvar*, stdp	Set *newvar* = standard error of the linear predictor.	2.12, 3.16
predict *newvar*, stdf	Set *newvar* = standard error of a forecasted value.	2.12, 3.16
predict *newvar*, xb	Set *newvar* = linear predictor.	2.12, 3.16
vce	Display variance–covariance matrix of last model.	4.18

Command Prefixes

Syntax	Function	Section
by *varlist*:	Repeat following command for each unique value of *varlist*.	1.3.6
sw	Fit a model with either the forward, backward or stepwise algorithm. N.B. sw is not followed by a colon.	3.17.1
xi:	Execute the following estimation command with categorical variables like i.*catvar* and i.*catvar1* * i.*catvar2*.	5.10, 5.23

Logical and Relational Operators and System Variables (See Stata User's Manual)

Operator or Variable	Meaning	Section
.	missing value	5.32.2
1	true	7.7
0	false	7.7
>	greater than	1.4.11
<	less than	1.4.11
>=	greater than or equal to	1.4.11
<=	less than or equal to	1.4.11
==	equal to	1.4.11
~=	not equal to	1.4.11
&	and	1.4.11
|	or	1.4.11
~	not	1.4.11
_n	Record number of current observation. When used with the *by id:* prefix, _n is reset to 1 whenever the value of *id* changes and equals k at the kth record with the same value of *id*.	7.11, 11.5
_N	Total number of observations in the data set. When used with the *by id:* prefix, _N is the number of records with the current value of *id*.	2.12, 11.5
varname[*expression*]	The value of variable *varname* in observation *expression*.	7.11

Functions (See Stata User's Guide)

Operator etc.	Meaning	Section
chi2tail(*df*, *var*)	Probability that a χ^2 statistic with *df* degrees of freedom will exceed *var*.	7.7
int(*var*)	Truncate *var* to an integer.	8.9
invttail(*df*, α)	Critical value of size α for a *t* distribution with *df* degrees of freedom.	2.12
recode(*var*, x_1, x_2, ..., x_n)	Missing if *var* is missing; x_1 if $var \le x_1$; x_i *if* $x_{i-1} < var \le x_i$ *for* $2 \le i < n$; x_n *otherwise*.	7.7
round(*x*, 1)	Round *x* to nearest integer.	8.9
ttail(*df*, *var*)	Probability that a *t* statistic with *df* degrees of freedom exceeds *var*.	2.20

Additional Options for the graph, ksm and sts graph Commands (insert after comma)

Option	Function	Section
b2title("*text*")	Add a title to the x-axis of a graph. (Recommended with *sts graph* command.)	6.9
gap(#)	Set the y axis # spaces from its title.	2.12
l1title("*text*")	Add "*text*" as title for the y-axis. Note that the default titles for both the x- and y-axes are given by the variable labels of the plotted variables.	4.18
noborder	Omit border from graph.	6.9
r1title("*text*")	Add "*text*" as title to the right vertical axis.	4.11
rlabel(#,...,#)	Add numeric labels to a vertical axis on the right of the graph.	4.11
title("*text*")	Add "*text*" as title to the x-axis of graph.	9.3
xlabel(#,...,#)	Add specific numeric labels #,...,# to the x-axis.	2.12
xline(#,...,#)	Add vertical grid lines at values #,...,#.	2.12
xlog	Plot the x-axis on a logarithmic scale.	11.2
xscale(#1,#2)	Specify the range of the x-axis to be not less than from #1 to #2.	2.20
xtick(#,...,#)	Add tick marks to the x-axis at #,...,#.	2.18
ylabel(#,...,#)	Add specific numeric labels #,...,# to the y-axis.	2.12
yline(#,...,#)	Add horizontal grid lines at values #,...,#.	2.12
yscale(#1,#2)	Specify the range of the y-axis to be not less than from #1 to #2.	2.20
ytick(#,...,#)	Add tick marks to the y-axis at #,...,#.	2.18

References

Armitage, P. and Berry, G. *Statistical Methods in Medical Research*. Oxford: Blackwell Science, Inc., 1994.

Bartlett, M.S. Properties of sufficiency and statistical tests. *P. R. Soc. Lond. A Mat.* 1937; **160**:268–82.

Bernard, G.R., Wheeler, A.P., Russell, J.A., Schein, R., Summer, W.R., Steinberg, K.P., et al. The effects of ibuprofen on the physiology and survival of patients with sepsis. The Ibuprofen in Sepsis Study Group. *N. Engl. J. Med.* 1997; **336**:912–8.

Brent, J., McMartin, K., Phillips, S., Burkhart, K.K., Donovan, J.W., Wells, M., et al. Fomepizole for the treatment of ethylene glycol poisoning. Methylpyrazole for Toxic Alcohols Study Group. *N. Engl. J. Med.* 1999; **340**:832–8.

Breslow, N.E. and Day, N.E. *Statistical Methods in Cancer Research: Vol. 1 – The Analysis of Case-Control Studies*. Lyon, France: IARC Scientific Publications, 1980.

Breslow, N.E. and Day, N.E. *Statistical Methods in Cancer Research: Vol. II – The Design and Analysis of Cohort Studies*. Lyon, France: IARC Scientific Publications, 1987.

Clayton, D. and Hills, M. *Statistical Models in Epidemiology*. Oxford: Oxford University Press, 1993.

Cleveland, W.S. Robust locally weighted regression and smoothing scatterplots. *J. Am. Stat. Assoc.* 1979; **74**:829–36.

Cleveland, W.S. *Visualizing Data*. Summit, N.J.: Hobart Press, 1993.

Cochran, W.G. and Cox, G.M. *Experimental Designs, 2nd Ed.* New York: Wiley, 1957.

Cook, R.D. Detection of influential observations in linear regression. *Technometrics* 1977; **19**:15–18.

Cook, R.D. and Weisberg, S. *Applied Regression Including Computing and Graphics*. New York: Wiley, 1999.

Cox, D.R. Regression models and life-tables (with discussion). *J. R. Stat. Soc. Ser. B* 1972; **34**:187–220.

Cox, D.R. and Hinkley, D.V. *Theoretical Statistics*. London: Chapman and Hall, 1974.

Cox, D.R. and Oakes, D. *Analysis of Survival Data*. London: Chapman and Hall, 1984.

Cox, D.R. and Snell, E.J. A general definition of residuals. *J. R. Stat. Soc. Ser. B* 1968; **30**:248–75.

Crowder, M.J. and Hand, D.J. *Analysis of Repeated Measures*. London: Chapman and Hall, 1990.

Diggle, P., Liang, K.-Y., and Zeger, S.L. *Analysis of Longitudinal Data*. Oxford: Oxford University Press, 1994.

Draper, N. and Smith, H. *Applied Regression Analysis, 3rd Ed.* New York: John Wiley, 1998.

Dupont, W.D. Sequential stopping rules and sequentially adjusted P values: does one require the other? *Control. Clin. Trials* 1983; **4**:3–10.

Dupont, W.D. Sensitivity of Fisher's exact test to minor perturbations in 2×2 contingency tables. *Stat. Med.* 1986; **5**:629–35.

Dupont, W.D. and Page, D.L. Risk factors for breast cancer in women with proliferative breast disease. *N. Engl. J. Med.* 1985; **312**:146–51.

Dupont, W.D. and Page, D.L. Relative risk of breast cancer varies with time since diagnosis of atypical hyperplasia. *Hum. Pathol.* 1989; **20**:723–5.

Dupont, W.D. and Plummer, W.D. Power and sample size calculations: a review and computer program. *Control. Clin. Trials* 1990; **11**:116–28.

Dupont, W.D. and Plummer, W.D. Power and sample size calculations for studies involving linear regression. *Control. Clin. Trials* 1998; **19**:589–601.

Dupont, W.D. and Plummer, W.D. Exact confidence intervals for odds ratio from case-control studies. *Stata Technical Bulletin* 1999; **52**:12–16.

Eisenhofer, G., Lenders, J.W., Linehan, W.M., Walther, M.M., Goldstein, D.S., and Keiser, H.R. Plasma normetanephrine and metanephrine for detecting pheochromocytoma in von Hippel–Lindau disease and multiple endocrine neoplasia type 2. *N. Engl. J. Med.* 1999; **340**:1872–9.

Fleiss, J.L. *Statistical Methods for Rates and Proportions, 2nd Ed.* New York: John Wiley, 1981.

Fleming, T.R. and Harrington, D.P. *Counting Processes and Survival Analysis.* New York: Wiley-Interscience, 1991.

Framingham Heart Study. *The Framingham Study – 40 Year Public Use Data Set.* Bethesda, MD: National Heart, Lung, and Blood Institute, NIH, 1997.

Greenwood, M. *The Natural Duration of Cancer.* Reports on Public Health and Medical Subjects, No. 33. London: His Majesty's Stationery Office, 1926.

Grizzle, J.E. Continuity correction in the χ^2 test for 2×2 tables. *The American Statistician* 1967; **21**:28–32.

Gross, C.P., Anderson, G.F. and Rowe, N.R. The relation between funding by the National Institutes of Health and the burden of disease. *N. Engl. J. Med.* 1999; **340**:1881–7.

Hamilton, L.C. *Regression with Graphics: A Second Course in Applied Statistics.* Pacific Grove, CA: Brooks/Cole Pub. Co., 1992.

Hennekens, C.H. and Buring, J.E. *Epidemiology in Medicine.* Boston, MA: Little, Brown and Company, 1987.

Hosmer, D.W. and Lemeshow, S. A goodness-of-fit test for the multiple logistic regression model. *Commun. Stat.* 1980; **A10**:1043–69.

Hosmer, D.W. and Lemeshow, S. *Applied Logistic Regression.* New York: Wiley, 1989.

Huber, P.J. The behavior of maximum likelihood estimates under non-standard conditions. *Proceedings of the Fifth Berkeley Symposium on Mathematical Statistics and Probability.* Berkeley, CA: University of California Press, 1967; 221–3.

Kalbfleisch, J.D. and Prentice, R.L. *The Statistical Analysis of Failure Time Data.* New York: Wiley, 1980.

Kaplan, E.L. and Meier, P. Nonparametric estimation from incomplete observations. *J. Am. Stat. Assoc.* 1958; **53**:457–81.

Kay, R. Proportional hazard regression models and the analysis of censored survival data. *Appl. Statist.* 1977; **26**:227–37.

Kruskal, W.H. and Wallis, W.A. Use of ranks in one-criterion variance analysis. *J. Am. Stat. Assoc.* 1952; **47**:583–621.

Lang, C.C., Stein, C.M., Brown, R.M., Deegan, R., Nelson, R., He, H.B., et al. Attenuation of isoproterenol-mediated vasodilatation in blacks. *N. Engl. J. Med.* 1995; **333**: 155–60.

Lawless, J.F. *Statistical Models and Methods for Lifetime Date.* New York: Wiley, 1982.

Levy, D., National Heart Lung and Blood Institute., Center for Bio-Medical Communication. *50 Years of Discovery: Medical Milestones from the National Heart, Lung, and Blood Institute's Framingham Heart Study.* Hackensack, N.J.: Center for Bio-Medical Communication Inc., 1999.

Liang, K.-Y. and Zeger, S. Longitudinal data analysis using generalized linear models. *Biometrika* 1986; **73**:13–22.

Mann, H.B. and Whitney, D.R. On a test of whether one of two random variables is stochastically larger than the other. *Ann. Math. Stat.* 1947; **18**:50–60.

Mantel, N. Evaluation of survival data and two new rank order statistics arising in its consideration. *Cancer Chemother. Rep.* 1966; **50**:163–70.

Mantel, N. and Greenhouse, S.W. What is the continuity correction? *The American Statistician* 1968; **22**:27–30.

Mantel, N. and Haenszel, W. Statistical aspects of the analysis of data from retrospective studies of disease. *J. Natl. Cancer Inst.* 1959; **22**:719–48.

Marini, J.J. and Wheeler, A.P. *Critical Care Medicine: The Essentials. 2nd Ed.* Baltimore: Williams & Wilkins, 1997.

McCullagh, P. and Nelder, J.A. *Generalized Linear Models.* New York: Chapman and Hall, 1989.

O'Donnell, H.C., Rosand, J., Knudsen, K.A., Furie, K.L., Segal, A.Z., Chiu, R.I., et al. Apolipoprotein E genotype and the risk of recurrent lobar intracerebral hemorrhage. *N. Engl. J. Med.* 2000; **342**:240–5.

Pagano, M. and Gauvreau, K. *Principles of Biostatistics, 2nd Ed.* Belmont, CA: Duxbury Thomson Learning, 2000.

Parl, F.F., Cavener, D.R. and Dupont, W.D. Genomic DNA analysis of the estrogen receptor gene in breast cancer. *Breast Cancer Res. Tr.* 1989; **14**:57–64.

Peto, R. and Peto, J. Asymptotically efficient rank invariant test procedures. *J. R. Stat. Soc. Ser. A* 1972; **135**:185–207.

Pregibon, D. Logistic regression diagnostics. *Ann. Stat.* 1981; **9**:705–24.

Robins, J., Breslow, N. and Greenland, S. Estimators of the Mantel–Haenszel variance consistent in both sparse data and large-strata limiting models. *Biometrics* 1986; **42**:311–23.

Rothman, K.J. and Greenland, S. *Modern Epidemiology.* Philadelphia: Lippincott-Raven, 1998.

Royall, R.M. *Statistical Evidence: A Likelihood Paradigm.* London: Chapman & Hall, 1997.

Satterthwaite, F.E. An approximate distribution of estimates of variance components. *Biometrics Bulletin* 1946; **2**:110–14.

Scholer, S.J., Hickson, G.B., Mitchel, E.F., and Ray, W.A. Persistently increased injury mortality rates in high-risk young children. *Arch. Pediatr. Adolesc. Med.* 1997; **151**:1216–9.

Searle, S.R. *Linear Models for Unbalanced Data.* New York: Wiley, 1987.

StataCorp. *Stata Statistical Software: Release 7.0.* College Station, TX: Stata Corporation, 2001.

Steel, R.G.D. and Torrie, J.H. *Principles and Procedures of Statistics: A Biometrical Approach, 2nd Ed.* New York: McGraw-Hill Book Co., 1980.

Student. The probable error of a mean. *Biometrika* 1908; **6**:1–25.

Therneau, T.M., Grambsch, P.M., and Fleming, T.R. Martingale-based residuals for survival models. *Biometrika* 1990; **77**:147–60.

Tuyns, A.J., Pequignot, G., and Jensen, O.M. Le cancer de l'oesophage en Ille-et-Vilaine en fonction des niveau de consommation d'alcool et de tabac. Des risques qui se multiplient. *Bull. Cancer* 1977; **64**:45–60.

Varmus, H. Evaluating the burden of disease and spending the research dollars of the National Institutes of Health. *N. Engl. J. Med.* 1999; **340**:1914–15.

Wald, A. Tests of statistical hypotheses concerning several parameters when the number of observations is large. *T. Am. Math. Soc.* 1943; **54**:426–82.

White, H. A heteroskedasticity-consistent covariance matrix estimator and a direct test for heteroskedasticity. *Econometrica* 1980; **48**:817–30.

White, H. Maximum likelihood estimation of misspecified models. *Econometrica* 1982; **50**:1–25.

Wilcoxon, F. Individual comparisons by ranking methods. *Biometrics Bulletin* 1945; **1**:80–3.

Woolf, B. On estimating the relationship between blood group and disease. *Ann. Hum. Genet.* 1955; **19**:251–3.

Xie, H.G., Stein, C.M., Kim, R.B., Xiao, Z.S., He, N., Zhou, H.H., et al. Frequency of functionally important beta-2 adrenoceptor polymorphisms varies markedly among African-American, Caucasian and Chinese individuals. *Pharmacogenetics* 1999; **9**:511–16.

Xie, H.G., Stein, C.M., Kim, R.B., Gainer, J.V., Sofowora, G., Dishy, V., et al. Human beta2-adrenergic receptor polymorphisms: no association with essential hypertension in black or white Americans. *Clin. Pharmacol. Ther.* 2000; **67**:670–5.

Yates, F. Contingency tables involving small numbers and the chi-square test. *J. R. Stat. Soc. Suppl.* 1934; **1**:217–35.

Zeger, S.L. and Liang, K.Y. Longitudinal data analysis for discrete and continuous outcomes. *Biometrics* 1986; **42**:121–30.

Index